NATURAL MEDICATIONS FOR PSYCHIATRIC DISORDERS

Considering the Alternatives

NATURAL MEDICATIONS FOR PSYCHIATRIC DISORDERS

Considering the Alternatives

Editors

David Mischoulon, M.D., Ph.D.

Assistant Professor of Psychiatry, Harvard Medical School
Department of Psychiatry, Massachusetts General Hospital
Boston, Massachusetts

Jerrold F. Rosenbaum, M.D.

Professor of Psychiatry, Harvard Medical School
Chief of Psychiatry, Massachusetts General Hospital
Boston, Massachusetts

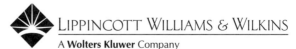

LIPPINCOTT WILLIAMS & WILKINS
A **Wolters Kluwer** Company
Philadelphia · Baltimore · New York · London
Buenos Aires · Hong Kong · Sydney · Tokyo

Acquisitions Editor: Charles W. Mitchell
Developmental Editors: Stacey L. Baze
Production Editor: Christiana Sahl
Manufacturing Manager: Benjamin Rivera
Cover Designer: Mark Lerner
Compositor: Lippincott Williams & Wilkins Desktop Division
Printer: Maple Press

Library of Congress Cataloging-in-Publication Data

Natural medications for psychiatric disorders : considering the alternatives /
edited by David Mischoulon, Jerrold F. Rosenbaum.
      p. ; cm.
   Includes bibliographical references and index.
   ISBN 0-7817-2954-8
   1. Mental illness—Alternative treatment. 2. Mental illness—Chemotherapy.
3. Naturopathy. 4. Alternative medicine. I. Mischoulon, David. II. Rosenbaum, J. F.
(Jerrold F.)
   [DNLM: 1. Mental Disorders—drug therapy. 2. Alternative Medicine.
3. Naturopathy. WM 402 N285 2002]
   RC480.5 .N285 2002
   616.89'1—dc21
                                                                    2001050583

Care has been taken to confirm the accuracy of the information presented and to describe generally accepted practices. However, the authors, editors, and publisher are not responsible for errors or omissions or for any consequences from application of the information in this book and make no warranty, expressed or implied, with respect to the currency, completeness, or accuracy of the contents of the publication. Application of this information in a particular situation remains the professional responsibility of the practitioner.

The authors, editors, and publisher have exerted every effort to ensure that drug selection and dosage set forth in this text are in accordance with current recommendations and practice at the time of publication. However, in view of ongoing research, changes in government regulations, and the constant flow of information relating to drug therapy and drug reactions, the reader is urged to check the package insert for each drug for any change in indications and dosage and for added warnings and precautions. This is particularly important when the recommended agent is a new or infrequently employed drug.

Some drugs and medical devices presented in this publication have Food and Drug Administration (FDA) clearance for limited use in restricted research settings. It is the responsibility of the health care provider to ascertain the FDA status of each drug or device planned for use in their clinical practice.

10 9 8 7 6 5 4 3 2 1

To Alisabet

—DM

To Lidia, Jed, Eliza, and Blake

—JFR

And to the Massachusetts General Hospital,
where there is no alternative to quality of care.

—DM and JFR

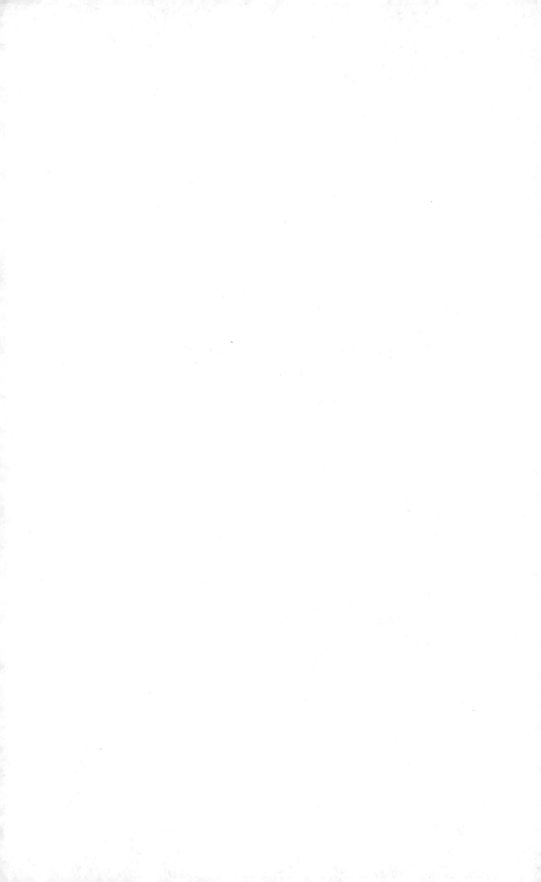

About the Editors

David Mischoulon, M.D., Ph.D., is an Assistant Professor of Psychiatry at Harvard Medical School and a staff psychiatrist in the Depression Clinical and Research Program at the Massachusetts General Hospital (MGH). He graduated from the combined M.D.–Ph.D. program at Boston University School of Medicine, where he earned a doctorate in biochemistry and authored several original papers in the area of liver biochemistry. He completed his General Medicine internship at Carney Hospital and his Psychiatry residency at Massachusetts General Hospital, where he served as Chief Resident in Psychopharmacology. Dr. Mischoulon has received research awards from the National Alliance for Research on Schizophrenia and Depression (NARSAD), from the American Psychiatric Association (APA), and from the National Center for Complementary and Alternative Medicine (NCCAM) at the National Institutes of Health. His areas of interest include research on the pharmacotherapy of depressive disorders, natural remedies for psychiatric disorders, and the treatment of depression in minority populations. He has authored more than 30 original articles, reviews, and book chapters, and he has also been an invited speaker at various academic sites around the country. In addition to his research and clinical activities, he is an active teacher and supervisor of psychiatric residents and medical students at MGH and Harvard Medical School. Dr. Mischoulon was recently named Associate Director of the Partners HealthCare Systems Center for Alternative Medicine in Psychiatry.

Jerrold F. Rosenbaum, M.D., is the Chief of Psychiatry at the Massachusetts General Hospital and a Professor of Psychiatry at Harvard Medical School. He received his undergraduate degree from Yale College and his medical degree from Yale School of Medicine. He completed his residency and fellowship in Psychiatry at MGH. Dr. Rosenbaum's clinical and consulting practice specializes in treatment-resistant mood and anxiety disorders, and he provides extensive consultation to colleagues on the management of these conditions. His research contributions include widespread participation in the design and conduct of clinical trials of new therapies; the design and implementation of trials to develop innovative treatments for major depression, treatment resistant depression, and panic disorder; studies of psychopathology, including comorbidity and subtypes; and studies of the longitudinal course and outcomes of those disorders. Dr. Rosenbaum has authored more than 300 original articles and reviews and has published over 12 books. He is recognized as one of the world's foremost authorities on mood and anxiety disorders, with a special emphasis on the pharmacotherapy of these conditions. He lectures widely on related topics, addressing thousands of practitioners annually in a variety of postgraduate educational venues. At MGH, he directs a department of over 500 clinicians and researchers, which has been ranked as the number one Department of Psychiatry in the United States by *U.S. News and World Report* for the past six years in a row (1). Dr. Rosenbaum also serves as the President and Executive Director of the MGH Mood and Anxiety Disorders Institute, which was established with a primary mission of enhancing the recognition, understanding, and treatment of those disorders. With his colleagues, he developed the MGH outpatient psychiatry service into a world-leading clinical and research center.

REFERENCES

1. America's best hospitals. *U.S. News and World Report*. 2001;131(3):105.

Contents

I. Treatment of Mood Disorders

II. Treatment of Anxiety and Sleep Disorders

III. Treatment of Other Disorders

IV. Polypharmacy and Side Effects Management

V. Afterword

Appendices

Contributing Authors

Jonathan E. Alpert, M.D., Ph.D. *Assistant Professor of Psychiatry, Harvard Medical School; Associate Director, Depression Clinical and Research Program, Massachusetts General Hospital, Boston, Massachusetts*

Robert H. Belmaker, M.D. *Hoffer-Vickar Professor of Psychiatry, Ben Gurion University of the Negev; Deputy Director, Beersheva Mental Health Center, Beersheva, Israel*

Jonathan Benjamin, M.D. *Associate Professor of Psychiatry, Ben Gurion University of the Negev, Beersheva; Chief of Psychiatry, Barzilai Medical Center, Ashkelon, Israel*

Kathryn M. Connor, M.D. *Assistant Professor of Psychiatry and Behavioral Sciences, Duke University Medical Center, Durham, North Carolina*

Jonathan R. T. Davidson, M.D. *Professor of Psychiatry, Duke University Medical Center, Durham, North Carolina*

Lindsay DeCecco, B.A. *Graduate Student, Department of School Psychology, University of Massachusetts, Amherst, Amherst, Massachusetts*

Steven Dentali, Ph.D. *President, Dentali Associates, Natural Products Consulting Services, Delray Beach, Florida*

Roberto A. Dominguez, M.D. *Professor, Department of Psychiatry and Behavioral Sciences, University of Miami School of Medicine, Miami, Florida*

Maurizio Fava, M.D. *Associate Professor of Psychiatry, Harvard Medical School; Director, Depression Clinical and Research Program, Department of Psychiatry, Massachusetts General Hospital, Boston, Massachusetts*

Leah Friedman, Ph.D. *Stanford University Medical School, Stanford, California*

Janet Kastelan, M.A. *Assistant Research Scientist, Aging and Dementia Research Center, Department of Psychiatry, New York University School of Medicine, New York, New York*

Pierre Le Bars, M.D., Ph.D. *Associate Professor of Psychiatry, New York University Medical Center, New York, New York*

Carol A. Locke, M.D. *Professor of Psychiatry, Harvard Medical School, Boston, Massachusetts; Founder, Omega Natural Health, Inc., Waltham, Massachusetts*

David Mischoulon, M.D., Ph.D. *Assistant Professor of Psychiatry, Harvard Medical School; Depression and Clinical Research Program, Department of Psychiatry, Massachusetts General Hospital, Boston, Massachusetts*

Andrew A. Nierenberg, M.D. *Associate Professor of Psychiatry, Harvard Medical School; Medical Director, Bipolar Programs; Associate Director, Depression Clinical and Research Program, Massachusetts General Hospital, Boston, Massachusetts*

Victor I. Reus, M.D., Ph.D. *Professor of Psychiatry, University of California, San Francisco; Attending Physician, Langley Porter Neuropsychiatric Institute, San Francisco, California*

Jerrold F. Rosenbaum, M.D. *Professor of Psychiatry, Harvard Medical School; Chief of Psychiatry, Massachusetts General Hospital, Boston, Massachusetts*

Hector Sabelli, M.D., Ph.D. *Director, Center for Creative Development, Chicago, Illinois*

Ziva Stahl, M.A. *Ministry of Health Mental Health Center; Faculty of Health Sciences, Ben Gurion University of the Negev, Beersheva, Israel*

Andrew L. Stoll, M.D. *Psychopharmacology Research Laboratory, McLean Hospital, Belmont, Massachusetts; Department of Psychiatry, Harvard Medical School, Boston, Massachusetts*

Owen M. Wolkowitz, M.D. *Professor of Psychiatry, University of California, San Francisco Medical Center; Director, Psychopharmacology Assessment Clinic, Langley Porter Psychiatric Institute, San Francisco, California*

Irina V. Zhdanova, M.D., Ph.D. *Research Associate Professor of Anatomy and Neurobiology, Boston University, Boston, Massachusetts*

Introduction

Although "alternative" or natural medications have been used for centuries (1), the popularity of these remedies in the United States and worldwide has increased dramatically over the last several years (2–5). News programs and the popular press routinely feature stories of natural medications, as well as of other alternative treatments, and most large bookstores have entire sections devoted to literature about these treatments. Studies suggest that 25% of people in the United States and up to 70% of the population worldwide seek and obtain non-traditional treatments (6). This represents an enormous market for the nutraceutical industry, as well as a growing field for academic and pharmaceutical research.

While many different types of natural treatments are available for almost any physical or medical problem, relatively few alternative medications exist for psychiatric disorders (1). Natural psychotropics have historically been limited to those treating mood disorders, anxiety disorders, and dementias. More recently, potential natural treatments for psychotic disorders and attention deficit disorders have begun to emerge, although evidence for these is still very premature.

Some of these alternative medications, such as St. John's wort, kava, valerian, ginkgo, and black cohosh, are derived from plants and herbs. Other medications, such as melatonin and dehydroepiandrosterone (DHEA), are natural hormones. Additional therapeutics include vitamins, such as the B-vitamin folic acid; amino acid derivatives, such as phenylethylamine and s-adenosyl methionine (SAMe); and omega-3 fatty acids, such as docosahexanoic acid (DHA) and eicosapentanoic acid (EPA), which are found in animals and fish. Homeopathy is also a popular alternative treatment modality.

Several factors may be contributing to the dramatic increase in the popularity of natural medications. In recent years, a growing trend for patients to be more proactive in their treatment, rather than assuming the more "traditional" passive stance when working with their physician, has been observed. This is reflected by the pharmaceutical companies' now common strategy of advertising prescription medications directly to patients—usually on television and in popular magazines—in the hopes that the consumers will ask their doctor about the products. Meanwhile, natural remedies are readily available at drugstores and natural food shops without a prescription, thus allowing patients to "prescribe" for themselves.

Portions of this chapter were previously published by the authors in modified form in Mischoulon D, Rosenbaum JF. The use of natural medications in psychiatry: a commentary. *Harvard Review of Psychiatry* 1999;6:279-283 and are being used with permission.

Some have suggested that dissatisfaction with the medical profession and orthodox medicine (7–10), particularly the increasingly rigid treatment delivery systems of managed care, may contribute to patients' dissent from conventional medicine and towards the independence that alternative treatments provide. Also, the number of non-physician practitioners has been increasing (11); many such practitioners recommend these treatments without consultation from their medical counterparts. Indeed, many such practitioners espouse views different from, and even adversarial to, those of typical physicians. Patients today may seek care from a variety of practitioners other than physicians, including chiropractors, acupuncturists, herbalists, and other healers. Bookstore shelves are stocked with books on the management of medical and psychological problems, and many of these books discourage patients from working with traditional medical doctors (7,8). Finally, the cost factor may also attract patients to alternative treatments, as many, though not all, of these over-the-counter substances are cheaper than their Food and Drug Administration (FDA)-sanctioned counterparts, particularly when several manufacturers are competing for customers.

Despite the growing popularity of alternative medicine, North America might be viewed as lagging behind many others in this movement. Most cultures outside the United States have embraced natural medications for centuries. Natural medications are routinely used throughout Asia, where many of these treatments were developed and which is today one of the largest markets and sources for alternative treatments (1). Asian physicians, when compared to those in the United States, are generally more accepting of, and better informed about, natural medications; they often prescribe them in combination with more conventional treatments. Most research studies on natural medications have originated in Europe (1), and European physicians routinely prescribe these remedies as well. South America historically has also embraced the use of natural medications, as well as other forms of therapy, for both medical and psychiatric problems (12). Hispanics in America often seek help from healers or spiritists in addition to, or in place of, their physician. They may also be hesitant to take standard medications and thus may prefer naturopathic medications.

Many individuals who opt to use these natural remedies are reticent to discuss them with their physician. This reticence may be due to a belief that "Western-trained" physicians do not believe such treatments are effective and that they may ridicule their use. Patients may also believe—often correctly—that physicians are not knowledgeable enough about these treatments to make useful suggestions. This is unfortunate, as the result is miscommunication between patients and their doctors, an effect that can, at times, have adverse consequences for treatment, as in cases in which drug-drug interactions may have toxic effects.

Whatever forces are driving the shift to alternative medications, the actual benefits of this approach to treatment are not clear because of the limited basic and clinical research data for natural medications. Manufacturers and suppliers, as well as the United States government, have generally avoided sponsoring clinical research; and these medications, with the exception of homeopathic remedies, are generally not regulated by the FDA (13). Consequently, little guidance from systematic study exists regarding optimal doses, contraindications, drug-drug interactions, and potential toxicities. Individual endorsements, anecdotal data, and case reports are found, but few well-designed, systematic studies address these questions or even the question of superiority to a placebo.

In addition, many alternative medications and treatments are quite expensive; since insurance companies by and large do not cover them, they may prove to be more costly in the long run and certainly less cost-effective than conventional remedies, particularly if they do not prove helpful. Also, because these medications are unregulated, preparations made by different companies vary in potency, quality, or purity of the preparation and hence in effectiveness. The buyer of natural remedies must indeed beware!

Another common misconception is that, just because a medication is "natural," it is automatically safe and may therefore be taken with impunity. While relatively few reports of serious adverse effects from these medications are heard—a large part of their appeal (1)—cases of toxicity have been recorded in some who have taken more than the recommended dosage (1,14). Likewise, there is a paucity of data regarding the safety and efficacy of combining alternative medications with the more conventional ones, although case reports about such interactions, including some potentially dangerous ones, are increasing, as various chapters in this volume will demonstrate.

Until recently, quality data on the safety and efficacy of alternative medications for psychiatric disorders have been relatively limited, and much of the available data have been in the form of case reports or uncontrolled, open clinical studies, often with small sample sizes (1). For example, St. John's wort, one of the most widely studied herbal psychotropics, has been compared mainly to doses of tricyclic antidepressants considered suboptimal by psychiatrists (15,16). Only recently has it been tested against the newer antidepressants that are more commonly used in the United States. Other natural medications have been studied in samples of between ten and 20 patients (1), and while some of the descriptive results are encouraging, these studies clearly show that, until larger controlled studies are available, we will not be able to say whether these medications work.

Because of the growing interest in natural treatments, clinicians are now being called upon to manage and offer recommendations to patients who use these treatments. Due to a lack of emphasis on alternative treatments in medical schools and residency programs (2), most physicians are not adequately trained in the proper uses for these medications. Furthermore, a lot of the information available about these remedies comes in the form of magazine articles, web pages, and books from the popular press; much of this material is biased, and it often lacks scientific evidence to support the claims that are made. We believe a reliable, scientific, yet clinically useful source that practitioners may use for reference in the office setting is needed. In assembling this monograph, we have sought to provide mental health clinicians with a clear and thorough understanding of the better-known natural, or "alternative," remedies for psychiatric disorders.

The goals of this book, therefore, are the following:

1. To provide a synthesis of the state of knowledge and published research data on the applications, clinical effectiveness, and safety of the better-studied natural psychotropics.
2. To allow the psychiatrist or the primary care physician to decide comfortably whether or not to prescribe natural psychotropics to certain patients and to recommend the appropriate doses.
3. To facilitate communication between health professionals and patients who are interested in alternative treatments.

In addition to being useful to physicians, we hope that the book may also be of value to psychologists, clinical social workers, and nurse practitioners who serve as psychotherapists or auxiliary psychopharmacologists. Because most alternative treatments are available without a prescription, these professionals frequently encounter patients who are using such remedies without the supervision of a physician. These clinicians may therefore benefit from having an accessible source of information that they can share with their patients.

Rather than trying to assemble an exhaustive textbook of all available natural psychotropics, we have restricted ourselves mostly to the better-studied natural remedies, which have a reasonable mass of peer-reviewed literature examining their claims. In putting together this volume, we have enlisted the participation of several academic physician–scientists who have carried out research with the various natural treatments reviewed here. These individuals are recognized leaders in the field of clinical research, and they have provided us with credible, cutting-edge information regarding the scientific rationale, effectiveness, and safety of various natural psychotropics.

We have organized the book into several sections covering different categories of disorders (e.g., mood disorders, anxiety disorders), and within each section we have dedicated individual chapters for each medication (or medications). No specific section covers psychotic disorders, but the preliminary evidence for the use of omega fatty acids in their treatment is mentioned in the chapters on omega-3 fatty acids and docosahexanoic acid (Chapters 2 and 3, respectively). We have also included several appendices for easy reference, providing rapidly accessible information about the indications, contraindications, doses, and drug-drug interactions for these remedies.

We hope that this book will provide a readable, yet thorough, synthesis that will help to fill in some of the knowledge gaps about natural psychotropic treatments in the medical and psychiatric community.

REFERENCES

1. Schulz V, Hansel R, Tyler VE. *Rational phytotherapy: a physicians' guide to herbal medicine*, 4th ed. Berlin: Springer, 2001.
2. Eisenberg DM, Kessler RC, Foster C, et al. Unconventional medicine in the United States: prevalence, costs, and patterns of use. *N Engl J Med* 1993;328:246–252.
3. Krippner S. A cross cultural comparison of four healing models. *Altern Ther Health Med* 1995;1: 21–29.
4. Whitmore SM, Leake NB. Complementary therapies: an adjunct to traditional therapies. *Nurse Pract* 1996;21:12–13.
5. Fisher P. The wheat and chaff in alternative medicine. *Lancet* 1997;349:1629.
6. National Institutes of Health Office of Alternative Medicine. Clinical Practice Guidelines in complementary and alternative medicine. An analysis of opportunities and obstacles. Practice and Policy Guidelines panel. *Archives in Family Medicine* 1997;6:149–154.
7. Mendelsohn RS. *Confessions of a medical heretic.* Chicago, IL: Contemporary Books, 1979.
8. Mendelsohn, RS. *How to raise a healthy child. . . in spite of your doctor.* New York: Ballantine Books, 1984.
9. Furnham A, Smith C. Choosing alternative medicine: a comparison of the beliefs of patients visiting a general practitioner and a homeopath. *Social Science & Medicine* 1988;26:685–689.
10. Furnham A, Bhagrath R. A comparison of health beliefs and behaviours of clients of orthodox and complementary medicine. *Br J Clin Psychol* 1993;32:237–246.
11. Weiner JP, Steinwachs DM, Williamson JW. Nurse practitioner and physician assistant practices in three HMOs: implications for future US health manpower needs. *Am J Public Health* 1986;76: 507–511.
12. Comas-Diaz L. Culturally relevant issues and treatment implications for Hispanics. In Koslow DR, Salett EP. *Crossing cultures in mental health.* Washington, D.C.: SIETAR International, 1989:31-48.
13. National Institutes of Health Office of Alternative Medicine. *Alternative medicine: expanding medical horizons.* Rockville, MD: National Institutes of Health, 1992.
14. Ernst E. Harmless herbs? A review of the recent literature. *Am J Med* 1998;104:170–178.
15. Vorbach EU, Hubner WD, Arnoldt KH. Effectiveness and tolerance of the hypericum extract LI 160 in comparison with imipramine. Randomized double blind study with 135 outpatients. *Nervenheilkunde* 1993;12:290–296.
16. Harrer G, Hubner WD, Podzuweit H. Effectiveness and tolerance of the hypericum preparation LI 160 compared to maprotiline. Multicentre double-blind study with 102 outpatients. *Nervenheilkunde* 1993;12:297-301.

David Mischoulon
Jerrold F. Rosenbaum

PART I

Treatment of Mood Disorders

1

St. John's Wort

A Critique of Antidepressant Efficacy and Possible Mechanisms of Action

Andrew A. Nierenberg, David Mischoulon, and Lindsay DeCecco

INTRODUCTION

People have used St. John's wort (*Hypericum perforatum*) to treat depression for centuries. Both the lay public and physicians in Europe perceive that St. John's wort (SJW) is effective for mild-to-moderate depression with a benign profile of adverse drug events, including lack of sedation. Studies show that SJW extracts are more effective than a placebo and that they are equally effective compared to active controls based on 15 double-blind, placebo-controlled studies and eight active comparator studies, all conducted in Europe since 1979.

In the United States, health food stores sell SJW flower bud extract, and, although it has been available, physicians rarely recommended that patients take it until recent extensive media coverage. Despite the growing popularity of SJW, more rigorous studies of both efficacy and toxicity are needed for Food and Drug Administration (FDA) approval and for physicians, patients, and third-party payers to accept SJW as a legitimate antidepressant with a reasonable risk-benefit ratio.

METAANALYSIS

In a metaanalysis that compared the efficacy of SJW to both a standard antidepressant and a placebo, similar results were found for both (1). Of the 23 randomized trials that were included in the study, 15 compared SJW to a placebo, and eight compared SJW to a standard antidepressant for a total of 1,757 outpatients with mild or moderately severe depressive disorders. Efficacy was defined either as a 50% decrease in a Hamilton Depression (HAMD; item-version unspecified) scale score or a final score of less than 10 or as a Clinical Global Impression (CGI) of much or very much improved. In the placebo-controlled trials, SJW was effective in 55.1% (Number of patients [N]=408) of the subjects, while the placebo was effective in 22.3% (N=422) of the subjects (pooled rate ratio [PRR], 2.67; 95% confidence interval [CI], 1.78 to 4.01). In the eight active comparator trials (six used single preparations of SJW, and two used combination preparations), SJW was as effective as standard antidepressants. A 63.9% (N=158) response rate was observed with single preparation SJW, compared to 58.5% (N=159) with antidepressants (PRR, 1.10; 95% CI, 0.93 to 1.31). In the two trials of SJW combination preparations, 88 responders (67.7%) were found compared with 66 responders (50%) with standard antidepressants (PRR, 1.52; 95% CI, 0.78 to 2.94). In these eight trials, 50 patients (19.8%) reported side effects from SJW with a 4.0% dropout rate; 84 patients (35.9%; PRR, 0.39; 95% CI, 0.23 to 0.68) treated with standard antidepressants reported side effects, with a 7.7% dropout rate.

Yet another metaanalysis suggests the acute efficacy of SJW in controlled trials but found none in severely or endogenously depressed patients; however, most studies have methodologic flaws. Currently no known studies of continuation or maintenance have been published (2). Vorbach et al., however, assessed the efficacy of SJW in severely depressed subjects (3). They compared the effects of Jarsin Ll 160 (1,800 mg) with imipramine (150 mg) in over 200 patients with severe depression and found no difference between the two antidepressants. The overall response rates, however, were only 35.3% and 41.2%, respectively; no placebo control group was included. All published studies were acute, lasting between 4 and 12 weeks without follow-up.

SJW was recently compared to the selective serotonin reuptake inhibitors (SSRIs). One double-blind, randomized study compared the effects of SJW (900 mg/day) to those of sertraline (75 mg/day) in 30 patients for 6 weeks (4). Clinical response was noted in 47% of patients receiving SJW and in 40% of those receiving sertraline. This difference was not statistically significant. Another randomized, double-blind study compared the effects of SJW to those of fluoxetine in 240 patients with mild-to-moderate depression (5). After 6 weeks of treatment, the mean endpoint HAMD scale scores were comparable for SJW and fluoxetine ($P<0.09$); the mean CGI score was significantly superior ($P<0.03$) on SJW, as was the responder rate ($P=0.005$). The incidence of adverse events was 23% with fluoxetine and 8% with SJW. Although SJW appeared to be superior in improving the responder rate, the authors noted that the main difference between the two treatments appeared to be tolerability. Additional studies comparing the effects of SJW to those of SSRIs for major depressive disorder (MDD) are currently underway in the United States.

In a study examining SJW treatment for menopausal symptoms, 111 women (43 to 65 years of age) received 12 weeks of treatment with SJW (Kira) at 900 mg/day. Climacteric complaints diminished or disappeared completely in the majority of women (76.4% by patient evaluation and 79.2% by physician evaluation) (6).

A recent study by Shelton et al. (7) suggested that SJW was not effective for the treatment of MDD. Two hundred adults with MDD received 12 weeks of SJW (up to 1200 mg/day) or a placebo. Investigators found that response rates did not differ between groups, although the remission rates were higher among the group that received SJW. However, the intent-to-treat analysis did not suggest a significant difference. Despite the discouraging data in the context of a well designed trial, several caveats are worth mentioning. The placebo remission rate was very low, which is unusual in depression trials. Also, no discontinuations secondary to nonresponse appeared to occur, which is unusual in depression trials as well. The average duration of the depressive episode was greater than 2 years, which suggests that SJW may be less effective for chronic depression but that it still may be effective for more acute depressive disorders. Likewise, the severity of depression was higher than that reported in other trials of SJW, which may only suggest that SJW is not as effective with more severe depressive states, an observation that was hinted in previous trials. SJW may still be an effective treatment for milder forms of depression, such as dysthymia and minor depression. To the authors' knowledge, this is only the first large-scale, well designed clinical trial of SJW for depression. More trials are necessary to appreciate better the implications of this study.

SIDE EFFECTS AND TOXICITY

Adverse drug events with SJW have generally been mild; patients have complained of dry mouth, dizziness, constipation, other unspecified gastrointestinal symptoms, and confusion. Fewer than 2% of patients discontinue intake of SJW because of side effects. In a postmarketing surveillance study, Woelk et al. (8) observed 3,250 patients treated with SJW by 633 physicians in routine clinical practice. Patients were monitored for side effects and for gross measures of response. Overall, 79% and 82% of patients rated themselves or were rated by physicians, respectively, as improved or symptom free. Only 2.4% of patients mentioned the side effects of gastrointestinal symptoms and allergic reactions, both of which were unspecified. Approximately 1.5% of patients stopped taking the drug because of these side effects.

Phototoxicity is thought to be associated with SJW, most commonly when used by veterinarians. Seigers et al. (9) studied the effects of several preparations of SJW on the susceptibility of human keratinocytes to ultraviolet (UV) radiation. They found that the extracts reduced the median lethal concentration (LC_{50}), but the reduction was less than that seen with psoralens, chlorpromazine, and pure SJW. The authors recommend that patients who take an overdose of SJW should be protected from UV radiation for 7 days, but this caution may not necessarily apply to those who are taking conventional doses. Brockmoller et al. (10) found that, while high doses of SJW (1,800 mg) caused minor increases in UV light sensitivity, no phototoxicity was detected.

When SJW was studied in a double-blind, placebo-controlled crossover trial in combination with alcohol, no difference between the active drug and the placebo was found in psychomotor performance, attention, or tests of driving in normal volunteers (11). SJW at a dose of 1,800 mg was found to be free of cardiac effects without changes in the heart rate, PR interval, QRS width, or QTc intervals (12).

Regarding drug-drug interactions, hyperforin has been shown to induce CYP-3A4 expression, but it has no effect on CYP-2D6 (13). Combinations of SJW products with warfarin, cyclosporin, oral contraceptives, theophylline, fenprocoumon, digoxin, and indinavir have led to reported interactions and reduced therapeutic activity (14–17). Proceeding with caution is therefore especially important in HIV-positive patients receiving protease inhibitors, as well as in transplant recipients. In addition, "serotonin syndrome" has been reported in cases where SJW was being taken concurrently with SSRIs (14,18,19). This adverse interaction may be due in part to the mild monoamine-oxidase inhibitor (MAOI) activity of SJW (20), so this combination is not recommended.

Cases of mania and hypomania secondary to SJW have been reported (14,21–25). Although the actual risk of a switch to mania in bipolar patients who take SJW is still unclear, physicians should warn bipolar patients about the risk of using SJW without supervision and without concomitant mood stabilizers.

ACTIVE INGREDIENTS OF SJW

Hypericin

Because SJW contains many different components, its antidepressant effect may likely have various pathways. Hypericin, believed by some to be one of the main active components, may inhibit monocyte cytokine production of interleukin-6 and perhaps interleukin 1β, resulting in a decrease in corticotropin-releasing hormone, which in turn reduces the production of cortisol, and regulating the hypothalamic-pituitary-adrenal axis (26) (Fig. 1.1). Hypericin also may inhibit the reuptake of serotonin, norepinephrine, and dopamine (27), and this may be followed by the downregulation of beta adrenoreceptors and increased 5-hydroxytryptamine-2 (5-HT2) and 5-HT1a receptor density (28). Finally, in addition, hypericin may have an affinity for γ-aminobutyric acid (GABA) receptors (29).

Hyperforin

Recent studies have suggested that the main active ingredient of SJW extracts may be hyperforin. Hyperforin ($C_{35}H_{52}O_4$), an acyl derivative of phoroglucinol, is one of the main constituents (2% to 4%) of hypericum. The new reports have suggested that it may function as a key component in the antidepressant effect of SJW (30–33).

Hyperforin was identified in therapeutically used alcoholic extracts of SJW (4.5% hyperforin). Initially, the specific effects of this constituent of the herb were detected in the peripheral organs using *in vitro* models and a hyperforin-enriched (38.8%) extract that was obtained by supercritical extraction of the herb via carbon dioxide (32). Hyperforin has been chemically isolated from the aerial parts of *H. perforatum* (34–36), in some instances with up to greater than

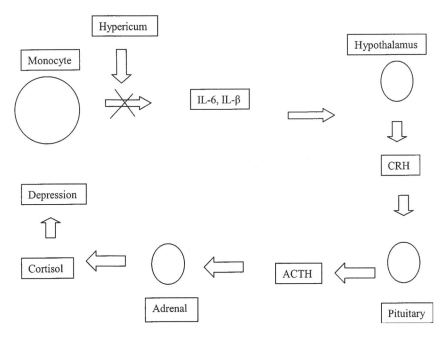

FIG. 1.1. Possible hypericum mechanism. Abbreviations: ACTH, adrenocorticotropic hormone; CRH, corticotropin-releasing hormone; IL, interleukin.

99.9% purity, by multistep protocols; sometimes, it is found in the form of furo-hyperforin, an oxygenated analogue of hyperforin (35).

Two clinical trials presented compelling evidence for a key antidepressant role for hyperforin. Laakmann et al. (30) performed a randomized, double-blind, placebo-controlled study of two different extracts of SJW on a sample of 147 patients. The two extracts varied in hyperforin content only (0.5% vs. 5%). At the end of the 6-week trial period, the patients who received the SJW extract with 5% hyperforin showed greater improvement in the mean HAMD scores (10.3±4.6 points) than the group that received the SJW extract with 0.5% hyperforin did (8.5±6.1 points); the latter group showed only slightly greater improvement than the placebo group (7.9±5.2 points).

A study by Schellenberg et al. (31) used quantitative electroencephalography (EEG) to show that the higher hyperforin content in SJW produces greater brain wave activity. In this study, 54 patients took either a placebo or one of the two SJW extracts with different levels of hyperforin (0.5% vs. 5%). Those who took the extract with 5% hyperforin showed greater changes in delta, theta, and alpha-1 brain wave activity after 8 days of treatment. One suggestion is that these EEG changes may have a relationship to the antidepressant effects of hyperforin, although this remains under investigation.

MECHANISMS OF ACTION OF HYPERFORIN

The authors of the previous studies proposed various mechanisms of antidepressant action for hyperforin, including the inhibition of the reuptake of serotonin, norepinephrine, and acetylcholine. Some studies support these postulated mechanisms, including the uptake inhibition of serotonin, dopamine, norepinephrine, GABA, and L-glutamate (36), although most evidence indicates that the serotonergic mechanisms might be the most critical.

Neurotransmitter Reuptake Mechanisms

Dimpfel et al. (37) used "Tele-Stereo-EEG," which consisted of continuous recording of intracerebral field potentials in the freely moving rat, to investigate the mechanism of action of hyperforin. Hyperforin produced changes of reproducible power increases within the alpha-1 band of the striatum. This early action was quite similar to that observed following the application of serotonin reuptake inhibitors (37), suggesting that hyperforin had an SSRI-like mechanism.

The antidepressant activities of the alcoholic hypericum extract (4.5% hyperforin) were compared to those of the CO_2 extract (38.8% hyperforin). Both had comparable antidepressant activity, but the ethanol extract potentiated dopaminergic behavioral responses, whereas these effects were less pronounced in the CO_2 extract–treated groups. Conversely, the serotoninergic effects of the CO_2 extract were more pronounced than those of the alcoholic extract. The authors therefore proposed that dopaminergic and serotoninergic mechanisms have a major role in the therapeutically observed antidepressant activities of SJW extracts and that the data particularly supported a serotonergic role for hyperforin (38).

Studies with the ethanolic extract of SJW and with isolated hyperforin indicated that hyperforin can inhibit serotonin-induced responses and the uptake of this neurotransmitter in the peritoneal cells. Based on the assumption that the effects of hyperforin were due to its actions on serotoninergic 5-HT3 and/or 5-HT4 receptors, further studies have been conducted to investigate its effects on the CNS. These efforts revealed hyperforin's antidepressant activity using the behavioral despair test and led to the working hypothesis that hyperforin and serotoninergic mechanisms were a major component in the antidepressant activities of alcoholic SJW extracts (32).

Kaehler et al. (39) tested whether hyperforin influenced the extracellular concentrations of neurotransmitters in the rat locus ceruleus. Hyperforin was found to enhance the extracellular levels of dopamine, norepinephrine, and serotonin, as well as that of the excitatory amino acid glutamate. The levels of the main serotonin metabolite 5-hydroxyindolacetic acid, as well as those of the amino acids GABA, taurine, aspartate, serine, and arginine, were not influenced. The authors suggested that the antidepressant property of hyperforin was due to enhanced concentrations of monoamines and glutamate in the synaptic cleft, probably as a consequence of uptake inhibition (39).

Receptor Downregulation

Hydroalcoholic SJW extract inhibited the synaptosomal uptake of serotonin, norepinephrine, and dopamine with comparable affinities, resulting in a significant downregulation of cortical β-adrenoceptors and 5-HT2 receptors after the subchronic treatment of rats. Hyperforin was identified as the unspecific reuptake inhibitor of SJW extracts for the three synaptosomal uptake systems. Moreover, the previously mentioned hyperforin-enriched (38%) CO_2 extract also led to a significant β-receptor downregulation after subchronic treatment (40).

Competitive and Uncompetitive Inhibition via Ionic Channels and Receptors

The effects of hyperforin on voltage-gated and ligand-gated ionic conductances were investigated with the whole-cell patch clamp and concentration clamp techniques on isolated hippocampal pyramidal neurons and on cerebellar Purkinje neurons of the rat. Hyperforin induced a rapidly stabilizing dose-dependent and time-dependent inward current. Hyperforin inhibited conductances of GABA, 2-(aminomethyl)phenylacetic acid (AMPA), and *N*-methyl-D-aspartate (NMDA). Hyperforin competitively inhibited AMPA-induced current (although not completely) and uncompetitively (and completely) inhibited NMDA receptor-activated ionic conductance. The authors postulate that hyperforin has a major role as a modulator of mechanisms involved in the control of neuronal ionic conductances, although its effects do not seem to be mediated by a single molecular mechanism of action (41).

Singer et al. (42) suggested that hyperforin may elevate intracellular sodium concentration, thus increasing sodium-hydrogen exchange, which is a known mechanism of serotonin uptake inhibition. Michaelis-Menten kinetics in synaptosomes of the mouse brain revealed that this type of inhibition appeared to be mainly noncompetitive (30).

Simmen et al. (43) found that low concentrations of hyperforin inhibited binding of various ligands to recombinant opioid and serotonin receptors expressed with the Semliki Forest virus system. The authors suggested that hyperforin may synergistically contribute to the antidepressant effect of SJW via this mechanism (43).

Synaptosomal Release: A Reserpine-Like Model

Gobbi et al. (44) proposed a reserpine-like mechanism of action for hyperforin; it, as well as SJW extracts containing other components, inhibited tritiated serotonin accumulation in cortical synaptosomes from the rat brain. The inhibitory effect, however, was not due to a direct blockade of the serotonin transporters because hyperforin did not inhibit tritiated citalopram binding. Hyperforin induced marked tritium release from superfused synaptosomes that had been previously loaded with tritiated serotonin, which suggests a mechanism similar to the releasing effect of reserpine (44).

PHARMACOKINETICS AND STABILITY

Biber et al. (45) investigated hyperforin pharmacokinetics in plasma. After the oral administration of 300 mg per kg SJW extract (WS 5572, containing 5% hyperforin) to rats, maximum plasma levels were reached after 3 hours, and the estimated half-life was 6 hours. Plasma levels of hyperforin could be detected for up to 24 hours in humans after the administration of film-coated tablets containing 300 mg SJW extracts representing 14.8 mg hyperforin. The maximum plasma levels were reached 3.5 hours after administration. The half-life was 9 hours, and mean residence time was 12 hours. The hyperforin pharmacokinetics were linear up to 600 mg of the extract. Doses of 900 to 1,200 mg of extract resulted in lower values for maximum concentration (C_{max}) and area under the curve (AUC) than those expected from linear extrapolation of data from lower doses. In a repeated- dose study, no accumulation of hyperforin in the plasma was observed. Using the observed AUC values from the repeated-dose study, the estimated steady-state plasma concentration of hyperforin after the normal therapeutic dose was approximately 100 ng per mL (45).

The stability of hyperforin is limited; sufficient shelf-life of the isolated compound can only be achieved by the hot maceration of dried flowers with eutanol G and storage in the absence of air (46). Because of the tendency of hyperforin to degrade, long-term storage at $-70°C$ under nitrogen is recommended (36). Additional polar hyperforin analogues have been detected by gradient high-performance liquid chromatography (HPLC) in SJW oils in which hyperforin had decomposed (46). Their function remains unelucidated.

SUMMARY

These studies suggest various possible mechanisms of action for hyperforin; it is likely a major—but not the only—antidepressive component of hypericum. The recently developed technology for isolating hyperforin should allow a more accurate characterization of the mechanisms of action of this compound.

The extracts of the flower from SJW, hypericum and hyperforin, have been shown to be effective antidepressants in controlled trials (better than the placebo and equal to active, albeit low-dose, antidepressant agents); they have demonstrated effectiveness (clinical improvement in the field in open studies); and they exhibit a benign side effect profile. More studies in the United States are underway, and the results of these trials are eagerly awaited.

REFERENCES

1. Linde K, Ramirez G, Mulrow CD, et al. St. John's wort for depression—an overview and meta-analysis of randomized clinical trials. *Br Med J* 1996;313:253–258.
2. Volz HP. Controlled clinical trials of hypericum extracts in depressed patients. *Pharmacopsychiatry* 1997;30:72–76.
3. Vorbach EU, Arnold KH, Hubner WD. Efficacy and tolerability of St. John's wort extract LI 160 versus imipramine in patients with severe depressive episodes according to ICD-10. *Pharmacopsychiatry* 1997;30:81–85.
4. Brenner R, Azbel V, Madhusoodanan S, et al. Comparison of an extract of hypericum (LI 160) and sertraline in the treatment of depression: a double-blind, randomized pilot study. *Clin Ther* 2000; 22:411–419.
5. Schrader E. Equivalence of St John's wort extract (Ze 117) and fluoxetine: a randomized, controlled study in mild-moderate depression. *Int Clin Psychopharmacol* 2000;15:61–68.
6. Grube B, Walper A, Wheatley D. St. John's Wort extract: efficacy for menopausal symptoms of psychological origin. *Adv Ther* 1999;16:177–186.
7. Shelton RC, Keller MB, Gelenberg A, et al. Effectiveness of St John's wort in major depression: a randomized controlled trial. *JAMA* 2001;285:1978–1986.
8. Woelk H, Burkard G, Grunwald J. Benefits and risks of the hypericum extract LI 160: drug monitoring study with 3250 patients. *J Geriatr Psychiatr Neurol* 1994;7:34–38.
9. Siegers CP, Biel S, Wilhelm KP. Phototoxicity caused by hypericum. *Nervenheilkunde* 1993; 12:320–322.
10. Brockmoller J, Reum T, Bauer S, et al. Hypericin and pseudohypericin: pharmacokinetics and effects on photosensitivity in humans. *Pharmacopsychiatry* 1997;30:94–101.
11. Schmidt U, Harrer G, Kuhn U, et al. Interaction of hypericum extract with alcohol. Placebo controlled study with 32 volunteers. *Nervenheilkunde* 1993;12:314–319.
12. Czekalla J, Hubner WD, Jager D. The effect of hypericum extract on cardiac conduction as seen in the electrocardiagram compared to that of imipramine. *Pharmacopsychiatry* 1997;30:86–88.
13. Moore LB, Goodwin B, Jones SA, et al. St. John's wort induces hepatic drug metabolism through activation of the pregnane X receptor. *Proc Natl Acad Sci U S A* 2000;97:7500–7502.
14. Fugh-Berman A. Herb-drug interactions. *Lancet* 2000;355:134–138.
15. Baede-van Dijk PA, van Galen E, Lekkerkerker JF. [Drug interactions of Hypericum perforatum (St. John's wort) are potentially hazardous.] *Ned Tijdschr Geneeskd* 2000;144:811–812.
16. Miller JL. Interaction between indinavir and St. John's wort reported. *Am J Health Syst Pharmacol* 2000;57:625–626.
17. Piscitelli SC, Burstein AH, Chaitt D, et al. Indinavir concentrations and St John's wort. *Lancet* 2000;355:547–548.
18. Prost N, Tichadou L, Rodor F, et al. St. Johns wort-venlafaxine interaction. *Presse Med* 2000;29: 1285–1286.
19. Beckman SE, Sommi RW, Switzer J. Consumer use of St. John's wort: a survey on effectiveness, safety, and tolerability. *Pharmacotherapy* 2000;20:568–574.
20. Bladt S, Wagner H. MAO inhibition by fractions and constituents of hypericum extract. *Nervenheilkunde* 1993;12:349–352.
21. Barbenel DM, Yusufi B, O'Shea D, Bench CJ. Mania in a patient receiving testosterone replacement postorchidectomy taking St John's wort and sertraline. *J Psychopharmacol* 2000;14:84–86.
22. Moses EL, Mallinger AG. St. John's wort: three cases of possible mania induction. *J Clin Psychopharmacol* 2000;20:115–117.
23. Nierenberg AA, Burt T, Matthews J, Weiss AP. Mania associated with St. John's wort. *Biol Psychiatr* 1999;46:1707–1708.
24. Schneck C. St. John's wort and hypomania. *J Clin Psychiatr* 1998;59:689.
25. O'Breasail AM, Argouarch S. Hypomania and St John's wort. *Can J Psychiatr* 1998;43:746–747.
26. Thiele B, Ploch M, Brink I. Modulation of cytokine expression by hypericum extract. *Nevenheilkunde* 1993;12:353–356.
27. Müller W, Rossol R. Effects of hypericum extract on the expression of serotonin receptors. *Nervenheilkunde* 1993;12:357–358.
28. Teufel-Mayer R, Gleitz J. Effects of long-term administration of hypericum extracts on the affinity and density of the central serotonergic 5-HT1 A and 5-HT2 A receptors. *Pharmacopsychiatry* 1997; 30:113–116.
29. Schulz V, Hansel R, Tyler VE. *Rational phytotherapy: a physicians' guide to herbal medicine*, 4th ed. Berlin: Springer, 2001.

30. Laakmann G, Schule C, Baghai T, et al. St. John's Wort in mild to moderate depression: the relevance of hyperforin for the clinical efficacy. *Pharmacopsychiatry* 1998;31:54–59.
31. Schellenberg R, Sauer S, Dimpfel W. Pharmacodynamic effects of two different hypericum extracts in healthy volunteers measured by quantitative EEG. *Pharmacopsychiatry* 1998;31:44–53.
32. Chatterjee SS, Bhattacharya SK, Wonnermann M, et al. Hyperforin as a possible antidepressant component of hypericum extracts. *Life Sci* 1998;63:499–510.
33. Firenzuoli F, Gori L. Is the antidepressant effect of hypericum extracts depending on their hyperforin content? *Forsch Komplementarmed* 1999;6:27–28.
34. Erdelmeier CA. Hyperforin, possibly the major non-nitrogenous secondary metabolite of Hypericum perforatum L. *Pharmacopsychiatry* 1998;31:2–6.
35. Verotta L, Appendino G, Belloro E, et al. Furohyperforin, a prenylated phloroglucinol from St. John's wort. *J Nat Prod* 1999;62:770–772.
36. Orth HC, Rentel C, Schmidt PC. Isolation, purity analysis and stability of hyperforin as a standard material from Hypericum perforatum L. *J Pharm Pharmacol* 1999;51:193–200.
37. Dimpfel W, Schober F, Mannel M. Effects of a methanolic extract and a hyperforin-enriched CO2 extract of St. John's Wort (Hypericum perforatum) on intracerebral field potentials in the freely moving rat (Tele-Stereo-EEG). *Pharmacopsychiatry* 1998;31:30–35.
38. Bhattacharya SK, Chakrabarti A, Chatterjee SS. Activity profiles of two hyperforin-containing hypericum extracts in behavioral models. *Pharmacopsychiatry* 1998;31:22–29.
39. Kaehler ST, Sinner C, Chatterjee SS, et al. Hyperforin enhances the extracellular concentrations of catecholamines, serotonin and glutamate in the rat locus coeruleus. *Neurosci Lett* 1999;262:199–202.
40. Muller WE, Singer A, Wonnemann M, et al. Hyperforin represents the neurotransmitter reuptake inhibiting constituent of hypericum extract. *Pharmacopsychiatry* 1998;31:16–21.
41. Chatterjee S, Filippov V, Lishko P, et al. Hyperforin attenuates various ionic conductance mechanisms in the isolated hippocampal neurons of rat. *Life Sci* 1999;65:2395–2405.
42. Singer A, Wonnemann M, Muller WE. Hyperforin, a major antidepressant constituent of St. John's Wort, inhibits serotonin uptake by elevating free intracellular Na^{+1}. *J Pharmacol Exp Ther* 1999;290: 1363–1368.
43. Simmen U, Burkard W, Berger K, et al. Extracts and constituents of hypericum perforatum inhibit the binding of various ligands to recombinant receptors expressed with the semliki forest virus system. *J Recept Signal Transduct Res* 1999;19:59–74.
44. Gobbi M, Valle FD, Ciapparelli C, et al. Hypericum perforatum L. extract does not inhibit 5-HT transporter in rat brain cortex. *Naunyn Schmiedebergs Arch Pharmacol* 1999;360:262–269.
45. Biber A, Fischer H, Romer A, et al. Oral bioavailability of hyperforin from hypericum extracts in rats and human volunteers. *Pharmacopsychiatry* 1999;31:36–43.
46. Maisenbacher P, Kovar KA. Analysis and stability of Hyperici oleum. *Planta Med* 1992;58:351–354.

2

Omega-3 Fatty Acids in Mood Disorders

A Review of Neurobiologic and Clinical Actions

Andrew L. Stoll and Carol A. Locke

INTRODUCTION TO OMEGA-3 FATTY ACIDS:
ORIGIN AND CHEMISTRY

The omega-3 fatty acids, along with their counterparts, the omega-6 fatty acids, are a group of crucial naturally occurring lipids, which collectively are termed essential polyunsaturated fatty acids (PUFA) (1,2). The following are three predominant, naturally occurring omega-3 fatty acids: docosahexanoic acid (DHA), eicosapentanoic acid (EPA), and α-linolenic acid (ALA). The first two are known as the long-chain omega-3 fatty acids and are found primarily in fish oil and other marine sources (particularly in cold-water and oily fish, such as anchovies, mackerel, and salmon) (3). The last, a shorter-chain fatty acid, is an omega-3 fatty acid obtained from certain species of land-based plants (flaxseed, purslane, and others) (4,5). The modern diet in Western nations is now largely depleted of omega-3 fatty acids (6).

Omega-6 fatty acids, such as the 18-carbon linoleic acid (LA) and the 20-carbon arachidonic acid (AA), are derived primarily from vegetable oils and are ubiquitous in the food supply of Western countries (1,6,7). The chemical structures of the PUFAs and related lipids are shown in Fig. 2.1.

Vertebrate animal species cannot desaturate, or add a double bond to, fatty acids before the ninth carbon atom from the lipophilic end of the carbon chain (8). Thus, the omega-3 and the omega-6 fatty acids, with double bonds beginning at the third and sixth carbon atoms, respectively, must be obtained from the diet (hence the term "essential"). The origin of the long-chain omega-3 fatty acids is photosynthesis within the chloroplasts of marine phytoplankton (9). The EPA and DHA are then passed through the food web, ultimately to humans.

The major differences among the various omega-3 fatty acids are the length of the carbon chain and the number of double bonds (Fig. 2.1). DHA has a 22-carbon chain with six double bonds, EPA has a 20-carbon chain with five double bonds, and ALA has an 18-carbon chain with three double bonds (1). In the omega-3 fatty acids, the double bonds recur every third carbon atom, and *in vivo*, humans can theoretically convert one omega-3 fatty acid into another. The rate-

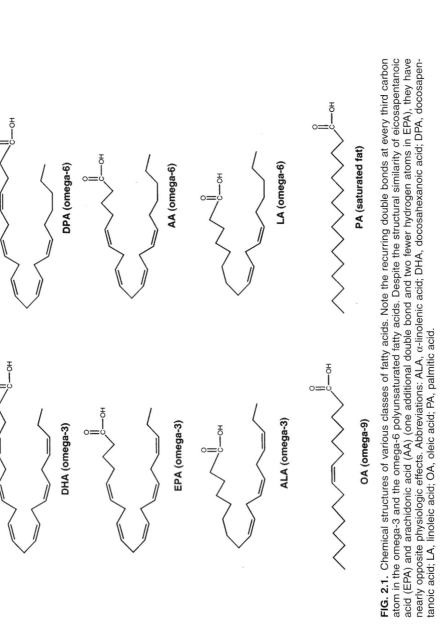

FIG. 2.1. Chemical structures of various classes of fatty acids. Note the recurring double bonds at every third carbon atom in the omega-3 and the omega-6 polyunsaturated fatty acids. Despite the structural similarity of eicosapentanoic acid (EPA) and arachidonic acid (AA) (one additional double bond and two fewer hydrogen atoms in EPA), they have nearly opposite physiologic effects. Abbreviations: ALA, α-linolenic acid; DHA, docosahexanoic acid; DPA, docosapentanoic acid; LA, linoleic acid; OA, oleic acid; PA, palmitic acid.

limiting step in the conversion process involves the enzyme Δ-6 desaturase, and thus the process of elongation is limited, with some conversion of ALA to EPA occurring, but little of EPA or ALA to DHA (10).

MEMBRANE EFFECTS OF THE OMEGA-3 FATTY ACIDS

Among the major biologic functions of the omega-3 fatty acids is their role in cell membranes. The omega-3 fatty acids are incorporated into the phospholipids that comprise the lipid bilayer surrounding every cell, as well as the organelles within cells (e.g., mitochondria) (1). The unique chemical structure of the omega-3 fatty acids is what produces their specific biologic effects within the membranes. The term polyunsaturated denotes the presence of two or more double bonds in the fatty acid molecule. The presence of multiple double bonds in the carbon chain produces a more highly folded and flexible molecule than those seen in more saturated fatty acids (Fig. 2.2) (11). The inherent flexibility and other

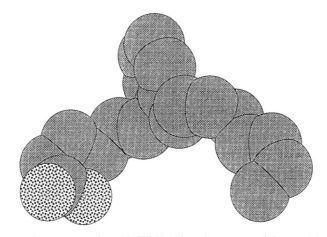

Eicosapentanoic acid (EPA): 20 carbon omega-3 fatty acid

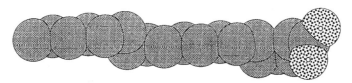

Palmitic acid: 18 carbon saturated fatty acid

FIG. 2.2. Three-dimensional space-filling models of the chemical structures of an omega-3 polyunsaturated fatty acid (EPA) and a saturated fat (palmitic acid). The presence of multiple double bonds in the polyunsaturated fatty acid leads to a very kinked and flexible molecule. This flexibility permits increased molecular motion, which is why polyunsaturated oils are liquid at room temperature and produce a more fluid cell membrane. The saturated fat, with no double bonds, is a straight and rigid molecule. Saturated fats are solids at room temperature and tend to produce less fluid cell membranes.

physical properties of PUFAs is why these oils are liquids at room temperature, in contrast to saturated fats, which are solids at room temperature. This difference in melting point between the PUFAs and more saturated fatty acids explains why membranes with a high content of omega-3 fatty acids are more fluid at a given body temperature when compared with membranes containing high concentrations of saturated fatty acids (11). This difference in membrane fluidity is thought to have significant biologic consequences, particularly on the conformation and the activities of proteins intrinsic to the lipid membrane, such as neurotransmitter receptors and enzymes regulating signal transduction in neurons (12).

OMEGA-3 FATTY ACIDS AND SIGNAL TRANSDUCTION

Omega-3 fatty acid-containing phospholipids within the inner leaflet of the lipid bilayer appear to dampen abnormal intracellular signal transduction (13). They accomplish this by inhibiting the G-protein–mediated and phospholipase C–mediated hydrolysis of crucial membrane phospholipids, such as phosphatidylinositol (PI), into the second messenger molecules inositol triphosphate (IP_3) and diacylglycerol (DAG) (13,14) (Fig. 2.3). This effect has been demonstrated in neutrophils in the periphery (13), and it presumably occurs in brain as well. The established mood stabilizers, lithium and valproate, also appear to inhibit different aspects of signal transduction related to the PI system (14) (Fig. 2.3). Thus, one possible mechanism for the apparent mood-stabilizing and antidepressant action of the omega-3 fatty acids is this effect on signal transduction.

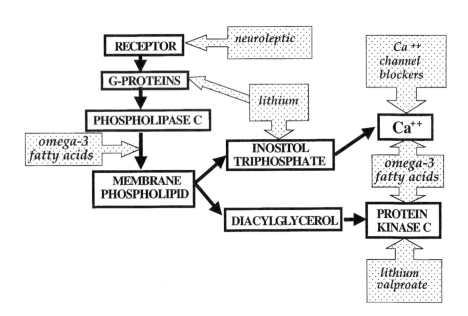

Calcium is another crucial intracellular signaling agent, the concentration of which is tightly regulated by cells (14,15) (Fig. 2.3). Omega-3 fatty acids modulate the influx of calcium ions through the L-type calcium channel (16,17). Some have suggested that this effect is the result of phospholipase A2–mediated hydrolysis of omega-3 fatty acids containing phospholipids into free omega-3 fatty acids. The free omega-3 fatty acids appear to interact with the L-type calcium channel, blocking the influx of calcium. The cardioprotective effects of the omega-3 fatty acids are thought to be mediated, in part, by this interaction with calcium channels and also possibly via omega-3 fatty acid regulation of sodium and potassium channels (16,17). Since L-type calcium channel blockers, such as verapamil and nimodipine, appear to have efficacy in the treatment of mania and possibly rapid cycling (15,18), omega-3 fatty acids may exert their mood-stabilizing effect, in part, via this calcium flux inhibition.

Omega-3 fatty acids also directly reduce the activity of protein kinase C (PKC) (19). PKC, a ubiquitous enzyme responsible for activating many crucial cellular responses, can be considered a third messenger molecule (20). PKC inhibition has been one of the more recently suggested mechanisms of action for valproate in bipolar disorder (21).

OMEGA-3 FATTY ACID ACTION IN IMMUNE AND INFLAMMATORY PATHWAYS

In addition to the important regulatory role of omega-3 fatty acids in signal transduction and as a component of cell membranes, they are crucial to inflammatory and immune pathways. A large body of data now supports inflammatory mechanisms in the pathophysiology of mood disorders (22–24). Specifically, an

---

FIG. 2.3. Recent research suggests that all of the currently available mood-stabilizing drugs appear to have inhibitory effects on neuronal signal transduction systems and that this inhibitory effect on cell-signaling pathways may be crucial to their mechanism of action in bipolar patients. An understanding of the crucial signal transduction pathway associated with the membrane phospholipid phosphatidylinositol is highly relevant to recently proposed mechanisms of action for mood-stabilizing drugs. The phosphatidylinositol system is the signal transduction pathway for a number of psychiatrically relevant neurotransmitter systems, such as the serotonin-2 receptor. When activated by an appropriate ligand-receptor interaction, receptor-linked G-proteins activate phospholipase C (and possibly other phospholipases). Phospholipase C activation leads to the hydrolysis of phosphatidylinositol into the second messenger molecules, diacylglycerol (DAG) and inositol triphosphate (IP_3). Diacylglycerol remains largely membrane bound due to its lipophilic structure and activates the third messenger enzyme, protein kinase C (PKC). PKC phosphorylates a number of cellular proteins (thus changing their structure and function), including DNA transcription factors. IP_3, which is hydrophilic, diffuses into the cytoplasm where it binds to a specific receptor on the endoplasmic reticulum. The IP_3-receptor interaction leads to rapid Ca^{2+} release from the endoplasmic reticulum. Ca^{2+} is another cellular messenger that activates a number of cellular processes. Using the model of suppression of neuronal signal transduction described above, new mood stabilizing agents can be rationally developed. One promising group of compounds are the omega-3 fatty acids, which are obtained from marine or plant sources. Omega-3 fatty acids have biochemical actions in common with conventional mood stabilizers, but they also inhibit other aspects of signal transduction in addition to their well described effects on membranes.

overactivity of inflammatory and immune responses has been documented in major depression.

EPA, with its 20-carbon chain, is converted directly to the 20-carbon eicosanoids (1). Eicosanoid is an umbrella term for several classes of hormone-like cell-signaling molecules, including the prostaglandins, prostacyclins, thromboxanes, and leukotrienes. Eicosanoids are present in every organ system, including the central nervous system; and they regulate inflammatory and immune function (1,22).

Omega-6 fatty acids, particularly AA, generally are antagonistic to omega-3 (EPA) action in the immune and inflammatory systems (1). Indirect evidence suggests that the rapid brain expansion phase of human evolution was accompanied, or even driven forward, by a dietary ratio of omega-6 to omega-3 fatty acids that was close to 1 to 1 (25–27). Under these optimal conditions, the omega-6 fatty acid AA competes with the omega-3 fatty acid EPA to achieve balanced immune and inflammatory function. However, the widespread use of omega-6–containing vegetable oils and the dramatic decline in the consumption of foods with omega-3 fatty acids in both the United States and other developed Western nations has resulted in a highly skewed ratio of omega-6 to omega-3 fatty acids (28–30). This overabundance of omega-6 fatty acids has shifted our eicosanoid-dependent inflammatory and immune pathways into an activated, proinflammatory state.

Like EPA, AA is converted to a series of eicosanoids (1). The balance of the precursor omega-6 (AA) and the omega-3 (EPA) fatty acids determines the activity of immune and inflammatory pathways. Eicosanoids from arachidonic acid (omega-6) have rapid and powerful inflammatory actions in the body (1). Eicosanoids derived from EPA (omega-3) are created more slowly, and their actions are often moderate in comparison to the omega-6–derived eicosanoids. EPA and AA are

---

TABLE 2.1. *Potential mechanisms of action of omega-3 fatty acids in mood disorders*

EPA, acting in the phospholipid cell membrane's inner leaflet, inhibits the action of the phosphatidylinositol-specific phospholipase C signal transduction pathway in humans, reducing the generation of second messenger molecules.

EPA competes with arachidonic acid, its omega-6 counterpart, at multiple sites in the body. High amounts of EPA will reduce the synthesis of arachidonic acid–derived eicosanoids, thereby reducing the formation of specific proinflammatory cytokines. Certain cytokines (IL-2, IL-6, and others), as a component of an exaggerated inflammatory response, can induce depression through unknown mechanisms.

DHA, and to a lesser extent EPA, are incorporated into the cell membrane, where they affect the physical structure and increase the fluidity of the membrane. This in turn leads to changes in the structure and function of various cell structures, particularly transmembrane proteins, such as receptors for neurotransmitters.

EPA, DHA, and eicosanoids can directly activate nuclear receptors, such as peroxisomal proliferator-activated receptors, leading to changes in gene expression and energy balance, possibly affecting mood.

DHA, EPA, and α-linolenic acid all affect calcium, sodium, and potassium ion channels, which are crucial for regulating neuronal activity.

EPA and various EPA-derived eicosanoids may directly affect mood via specific receptors in the brain.

Direct omega-3 inhibition of the eicosanoid-producing enzyme cyclooxygenase 2.

Abbreviations: DHA, docosahexanoic acid; EPA, eicosapentanoic acid; IL, interleukin.

intended to exist in balance; but, without sufficient EPA, AA and its progeny will monopolize the eicosanoid-associated systems throughout the body, thereby increasing the risk for intense, unchecked inflammatory responses. Such an imbalance toward the omega-6 eicosanoids causes white blood cells to release potent immune-activating cytokines (1,22–24). Cytokines are small peptide hormones, such as interleukins (IL), interferons, and tumor necrosis factor, that directly mediate inflammation and immunity. Excess cytokine activity has been observed in major depression (22–24), as this chapter discusses later.

Many other possible mechanisms of action have been suggested for the omega-3 fatty acids in mood disorders (Table 2.1).

GENERAL HEALTH EFFECTS OF THE OMEGA-3 FATTY ACIDS

Omega-3 fatty acids are involved in the functioning of virtually every organ system in the human body. Thus, the finding that omega-3 fatty acid deficiency states, so prevalent in Western nations, are associated with a variety of disease states is not surprising, and omega-3 fatty acid supplementation is associated with prophylactic or therapeutic benefits in a number of major disease categories of the West (7,29). For example, one well established and replicated finding is that the omega-3 fatty acids from fish oil promote cardiovascular health (30–32). Adequate omega-3 fatty acid consumption is associated with an approximately 30% reduction in the incidence of first myocardial infarctions and with a 30% reduction in sudden cardiac death if a heart attack occurs (30–32). Some controlled studies demonstrate an omega-3 fatty acid benefit in rheumatoid arthritis (33), Crohn disease (34), and other inflammatory illnesses (35). With all of these data, the fact that the omega-3 fatty acids are not used more often in the typical primary care setting or cardiology office may seem surprising. One possible reason is the lack of corporate-sponsored research and marketing because the well described omega-3 fatty acid chemical structure cannot be patented. Another explanation may be related to the state of nutritional science, a discipline that was long ago cast outside of medicine. As a result, nutritional studies have been traditionally omitted or are covered only superficially in medical schools, and many physicians continue to underestimate the importance of nutrition as a foundation of health and preventive medicine.

OMEGA-3 FATTY ACIDS IN BIPOLAR DISORDER

The authors' group's initial interest in omega-3 fatty acids for bipolar disorder was based on the similarity between the biochemical actions of the omega-3 fatty acids and the established and putative mood stabilizers (14). The shared property of inhibition of signal transduction is particularly striking. The hypothesis that an omega-3 fatty acid formulation derived from fish oil would be an effective mood stabilizer was tested recently in a 4-month, prospective, double-blind, parallel design, placebo-controlled trial (36). High-dose omega-3 fatty acids (6.2 g of EPA and 3.4 g of DHA per day) were compared to a placebo (olive oil) in bipolar patients who had experienced a recent manic or hypomanic episode. This high dose was chosen on the basis of previously reported controlled studies in rheumatoid arthritis and other medical disorders. The omega-3 fatty acid formulation used in the study was supplied by the National Institutes of Health in 1,000-mg capsules containing 70% omega-3 fatty acids, with a ratio of EPA to DHA of nearly 2 to 1.

Participating subjects were men and women, 18 to 65 years old, who met the Diagnostic and Statistical Manual of Mental Disorders, fourth edition (DSM-IV) (37) criteria for bipolar disorder (types I or II) and who were free of significant medical and psychiatric comorbidity. Forty percent of the study cohort had displayed rapid-cycling symptoms in the year prior to enrollment in the study. Subjects were enrolled regardless of current mood state if they met the other inclusion criteria. Patients were permitted to continue therapy with their outpatient psychiatrist or psychotherapist and were maintained (at constant dosages) on the medications they were receiving at study entry.

The main outcome measures were chosen *a priori* to be the overall response to treatment and the time patients remained in the study. Response to treatment was defined as not meeting the Structured Clinical Interview for DSM-IV diagnosis (SCID) (38) criteria for a mood episode, a reduction in the corresponding rating scale scores, and a lack of illness recurrence. Patients remained in the study unless mood symptoms were of a sufficient severity to require a change in medication. Hence, duration in the study represented an overall measure of treatment efficacy.

The study was originally intended to run 9 months per patient. However, the study was terminated after an interim data analysis at the 4-month mark revealed marked differences between the omega-3 fatty acid and placebo groups. The decision to end the study early was also influenced by a shortage of study drugs, which would have forced a premature termination of the study at approximately the 6-month point.

For nearly every outcome measure, the omega-3 fatty acid group performed better than the placebo group. For example, nine of 14 (64.3%) patients treated with omega-3 fatty acids responded to treatment, compared to three of 16 (18.8%) placebo-treated subjects ($P=0.02$; Fisher). In addition, the duration of remission was significantly greater in the omega-3 fatty acid–treated group when compared to the placebo group ($P=0.002$; Mantel-Cox; Fig. 2.4). The time to a 50% rate of recurrence of illness was only 65 days for the placebo group, reflecting the unstable nature of the study population; the omega-3 group did not reach the 50% rate of recurrence.

The most common adverse effect in both the omega-3 and olive oil groups was mild gastrointestinal distress, generally involving loose stools. Of the patients with adverse effect data at week 4 of the trial, nine of 14 omega-3–treated subjects (64.3%) complained of mild gastrointestinal side effects, while nine of 17 placebo-treated subjects (52.9%) experienced gastrointestinal

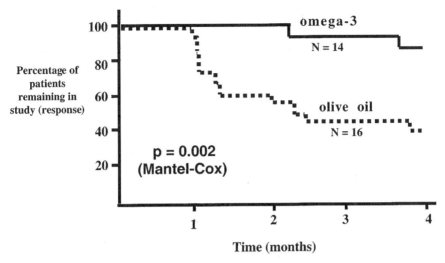

FIG. 2.4. Double-blind comparison of the clinical response to omega-3 fatty acids versus placebo treatment in patients with bipolar disorder, using Kaplan-Meier survival statistics. Note the poor response of the placebo-treated patients, where more than 50% either had not responded or had relapsed by the end of the 4-month study. In contrast, only two of 14 omega-3 fatty acids subjects failed to respond during the 4-month study period. Abbreviation: N, number of patients.

side effects (*P*=not significant; Fisher). No other adverse effects appeared with significant frequency or severity, and overall the patients tolerated the trial well.

Eight patients entered the pilot study receiving no other mood-stabilizing drugs. Four patients received the omega-3 fatty acids, and four patients received placebo. These patients either could not tolerate or did not respond to typical mood stabilizers. These patients were fully informed of the risks of placebo treatment in bipolar disorder. Even with this small cohort of patients, the four omega-3 fatty acid–treated patients experienced a statistically significant longer period of remission than the placebo group (*P*=0.04; Mantel-Cox).

Methodologic strengths of this study include the prospective, double-blind, placebo-controlled design, as well as the 4-month study duration. All patients had experienced a recent hypomanic or manic episode, creating a high-risk cohort of study patients. This study also examined two distinct aspects of clinical improvement. The specific rating scales for mania and depression, as well as the global rating scales, measured symptom improvement, and the SCID determined whether syndromic recovery or recurrence had occurred. Syndromic recovery and recurrence criteria are more stringent than symptom changes, and they may be more appropriate measures for the long-term assessment of the clinical course of a patient with bipolar disorder (39).

Methodologic problems in this study included the lack of long-term follow-up on the study drug, the differing mood states permitted at study entry, as well as the inherent heterogeneity present in any sample of bipolar patients. In this pilot study, additional heterogeneity was introduced by the use of both bipolar I and bipolar II patients. Moreover, this study did not control for concomitant pharmacotherapy.

Since this study was completed, the authors have had 3 years of clinical experience using various omega-3 fatty acid preparations in the open-label treatment of more than 150 patients with bipolar disorder. No controlled dose-response studies have yet been performed; however, the high dose of omega-3 fatty acids used in the controlled bipolar trial appears to be unnecessary in most patients. In addition, whether EPA, DHA, ALA, or all three omega-3 fatty acids are active is not clear at this time. However, based on a small number of neurochemical studies in animals, biochemical data in humans with major depression, and anecdotal evidence, EPA is the most likely omega-3 fatty acid to be clinically active in mood disorders. In addition, a recently presented double-blind controlled study in schizophrenia reported that EPA was effective and that DHA was not (40). Therefore, until more definitive data are reported, a simple and direct method for calculating dosage is simply to use the EPA content of the omega-3 supplement. A dosage of 1.5 to 6 g per day is often adequate with EPA. Some clinicians prefer to use the total omega-3 content (EPA plus DHA plus other omega-3 fatty acids) when determining dosage.

Omega-3 fatty acids are free from toxicity and serious side-effects (2,7,41). Table 2.2 describes some of the more common, generally benign side effects, as

TABLE 2.2. *Potential adverse effects of fish oil*

Adverse effect	Comments
Gastrointestinal disturbance	Benign and generally seen only at high doses. Diarrhea more common than nausea.
	Divide the dose to b.i.d. or t.i.d.; lower the dose; take the supplements with food and/or ginger root (for nausea); Daikon radish can reduce or eliminate GI disturbance.
Fishy aftertaste (repeat)	Due mainly to rancidity of fatty acids through oxidation.
	High-quality formulations are concentrated through one or more distillation steps and are processed and encapsulated under nitrogen to reduce oxidation. Such processing methods diminish or eliminate any unpleasant aftertaste.
	Divide the dose to b.i.d. or t.i.d., take all of the supplement at bedtime, or lower the dose to reduce or eliminate repeat.
Hypervitamosis A	Only seen if cod or another fish liver oil is used at higher dose. Use only fish body oils.
Impaired platelet function	No published cases of abnormal bleeding have been reported; unlike aspirin, omega-3 fatty acids inhibit platelets only moderately and transiently.
	Monitor closely and use a lower dose if receiving anticoagulants, such as warfarin or nonsteroidal antiinflammatory drugs. Low-dose aspirin used for the prevention of myocardial infarction appears safe in combination with omega-3 fatty acids.
Contamination with heavy metals or organochlorine carcinogens	*Not* an issue with highly concentrated fish oils because the distillation process used to concentrate the omega-3 fatty acids separates the oil from any potential contaminants.
	Small, nonpredatory species of fish with short life spans and those from nonpolluted waters are preferred.

well as strategies to mitigate these adverse effects. Omega-3 fatty acids appear to behave much like lamotrigine in their action in bipolar disorder (42). That is, the omega-3 fatty acids from fish oil appear to be moderate-to-strong antidepressant compounds with moderate mood-stabilizing features. Some patients appear to respond to the omega-3 fatty acids in monotherapy, but generally the fatty acids are used as adjuncts to ongoing mood stabilizer therapy. No negative interactions have been reported between the omega-3 fatty acids and psychotropic drugs or electroconvulsive therapy (43).

Cases of hypomania or mania induction are reported with omega-3 fatty acids (43–45). From the available anecdotal evidence, ALA from flaxseed oil appears to be more likely to induce abnormal mood elevation than EPA, and EPA more likely than DHA (43–45). However, without controlled data, to conclude definitively that the omega-3 fatty acids were responsible for the reported mood elevation is impossible, since patients with bipolar disorder are at risk for switching spontaneously, regardless of treatment (46). Mania and hypomania induction have been reported with a wide variety of treatments. Possibly, any agent that elevates mood introduces some risk of pathologic mood elevation. In addition, mood stabilizers likely exist along a spectrum of antimanic and antidepressant capacity. Agents such as valproate and conventional neuroleptics appear to have stronger antimanic than antidepressant action, while putative mood stabilizers, such as lamotrigine and omega-3 fatty acids, may have relatively greater mood-elevating effects.

Numerous possible mechanisms of action exist for the omega-3 fatty acids in bipolar disorder (Table 2.1), as the previous section describes. Whether the administration of concentrated fish oil supplements is producing a specific pharmacologic effect or whether it is merely replacing the known widespread deficiency of omega-3 fatty acids in Western countries is unclear at this time. Notwithstanding the unanswered questions, the omega-3 fatty acid preparations, particularly those derived from fish oil, are attractive adjuncts in patients with bipolar disorder. Currently, at least three placebo-controlled clinical trials are underway in an effort to confirm or refute the findings from the bipolar study.

OMEGA-3 FATTY ACIDS IN UNIPOLAR MAJOR DEPRESSION

The notion that omega-3 fatty acids may be effective antidepressants in unipolar depression predates the bipolar work by a number of years (7,22,44). Despite the current lack of double-blind, placebo-controlled trials in patients with unipolar depressive illness, compelling data exist that link omega-3 fatty acids to the etiology, pathophysiology, and treatment of major depression. Table 2.3 lists six lines of evidence supporting a role for the omega-3 fatty acids in major depression.

The Epidemiology of Major Depression and Omega-3 Fatty Acids

Recently, Hibbeln (47) reported his findings of a strong relationship between the amount of fish a given country consumes and the rates of major depression within that country. For example, countries such as Japan, Korea, and Taiwan

TABLE 2.3. *Six lines of evidence supporting a role for the omega-3 fatty acids in unipolar major depression*

Epidemiologic data links low omega-3 fatty acid (fish) intake and high rates of major depression.

Neurochemical studies of omega-3 fatty acids in animals have reported findings consistent with antidepressant action.

Biochemical analyses of the blood of patients with major depression indicate omega-3 fatty acid depletion.

Abnormalities in the omega-3–dependent eicosanoid and cytokine pathways during major depression are consistent with omega-3 fatty acid depletion.

Strong antidepressant effects of the omega-3 fatty acids were observed in the recent double-blind, placebo-controlled study of omega-3 fatty acids in bipolar disorder. Nearly all compounds with antidepressant effects in bipolar disorder exhibit antidepressant effects in unipolar depression.

Mood-elevating effects of omega-3 fatty acids have been reported in preliminary uncontrolled or open-label clinical studies in patients with unipolar depression and other neuropsychiatric disorders.

---

have among the highest levels of fish consumption and the lowest rates of major depression. The correlation appears strong, despite potential culture-specific underreporting of major depression in these Asian countries.

Hibbeln has also recently published a larger and more impressive data set indicating an even more robust association between the rates of postpartum depression and fish consumption among a large number of countries (48). Thus, the high fish-consuming nations exhibited the lowest rates of postpartum depression. A sound scientific rationale exists for this association between low omega-3 fatty acid consumption and the high rates of postpartum depression. High amounts of long-chain omega-3 fatty acids are required by the developing fetus and newborn, which they receive through the placenta and breast milk, respectively (49–51). The baby's ability to import and incorporate omega-3 fatty acids appears to outweigh the mother's ability to retain these compounds. If the mother has a diet low in omega-3 oils and a resultant low level of omega-3 fatty acids in her body, she is at risk for experiencing depletion of omega-3 fatty acids during pregnancy and breast feeding (52,53). A low brain and body omega-3 fatty acid content presumably leads to a greater risk of becoming depressed through some as yet unknown pathophysiologic mechanism.

Neurochemical Studies in Animals

The omega-3 fatty acids have fundamental structural and functional roles in the developing and mature nervous system (50,51,54). Several groups of investigators have recently documented interactions between omega-3 fatty acids and the neurotransmitters relevant to major depression. For example, Delion et al. (55) reported that omega-3 fatty acid deficiency in rats was associated with an increase in serotonin-2 receptor density but a normal concentration of serotonin in the frontal cortex (but not in the other brain regions studied). In addition, they observed a decrease in frontal cortex dopamine-2 receptor density and reduced dopamine levels. The direction of the changes in these neurotransmitter systems is consistent with some animal and human models of major depression. In more recent work, the same group of researchers reported that a high omega-3 fatty acid diet in rats produced an increase in frontal cortex dopamine (56). Other research groups have documented interactions of omega-3 fatty acid with peripheral serotonin function. For example, Pakala et al. (57) reported that EPA and DHA each modulated serotonin's effect on the platelets and that the combination of EPA and DHA was synergistic.

Another potential mechanism for the mood-elevating and mood-stabilizing effects of the omega-3 fatty acids may involve the direct biophysical effects of omega-3 fatty acids on the membrane environment of crucial monoamine receptors. Specifically, a high concentration of polyunsaturated fatty acids in a lipid bilayer reduces the membrane order, rendering it more fluid (11). This altered lipid environment may have important effects on the structure and function of proteins (e.g., receptors) embedded in the membrane. Heron et al. (12) measured serotonin receptor binding under varying membrane fluidity conditions. Specifically, isolated mouse brain synaptosomes were chemically modified with exogenous lipids to alter their fluidity. The researchers observed that serotonin binding was reduced as the fluidity of the membranes increased. Whether this finding is relevant to major depression in humans is unclear. However, this indicates that altering the lipid environment of a serotonin receptor can change its functioning. Conceivably, the neuronal membranes of a depressed patient who is deficient in long-chain omega-3 fatty acids would exhibit altered fluidity, which may influence the serotonin function and thus may contribute to the neurobiologic changes that cause major depression.

Biochemical studies have revealed that the ingestion of omega-3 fatty acids leads to the incorporation of these polyunsaturated compounds into membrane phospholipids (58), including those crucial for cell signaling, such as phosphatidylinositol (13,59). Increased concentrations of omega-3 fatty acids in membrane phospholipids appear to suppress phosphatidylinositol-associated signal transduction pathways (13). The precise mechanism for this effect remains unclear. However, as was previously noted, the incorporation of the polyunsaturated omega-3 fatty acids into the lipid bilayer of the cell membrane alters the physical and chemical properties of the membrane (11,58,59), possibly producing membrane phospholipids (e.g., omega-3 containing phosphatidylinositol) that are more resistant to hydrolysis by phospholipases. This could result in the reduced generation of the second messenger molecules DAG and IP_3, thereby producing less activation of downstream intracellular signaling molecules, such as PKC and calcium ions (14). The phosphatidylinositol-associated signal transduction pathway is used in many neurotransmitter systems, including the serotonin-2 receptor, which is linked to major depression, anxiety, sexual functioning, sleep, and many other neurobiologic functions (60). Many conventional mood stabilizers and antidepressants also affect signal transduction associated with the serotonin system in a manner similar to the omega-3 fatty acids (14).

One potentially crucial effect of all three omega-3 fatty acids on brain function is their modulation of sodium, potassium, and calcium channels (61). This omega-3 fatty acid alteration in ion channel activity produces antiarrhythmic effects in animal models of cardiac arrhythmias and sudden death (61). Omega-3 fatty acid modulation of ion channel function may also have strong effects on the brain, which, like the heart, is an electrochemically excitable tissue. In fact, emerging data now suggest that omega-3 fatty acids have anticonvulsant and antikindling properties (62,63). These actions are highly relevant to the possible mood effects of the omega-3 fatty acids, since most, if not all, currently used mood stabilizers modulate calcium or sodium ion channels and exhibit antikindling or anticonvulsant effects (14).

Biochemical Analyses of the Blood of Patients with Major Depression

A number of recent studies document a depletion of omega-3 fatty acids in patients with major depression (64–68). Table 2.4 presents the major findings from each study. In most of these studies, depletion of EPA, rather than DHA or ALA, was correlated with clinical variables. In contrast to these recent studies, two older, less well designed studies from one group of investigators (69,70) found that the EPA and DHA content of erythrocytes and plasma choline phosphoglycerides were actually higher in patients with endogenous depression than in their control subjects. Although reconciling these contrasting findings is difficult, the consistency and extent of the more recent data suggesting an association between omega-3 depletion in the blood and major depression are compelling.

Omega-3 Fatty Acids and Inflammatory Mechanisms in Major Depression

Another plausible mechanism for the association of omega-3 deficiency and major depression concerns the central nervous system and its inflammatory and immune pathways. Substantial data support an immunologic component in the etiology of mood disorders (22–24,29,71,72). Overactivity of the inflammatory response has been documented; and omega-3 fatty acids, particularly EPA, may dampen such overactivity. For example, investigators have reported a higher expression of T-cell activation markers (23) in patients with major depression. Excessive secretion of macrophages has also been postulated to contribute to major depression (22,71). Similarly, overactivity of the acute phase protein response has been demonstrated in major depression and mania (72).

How can an overactive immune and inflammatory response influence mood? One explanation may be the effect of the inflammatory process on the levels of neurotransmitters, especially serotonin. For example, the inflammatory response observed in major depression has been associated with a decreased availability of serum tryptophan (73,74). Another potential mechanism linking inflamma-

TABLE 2.4. *Biochemical analyses of the blood of patients with major depression*

Investigators*	Methods and findings
Adams et al. 1996 (65)	N=20 patients with moderate or severe unipolar major depression. The mean plasma and erythrocyte PUFA concentrations in the depressed patients were no different than in normal controls. A statistically significant negative correlation was observed between erythrocyte phospholipid EPA content and the severity of depressive symptoms in the depressed group. Lower EPA values were associated with more severe depressive symptoms. The ratio of omega-6 (AA) to omega-3 (EPA) in the erythrocytes displayed an even stronger correlation, with a high ratio of omega-6 to omega-3 associated with a more severe depressive syndrome.
Maes et al. 1996 (66)	36 patients with major depression, compared to 2 control groups (14 patients with minor depression and 24 normal subjects). Patients with major depression had significantly higher ratios of omega-6 (AA) to omega-3 (EPA) in serum phospholipids and cholesterol esters than either control group.
Peet et al. 1998 (67)	A statistically significant negative correlation was observed between EPA and the severity of the depressive symptoms. 15 patients with unipolar major depression, compared to 15 normal controls. Omega-3 fatty acids were substantially depleted in the patients with major depression. In this study, DHA was more depleted than EPA. Significant depletions in omega-6 and omega-9 fatty acids were also detected. A corresponding increase in the erythrocyte membrane concentration of saturated fat was observed.
Edwards et al. 1998 (68) (same group of investigators as Peet et al)	10 patients with major depression compared to 14 normal controls. Both EPA and DHA, but not ALA, were depleted. A significant negative correlation between erythrocyte membrane omega-3 content and the severity of the depressive symptoms was observed.
Hibbeln 1998 (69)	No significant difference in omega-6 content was observed between the depressed patients and the controls. 50 patients hospitalized for suicidal behavior. The 20 suicidal subjects *without* major depression showed a statistically significant negative correlation between plasma EPA and the severity of their suicidal ideation and other psychiatric symptoms. Plasma DHA and ALA showed no such correlation. Surprisingly, the 30 suicidal patients with major depression did not exhibit any significant correlation between plasma fatty acids and depressive symptoms.
Ellis et al. 1977 (70) Fehily et al. 1981 (71) (same group of investigators as Ellis et al.)	Patients with "endogenous depression" were compared to normal controls. The EPA and DHA content of erythrocytes and plasma choline phosphoglycerides were *higher* in the depressed patients.

*See chapter references for reference information.

Abbreviations: AA, arachidonic acid; ALA, α-linolenic acid; DHA, docosahexanoic acid; EPA, eicosapentanoic acid; PUFA, polyunsaturated fatty acids.

tion with mood dysregulation is the appearance of excess cytokine activity stimulating the hypothalamus to release corticotrophin-releasing factor, which then stimulates the pituitary and adrenal glands to release adrenocorticotropic hormone and the corticosteroids, respectively (75). Corticosteroids can cause either depression or mania and can also impair immunity (76). The proinflammatory cytokines, particularly IL-1β, IL-6, and tumor necrosis factor, may also be activated in the presence of various stressors, such as cancer or a heart attack (22). This may explain, in part, the increase in depression observed in certain cancers or after a stroke or heart attack.

Although speculative, the inflammatory theory of depression may unify a host of observations that were previously unexplained (22a). It is also consistent with the theory that the soaring rates of major depression in the 20th century are mediated by the rising ratios of omega-6 fatty acids relative to those of omega-3 in diets. EPA is especially important in reducing the inflammatory process and thus may be of particular interest for its antidepressant activity. Future studies should compare the antidepressant effects of EPA, DHA, and ALA individually.

Clinical Data Supporting Mood-Elevating Effects of Omega-3 Fatty Acids

Bipolar disorder and unipolar depression are distinct disorders, yet major depression occurs in patients with either illness. Historically, virtually every treatment that elevates mood in bipolar disorder can elevate mood in unipolar major depression and vice versa. Mood-elevating effects were the strongest finding in the controlled study of omega-3 fatty acids in bipolar disorder. However, confirming the assumption that the omega-3 fatty acids will be mood elevating in unipolar depression based on this paradigm must await controlled clinical trials.

In 1981, Rudin (45) published an open-label case series on the use of high dosages of flaxseed oil in psychiatric patients with a variety of diagnoses. He noted antidepressant effects, as well as a frequent occurrence of mania, that presumably was induced by the large dosage of α-linolenic acid used. With regard to other uncontrolled data, the authors have previously described treating 16 patients diagnosed with treatment-refractory unipolar major depression with omega-3 fatty acids (23). Five of the 16 patients responded at least partially; four of the five responders had a marked response to the addition of omega-3 oils to their ongoing antidepressant treatment. Although five of 16 (31%) may seem like a low rate of response to a treatment, keeping in mind that patients with treatment-resistant depression often have response rates well below this figure is important.

TYPICAL USAGE OF OMEGA-3 FATTY ACIDS
IN MOOD DISORDERS

Overview

The typical use of the omega-3 fatty acids in psychiatry is as adjuncts to conventional psychopharmacology, particularly in treatment-refractory patients.

Some patients do appear to respond to omega-3 fatty acids in monotherapy, and the double-blind, placebo-controlled data (37) from the small subgroup of medication-free bipolar patients (N=8) support this view. Despite these encouraging preliminary findings, enough data or clinical experience do not yet exist to say that the omega-3 fatty acids are truly effective antidepressants or mood stabilizers. Therefore, except under unusual circumstances, omega-3 fatty acids should be considered primarily as adjunctive treatments.

Fish Oil

Clinically, most patients seem to respond to between 1.5 to 6 g per day of EPA (or EPA plus DHA) from marine sources. However, the effective dosage appears to be highly individualized, and gradual titration is often required. In clinical trial settings, daily dosages of omega-3 fatty acids have safely exceeded 10 g per day. More than 5,000 research subjects have entered controlled trials of omega-3 fatty acids over the past two decades; these trials have used a range of omega-3 fatty acid dosages, trial lengths, and preparations in male and female patients with various disorders, different ages, and concomitant medications. A recent review of this literature revealed no serious adverse reactions in these trials (Daly B, Stoll A, Damico K, unpublished observations, 2000). Further supporting the safety of even high-dose omega-3 fatty acids is the apparent safety of the diet of traditional Arctic people, which may contain more than 16 g per day of EPA plus DHA (77). This amount of omega-3 fatty acids has been associated with a reduced risk of coronary artery disease and other common medical disorders of Western nations. Thus, even long-term use of large amounts of omega-3 fatty acids appears safe.

The number of omega-3 fatty acid capsules required per day is calculated based on the content of omega-3 fatty acids listed on the labels of these over-the-counter dietary supplements. One should read the labels carefully, as the amount of omega-3 per serving is listed, rather than the amount per capsule. Desirable qualities in an omega-3 supplement are listed in Table 2.5.

Flaxseed Oil

Flaxseed oil is produced by pressing the seeds of *Linum usitatissimmum*, which contains large quantities of ALA. For mood disorders, 3 to 5 g per day of ALA is a reasonable starting dosage. Flaxseed oil may be obtained in capsules, as with fish oil, or as a liquid. The liquid formulation is less expensive than the capsules, but some patients cannot tolerate the usually unpleasant taste of flaxseed oil. In addition, liquid flaxseed oil must be stored in the refrigerator, and it presents logistical difficulties when traveling. Whether the liquid or capsule form is used, one should calculate the dosage based on the concentration of omega-3 fatty acid listed on the label.

Some concern that flaxseed oil may present more risk than fish oil exists. For example, several cases of hypomania during omega-3 fatty acid treatment have been observed, particularly with flaxseed oil (44,46), but whether this was

TABLE 2.5. *Desirable characteristics of an omega-3 fatty acid supplement (fish oil)*

Characteristic	Comment
Highest concentration of omega-3 fatty acids	Supplements containing >90% omega-3 fatty acids are now available.
Highest concentration of EPA per capsule	Preliminary data suggest that EPA is the active mood agent of fish oil.
High ratio of EPA to DHA	Preliminary data suggest that EPA is the active mood agent of fish oil. Very little DHA is required by an older child or adult to maintain healthy tissue concentrations.
Low omega-6 fatty acid and saturated fat concentration	In unconcentrated formulations, the composition of the remaining non–omega-3 fatty acid in the oil becomes more important.
Low cholesterol concentration	The presence and concentration of cholesterol should be listed on the label.
Pharmaceutical-grade quality	Good Manufacturing Practices (GMP) are required for pharmaceutical grade products.
Omega-3 fatty acids supplement processed and encapsulated under nitrogen	Nitrogen preserves potency by preventing oxidation and rancidity of oil.
The source of the fish oil, including the type of fish used and the location of catch	Smaller species, such as sardines and anchovies, are shorter lived and lower on the food chain and therefore are less prone to the accumulation of environmental pollutants, such as mercury and poly-chlorinated biphenyls, when compared to longer-lived, predatory species, such as salmon and mackerel. Antarctic waters are among the least polluted bodies of water on earth. These factors are particularly important in brands that are not purified by distillation.
No cod liver oil	Avoid cod and other fish liver oils as the source of omega-3 fatty acids, since fish liver oil contains toxic amounts of vitamin A at higher dosages.
Presence of tocopherols (vitamin E) in the encapsulated oil as antioxidants	Very small amounts of vitamin E (<5 IU) can help prevent oxidation and can preserve the potency and freshness of the fish oil product.

Abbreviations: DHA, docosahexanoic acid; EPA, eicosapentanoic acid.

induced by the omega-3 fatty acid or whether it was merely part of the natural cycling of the patient's illness remains unclear. Other risks are associated with excessive consumption (more than 2–3 tablespoons per day) of flaxseed husks (not the oil), which contain cyanogenic nitrates and linamarin, naturally occurring molecules that inhibit iodine uptake by the thyroid gland and that have been associated with goiter (77).

IMPROVING THE SAFETY, EFFECTIVENESS, AND TOLERABILITY OF OMEGA-3 FATTY ACID SUPPLEMENTS

Taking regular antioxidant vitamins (e.g., vitamin C, 1,000 mg per day, and vitamin E, 800 IU per day) helps prevent omega-3 fatty acid oxidation in the body (78). *In vivo* oxidation of omega-3 fatty acids has the following two consequences: oxidation essentially destroys the omega-3 fatty acid molecule, and the oxidized omega-3 fatty acids can form lipid peroxides. However, with regard to oxidation, if excessive oxidation occurs, the body may become depleted of omega-3 fatty acids sooner. The lipid peroxides produced from oxidized omega-3 fatty acids are chemically reactive compounds that can damage cell membranes. Using water-soluble vitamin C with lipid-soluble vitamin E to prevent this has been suggested to work better than either antioxidant alone (79).

Taking omega-3 fatty acid supplements with a meal increases omega-3 absorption, probably through pancreatic enzyme action. The mitigation of common omega-3 fatty acid side effects is described in Table 2.2.

SUMMARY

Several compelling and independent lines of evidence support a role for the omega-3 fatty acids in the etiology, pathogenesis, and treatment of bipolar disorder and unipolar major depression. While DHA historically has been the major focus of many investigators due to its large structural role in the brain, EPA now merits a closer look. EPA is involved in a huge array of neuropsychiatrically relevant biochemical processes, and the bulk of the biochemical data in patients with unipolar depression indicates that EPA depletion is more highly correlated with depression severity than the other omega-3 fatty acids. Preliminary indications show that ALA may also possess antidepressant action. Future studies should examine the individual actions and effects of EPA, DHA, ALA, and various combinations of these oils. Dose-response studies, the effects of concomitant antioxidants, and possible positive and negative interactions of omega-3 fatty acids with conventional pharmacologic treatments also need to be performed. A definitive statement regarding the antidepressant and mood-stabilizing effects of the omega-3 fatty acids must await the results of forthcoming well designed studies (80).

ACKNOWLEDGMENTS

This work was supported, in part, by NIH RO-1 AT00161-01 and grants from the Stanley Foundation, the Poitras Charitable Foundation, and the Hirschhorn Foundation.

CONFLICT OF INTEREST STATEMENT

Dr. Stoll has research grants from the National Institutes of Health (NIH), Harvard Medical School, Janssen Pharmaceutica, the Stanley Foundation, the Poitras Foundation, and the Hirschhorn Foundation. He is on the Speaker's Bureau for Abbott Laboratories, Bristol Myers Squibb, Glaxo-Wellcome, Janssen, Lilly, Organon, Parke-Davis, Pfizer, SmithKline Beecham, and Wyeth-Ayerst. Dr. Stoll has been a consultant for Janssen, Eli Lilly, Parke-Davis, Pfizer, and CX Research (a distributor of nutriceutical products, including an omega-3 fatty acid supplement).

Dr. Locke is founder of Omega Natural Health, Inc., a nutraceutical company involved in the development of the omega-3 fatty acid product, OmegaBrite.

Dr. Locke is a consultant to CX Research on omega-3 fatty acid product development. Dr. Locke is a past consultant to Eli Lilly, Inc.

REFERENCES

1. Lands WEM. Biochemistry and physiology of n-3 fatty acids. *FASEB J* 1992;6:2530–2536.
2. Simopoulos AP, Leaf A, Salem N Jr. Workshop on the essentiality of and recommended dietary intakes for omega-6 and omega-3 fatty acids. *J Am Coll Nutr* 1999;18:487–489.
3. Stensby ME. Nutritional properties of fish oils. *World Rev Nutr Diet* 1969;11:46–105.
4. Simopoulos AP, Salem N Jr. Purslane: a terrestrial source of omega-3 fatty acids [letter]. *N Engl J Med* 1986;315:833.
5. Simopoulos AP, Norman HA, Gillaspy JE, Duke JA. Common purslane: a source of omega-3 fatty acids and antioxidants. *J Am Coll Nutr* 1992;11:374–382.
6. Leaf A, Weber PC. A new era for science in nutrition. *Am J Clin Nutr* 1987;45:1048–1053.
7. Hibbeln JR, Salem N. Dietary polyunsaturated fats and depression: when cholesterol does not satisfy. *Am J Clin Nutr* 1995;62:1–9.
8. Salem N, Ward GR. Are omega-3 fatty acids essential nutrients for mammals? In: Simopoulos AP, ed. *Nutrition and fitness in health and disease and in growth and development.* World Review of Nutrition and Dietetics, Vol. 72. Basel: Karger, 1993;72:128–147.
9. Cohen Z, Norman HA, Heimer YM. Microalgae as a source of omega-3 fatty acids. *World Rev Nutr Diet* 1995;77:1–31.
10. Salem N, Wegher B, Mena P, Uauy R. Arachidonic and docosahexaenoic acids are biosynthesized from their 18-carbon precursors in human infants. *Proc Natl Acad Sci U S A* 1996;93:49–54.
11. Barton PG, Gunstone FD. Hydrocarbon chain packing and molecular motion in phospholipid bilayers formed from unsaturated lecithins. *J Biol Chem* 1975;250:4470–4476.
12. Heron DS, Shinitzky M, Hershkowitz M, Samuel D. Lipid fluidity markedly modulates the binding of serotonin to mouse brain membranes. *Proc Natl Acad Sci U S A* 1980;77:7463–7467.
13. Sperling RI, Benincaso AI, Knoell CT, et al. Dietary omega-3 polyunsaturated fatty acids inhibit phosphoinositide formation and chemotaxis in neutrophils. *J Clin Invest* 1993;91:651–660.
14. Stoll AL, Severus E. Mood stabilizers: shared mechanisms of action at post synaptic signal transduction and kindling processes. *Harvard Rev Psychiatry* 1996;4:77–89.
15. Dubovsky SL, Thomas M, Hijazi A, Murphy J. Intracellular calcium signaling in peripheral cells of patients with bipolar affective disorder. *Eur Arch Psychiatry Clin Neurosci* 1994;243:229–234.
16. Pepe S, Bogdanov K, Hallaq H, et al. Omega-3 polyunsaturated fatty acid modulates dihydropyridine effects on L-type Ca^{2+} channels, cytosolic Ca^{2+}, and contraction in adult rat cardiac myocytes. *Proc Natl Acad Sci U S A* 1994;91:8832–8836.
17. Xiao YF, Gomez AM, Morgan JP, et al. Suppression of voltage-gated L-type Ca^{2+} currents by polyunsaturated fatty acids in adult and neonatal rat ventricular myocytes. *Proc Natl Acad Sci U S A* 1997;94:4182–4187.
18. Giannini AJ, Houser WL, Loiselle RH, Giannini MC. Antimanic effects of verapamil. *Am J Psychiatry* 1984;141:1602–1603.
19. Holian O, Nelsom R. Action of long chain fatty acids on protein kinase C activity: comparison of omega-6 and omega-3 fatty acids. *Anticancer Res* 1992;12:975–980.
20. Majerus PW, Ross TS, Cunningham TW, et al. Recent insights in phosphatidylinositol signaling. *Cell* 1990;63:459–465.
21. Chen G, Manji HK, Hawver DB, et al. Chronic sodium valproate selectively decreases protein kinase C alpha and epsilon in vitro. *J Neurochem* 1994;63:2361–2364.
22. Smith RS. Fatty acids, cytokines, and major depression. *Biol Psychiatry* 1998;43:313–314.
22a. Smith RS. The macrophage theory of depression. *Med Hypotheses* 1991;35:298–306.
23. Maes M, Stevens WJ, Declerck LS, et al. Significantly increased expression of T-cell activation markers (interleukin-2 and HLA-DR) in depression: further evidence for an inflammatory process during that illness. *Prog Neuropsychopharmacol Biol Psychiatry* 1993;17:241–255.
24. Maes M. Evidence for an immune response in major depression: a review and hypotheses. *Prog Neuropsychopharmacol Biol Psychiatry* 1995;19:11–38.
25. Eaton SB. Humans, lipids and evolution. *Lipids* 1992;27:814–820.
26. Chamberlain JG. The possible role of long-chain, omega-3 fatty acids in human brain phylogeny. *Perspect Biol Med* 1996;39:436–445.

27. Broadhurst CL, Cunnane SC, Crawford MA. Rift Valley lake fish and shellfish provided brain-specific nutrition for early Homo. *Br J Nutr* 1998;79:3–21.
28. Crawford MA, Gale MM, Woodford MH, Casped NM. Comparative studies on fatty acid composition of wild and domestic meats. *Int J Biochem* 1970;1:295–305.
29. Rudin DO. The dominant diseases of modernized societies as omega-3 essential fatty acid deficiency syndrome: substrate beriberi. *Medical Hypotheses* 1982;8:17–47.
30. Burr ML, Gilbert JF, Holliday RM, et al. Effects of changes in fat, fish, and fibre intakes on death and myocardial reinfarction: diet and reinfarction trial (DART). *Lancet* 1989;2:757–761.
31. De Lorgeril M, Renaud S, Mamelle N. Mediterranean alpha-linolenic acid rich diet in secondary prevention of coronary heart disease. *Lancet* 1994;343:1454–1459.
32. Valagussa F, Franzosi MG, Geraci E, et al. Dietary supplementation with n-3 polyunsaturated fatty acids and vitamin E after myocardial infarction: results of the GISSI-prevenzione trial. *Lancet* 1999;354:447–455.
33. Cleland LG, French JK, Betts WH, et al. Clinical and biochemical effects of dietary fish oil supplements in rheumatoid arthritis. *J Rheumatol* 1988;15:1471–1475.
34. Belluzzi A, Brignola C, Campieri M, et al. Effect of an enteric-coated fish-oil preparation on relapses in Crohn's disease. *N Engl J Med* 1996;334:1557–1560.
35. Robinson DR, Xu LL, Tateno S, Guo M, Colvin RB. Suppression of autoimmune disease by dietary n-3 fatty acids. *J Lipid Res* 1993;34:1435–1444.
36. Stoll AL, Severus E, Freeman MP, et al. Omega-3 fatty acids in bipolar disorder: a preliminary double-blind, placebo-controlled trial. *Arch Gen Psychiatry* 1999;56:407–412.
37. American Psychiatric Association. *Diagnostic and statistical manual of mental disorders*, 4th ed. Washington D.C.: American Psychiatric Association, 1994.
38. Spitzer R. *Structured clinical interview for DSM-IV*. Washington D.C.: American Psychiatric Association, 1994.
39. Tohen M, Hennen J, Zarate C Jr, et al. Two-year syndromal and functional recovery in 219 cases of first-episode major affective disorder with psychotic features. *Am J Psychiatry* 2000;157:220–228.
40. Peet M. *Eicosapentaenoic acid in schizophrenia*. Presented at the Annual meeting of the International Society for the Study of Fatty Acids and Lipids, Tsukuba, Japan, June 2000.
41. Sprecher H. Biochemistry of essential fatty acids. *Prog Lipid Res* 1981;20:13–22.
42. Calabrese JR, Fatemi SH, Woyshville MJ. Antidepressant effects of lamotrigine in rapid cycling bipolar disorder. *Am J Psychiatry* 1996;153:1236.
43. Stoll AL, Locke CA, Marangell LB, Severus WE. Omega-3 fatty acids and bipolar disorder: a review. *Prostaglandins Leukot Essent Fatty Acids* 1999;60:329–337.
44. Rudin DO. The major psychoses and neuroses as omega-3 essential fatty acid deficiency syndrome: substrate pellagra. *Biol Psychiatry* 1981;16:837–850.
45. Stoll AL, Damico K, Severus WE, Marangell LM. Are omega 3 fatty acids beneficial in depression but not mania? *Arch Gen Psychiatry* 2000;57:716–717.
46. Stoll Al, Mayer PV, Tohen M, et al. Antidepressant-associated mania: a controlled comparison to spontaneous mania. *Am J Psychiatry* 1994;151:1642–1645.
47. Hibbeln JR. Fish consumption and major depression. *Lancet* 1998;351:1213.
48. Hibbeln JR. Long-chain polyunsaturated fatty acids in depression and related conditions. In: Peet M, Glen I, Horrobin D, eds. *Phospholipid spectrum disorder*. Lancashire UK: Marius Press, 1999:195–210.
49. Al MD, Hornstra G, van der Schouw YT, Bulstra-Ramakers MT, Huisjes HJ. Biochemical EFA status of mothers and their neonates after normal pregnancy. *Early Hum Dev* 1990;24:239–248.
50. Neuringer M, Reisbick S, Janowsky J. The role of n-3 fatty acids in visual and cognitive development: current evidence and methods of assessment. *J Pediatr* 1994;125:S39–S49.
51. Uauy R, Hoffman DR. Essential fatty acid requirements for normal eye and brain development. *Semin Perinatol* 1991;15:449–455.
52. van Houwelingen AC, Ham EC, Hornstra G. The female docosahexaenoic acid status related to the number of completed pregnancies. *Lipids* 1999;34:S229.
53. Ziejdner EE, Houwelingen ACV, Kester ADM, Hornstra G. Essential fatty acid status in plasma phospholipids of mother and neonate after multiple pregnancy. *Prostaglandins Leukot Essent Fatty Acids* 1997;56:395–401.
54. Bourre JM, Bonneil M, Clement M, et al. Function of dietary polyunsaturated fatty acids in the nervous system. *Prostaglandins Leukot Essent Fatty Acids* 1993;48:5–15.
55. Delion S, Chalon S, Guilloteau D, et al. alpha-Linolenic acid dietary deficiency alters age-related changes of dopaminergic and serotonergic neurotransmission in the rat frontal cortex. *J Neurochem* 1996;66:1582–1591.

56. Chalon S, Delion-Vancassel S, Belzung C, et al. Dietary fish oil affects monoaminergic neurotransmission and behavior in rats. *J Nutr* 1998;128:2512–2519.
57. Pakala R, Pakala R, Radcliffe JD, Benedict CR. Serotonin-induced endothelial cell proliferation is blocked by omega-3 fatty acids. *Prostaglandins Leukot Essent Fatty Acids* 1999;60:115–123.
58. Bourre JM, Bonneil M, Clement M, et al. Function of dietary polyunsaturated fatty acids in the nervous system. *Prostaglandins Leukot Essent Fatty Acids* 1993;48:5–15.
59. Fowler KH, McMurray DN, Fan YY, et al. Purified dietary n-3 polyunsaturated fatty acids alter diacylglycerol mass and molecular species composition in concanavalin A-stimulated murine splenocytes. *Biochim Biophys Acta* 1993;1210:89–96.
60. Shih JC, Chen KJS, Gallaher TK. Molecular biology of serotonin receptors: a basis for understanding and addressing brain function. In: Bloom FE, Kupfer DJ, eds. *Psychopharmacology: the fourth generation of progress.* New York: Raven, 1995:422–424.
61. Kang JX, Leaf A. Antiarrhythmic effects of polyunsaturated fatty acids. Recent studies. *Circulation* 1996;94:1774–1780.
62. Yehuda S, Carasso RL, Mostofsky DI. Essential fatty acid preparation (SR-3) raises the seizure threshold in rats. *Eur J Pharmacol* 1994;254:193–198.
63. Voskuyl RA, Vreugdenhil M, Kang JX, Leaf A. Anticonvulsant effect of polyunsaturated fatty acids in rats, using the cortical stimulation model. *Eur J Pharmacol* 1998;341:145–152.
64. Adams PB, Lawson S, Sanigorski A, Sinclair AJ. Arachadonic acid to eicosapentaenoic acid ratio in blood correlates positively with clinical symptoms of depression. *Lipids* 1996;31:S157–S161.
65. Maes M, Smith R, Christophe A, et al. Fatty acid composition in major depression: decreased omega-3 fractions in cholesteryl esters and increased C20:4 omega 6/C20:5 omega 3 ratio in cholesteryl esters and phospholipids. *J Affect Disord* 1996;38:35–46.
66. Peet M, Murphy B, Shay J, Horrobin D. Depletion of omega-3 fatty acid levels in red blood cell membranes of depressive patients. *Biol Psychiatry* 1998;43:315–319.
67. Edwards R, Peet M, Shay J, Horrobin D. Omega-3 polyunsaturated fatty acid levels in the diet and in red blood cell membranes of depressed patients. *J Affect Disord* 1998;48:149–155.
68. Hibbeln JR. *Essential fatty acid status and markers of serotonin neurotransmission in alcoholism and suicide.* Presented at the NIH Workshop on Omega-3 Fatty Acids and Psychiatric Disorders, Washington, D.C., September 2–3, 1998.
69. Ellis FR, Sanders TAB. Long chain polyunsaturated fatty acids in endogenous depression. *J Neurol Neurosurg Psychiatry* 1977;40:168–169.
70. Fehily AMA, Bowey OAM, Ellis FR, et al. Plasma and erythrocyte membrane long chain polyunsaturated fatty acids in endogenous depression. *Neurochem Int* 1981;3:37–42.
71. Maes M, Smith RS. Fatty acids, cytokines, and major depression. *Biol Psychiatry* 1998;43:313–314.
72. Maes M, Delange J, Ranjan R, et al. Acute phase proteins in schizophrenia, mania, and major depression: modulation by psychotropic drugs. *Psychiatry Res* 1997;66:1–11.
73. Song C, Lin A, Bonaccorso S, et al. The inflammatory response system and the availability of plasma tryptophan in patients with primary sleep disorders and major depression. *J Affect Disord* 1998;49:211–219.
74. Maes M, Verkerk R, Vandoolaeghe E, et al. Serotonin-immune interactions in major depression: lower serum tryptophan as a marker of an immune-inflammatory response. *Eur Arch Psychiatry Clin Neurosci* 1997; 247:154–161.
75. Kling MA, Perini GI, Demitrack MA, et al. Stress-responsive neurohormonal systems and the symptom complex of affective illness. *Psychopharm Bull* 1989;25:312–318.
76. Brown ES, Khan DA, Nejtek VA. The psychiatric side effects of corticosteroids. *Ann Allergy Asthma Immunol* 1999;83:495–503.
77. Simopoulos AP, Robinson J. *The omega diet.* New York: Harper Collins, 1999.
78. Allard JP, Kurian R, Aghdassi E, et al. Lipid peroxidation during n-3 fatty acid and vitamin E supplementation in humans. *Lipids* 1997;32:535–541.
79. Mahadik SP, Scheffer RE. Oxidative injury and potential use of antioxidants in schizophrenia. *Prostaglandins Leukot Essent Fatty Acids* 1996;55:45–54.
80. Stoll AL. *The omega-3 connection.* New York: Simon & Schuster, 2001.

3

Docosahexanoic Acid in the Prevention and Treatment of Depression

Maurizio Fava and David Mischoulon

INTRODUCTION

Docosahexanoic acid (DHA) is an omega-3 (ω3), long-chain (22-carbon, with six polyunsaturated bonds) essential fatty acid (EFA). Therefore, it is designated as 22:6-ω-3 (Table 3.1). It is the most abundant fat in the brain and retina, as well as in human breast milk (1). It is found in eggs, red meat, cold-water fish, and animal organ meats (2,3). Several investigators have hypothesized that deficiency of DHA may play a role in the development of major depression, as well as of other psychiatric disorders (4–7). Evidence for this hypothesis will be reviewed in this chapter.

DHA AND OMEGA-3 FATTY ACIDS IN THE CENTRAL NERVOUS SYSTEM

In the brain, EFAs, such as DHA, are a major determinant of fluidity in synaptic membranes (7), and up to 45% of fatty acids in the synaptic membrane are EFAs (8). This suggests that DHA may play a role in signal transduction, particularly because it seems to be specialized for neuronal membrane function (9), and evidence demonstrates that deficiency of DHA in the central nervous system (CNS) may result in neurologic and psychiatric pathosis.

Deficient dietary intake of DHA during critical periods in brain development has been postulated to explain geographic differences in the incidence of multiple sclerosis (MS) (10). Indeed, DHA levels have been found to be decreased in plasma (11) and have not been detected in the adipose stores in patients with MS (12). Hibbeln and associates (13–15) investigated serotonin and dopamine metabolism and their relationship to DHA and mood symptoms. They found that violent subjects had lower concentrations of the serotonin metabolite 5-hydroxyindole-acetic acid (5-HIAA) in the cerebrospinal fluid (CSF) than that found in the CSF

This chapter was previously published by the authors in modified form in the following: Mischoulon D, Fava M. Docosahexanoic acid and ω3 fatty acids in depression. *Psychiatr Clin North Am* 2000; 23:785–794 (used with permission).

TABLE 3.1. *Long-chain unsaturated fatty acids*

Name	Number of carbon atoms	Number of double bonds	Double bond position (ω)	Food source
Palmitoleic	16	1	7	Butter/seed oils
Oleic	18	1	9	Most fats
Linoleic	18	2	6	Seed fats
Linolenic	18	3	3	Soybean oil
Arachidonic	20	4	6	Peanut oil, lard
Eicosapentanoic	20	5	3	Fish oil
Docosahexanoic	22	6	3	Fish oil, eggs, red meats, organ meats

Unsaturated fatty acids are classified according to the position of the first double bond with respect to the methyl (CH3-) end of the molecule (designated as the ωcarbon). Omega-3 fatty acids include docosahexanoic acid, eicosapentanoic acid, and linolenic acid; ω6 fatty acids include linoleic acid and arachidonic acid; and ω9 fatty acids include oleic acid.

levels in nonviolent subjects. Plasma DHA was negatively correlated with CSF 5-HIAA only among violent subjects, suggesting that dietary essential fatty acids may affect neurotransmitter concentrations (15) and hence may play a role in the development of psychiatric pathosis in cases where deficiencies are present.

RELATIONSHIP BETWEEN DHA, OMEGA-3s, AND DEPRESSION

Indirect, but compelling, evidence exists for a specific link between DHA and depression. For example, ω3 fatty acid (FA) consumption is greater in China and Taiwan than in North America (16), and the rates of depression are tenfold greater in North America than in Taiwan (17). This may be explained by the fact that the average daily intake of DHA in the United States is currently 100 mg less than it was 50 years ago, perhaps due to more modest fish consumption than in other countries. Also, DHA levels in breast milk in the United States are the lowest in the world, and DHA is not routinely incorporated in infant formulas in the United States, as opposed to those distributed in Europe, Australia, and the Middle East. Since breast milk has a greater concentration of ω3 FAs than do formulas, decreased cortical concentration of DHA is observed in formula-fed infants (18–20). DHA deficits may affect the nervous system during early development and may lead to increased vulnerability to depression (4,21,22).

Specific investigation into the mood-altering effects of ω3 FAs showed that a cholesterol-lowering diet involving increased fish intake was associated with a decrease in depression (23); this may be explained by increased levels of ω3 FAs (5). Indeed, ω3 FAs in the normal diet were negatively correlated with scores on self-rating scales for depression (7). Edwards et al. (24) found an association between the severity of depression and lower levels of red blood cell membrane ω3 FAs. Furthermore, examination of DHA and ω3 levels in cases of depression have shown that serum total ω3 FAs were decreased in depressed individuals when compared to levels in healthy controls and in individuals with minor depression (6). Finally, depression severity was shown to correlate positively with the ratio of arachidonic acid (AA) to eicosapentanoic acid (EPA) (ω6/ω3) in plasma and red blood cell phospholipids (25), suggesting that a lower level of ω3 FAs and/or a high level of ω6 FAs may be associated with depression.

DHA deficiency may also have a potential role in the development of perinatal and postpartum depression (26). A single pregnancy has been shown to deplete maternal plasma DHA levels (27), and multiple pregnancies may cause a progressive decrease in maternal plasma DHA levels (27). Postpartum periods are associated with an increased risk of depressive relapse (28), and the drop in DHA levels may play a role in the development of depression.

Alcoholism may also have a relationship to DHA levels and depression. Chronic alcohol intoxication depletes long-chain ω3 FAs from neuronal membranes (29), and depression occurs more frequently in alcoholics than in opiate addicts (30). Hibbeln and Salem (13) therefore postulated that DHA supplementation may accelerate the resolution of depression among alcoholics.

Other types of psychiatric disorders, such as bipolar disorder and psychotic disorders, may also have a relationship with DHA and ω3 FAs. Stoll et al. (31) reported on ω3 supplementation in patients with bipolar disorder, suggesting that ω3 FAs may improve the short-term course of bipolar illness. Their double-blind, placebo-controlled trial with 30 patients diagnosed with bipolar disorder revealed that of those who received the ω3 mix, only one had a recurrence; subjects in this group also had a longer period of remission. EFA deficiencies may also have a relationship with psychotic disorders, such as schizophrenia (32–34). Omega-3 and ω6 mixtures may help alleviate psychotic symptoms, and case reports with EFAs have shown variable results when they are used alone or as an adjunct to antipsychotic medications (35).

Omega-3 FAs may also have a relationship with dementia (36). For example, reduced ω3 FA content has been demonstrated in the postmortem brain tissue of individuals with Alzheimer disease when compared to that of healthy controls (37), and diets high in fish may have a protective effect (38). One case report in which an individual with dementia demonstrated clinical improvement by increasing his intake of fish exists (39), but at this time no published studies exist on the use of ω3s in dementia.

What are the possible causes of DHA deficiency in depression? Long-term dietary deficiency or a change in dietary fat selection may be contributing factors. For example, low-fat diets can increase the ratios of ω6/ω3 FAs (40), and such ratios have been increasing over time (41); depression severity has been shown to correlate positively with the AA-to-EPA ratio (ω6/ω3) in plasma and red blood cell phospholipids (25,42). Also, wild and free-range animals have significantly more ω3 FAs in tissues than do currently produced commercial livestock (43,44), which may contribute to lower ω3 FAs in the U.S. diet. Other causes of DHA deficiency in depressed states include an insufficient capacity for elongation and desaturation of ω3 precursors; an increase in ω3 FA catabolism; and hyperactivity of the hypothalamic-pituitary-adrenal axis, causing degradation of polyunsaturates; finally, repeated stressors may increase long-term chain polyunsaturate degradation via peroxidation (4).

Based on previous research, one wonders whether the replenishment of DHA in DHA-deficient individuals and the administration of DHA in nondeficient individuals would be of use in ameliorating depressive symptoms. Limited evidence exists for the psychotropic effects of exogenous DHA. For example, DHA supplementation was shown to decrease stress-induced aggression in students (45). Studies of open treatment with phosphatidylserine prepared from bovine cortex (thus rich in DHA) showed reduced withdrawal and apathy scores compared to the placebo (corn oil) among 494 elderly patients (46), and it improved depressive symptoms in 11 elderly women (47).

POSSIBLE MECHANISMS OF ACTION

If DHA has an antidepressant effect, how might it work? Omega-3 FAs decrease secretion of inflammatory cytokines that can provoke, in humans, signs and symptoms similar to those of major depressive disorder (48). In depression, a positive correlation is found between serum zinc (an antioxidant and cofactor for synthesis of ω3) and the proportions of EPA and DHA (ω3) fractions in serum phospholipids, as well as an inverse relationship between serum zinc and the ω6/ω3 ratio in phospholipids (42). These relationships suggest that abnormal ω3 metabolism may upregulate the inflammatory response via the increased oxidative potential resulting from lower zinc levels, leading to depressive symptoms.

A relationship also appears to exist between ω3 FAs and CNS neurotransmitters. Increased ω3 FA levels cause increased membrane fluidity, leading to increased serotonin (5-HT) transport by endothelial cells (49), which might account for the alleviation of depressive symptoms. Interestingly, the successful administration of serotonergic antidepressants does not seem to affect any FA variables (42), suggesting that abnormal ω3 levels may, in fact, be a trait marker for depression rather than a direct cause of a mood disorder.

Although the relationship between DHA and dopaminergic systems is unknown, decreased DHA concentration in the frontal cortex and striatum of rats achieved through dietary manipulations can lead to a decrease in dopamine concentration and dopamine-2 (D2) receptor binding (13,15), which suggests that with increased DHA levels, the opposite might occur.

Omega-3 FAs may also interact with neuronal cell membrane receptors and second messengers involved in mood alteration. DHA induces the relaxation of vasculature *in vitro* through α-2 adrenergic receptors (50), and this activity may also contribute to its antidepressant effect. Diets enriched in ω3 lead to increased G-protein coupling to adenyl cyclase stimulated by glucagon (51), which may represent a step in a cascade mechanism of antidepressant action. Phosphatidylcholine species containing DHA stabilize protein kinase C, either potentiating or attenuating its activity (41), an effect considered similar to that of mood-stabilizing medications, such as lithium.

CURRENT USE OF DOCOSAHEXANOIC ACID AND OMEGA-3 FATTY ACIDS IN THE PSYCHIATRIC COMMUNITY

Typical commercially available preparations of ω3 fatty acid mixes may contain up to 1,000 mg of ω3 and 100 to 200 mg DHA per capsule. Suggested doses are 1 to 2 capsules per day. Currently, concentrated preparations of high-grade DHA are available. Indications for these preparations are still unclear; they may include mood elevation and balance, as well as general nutritional supplementation. ω3 FA supplements appear to be extremely safe. DHA and other ω3 FAs have a benign side effect profile, with dose-related unspecified gastrointestinal upset as their main side effect (31).

The effective dose of DHA for depression is not currently known. The Workshop on the Essentiality of and Recommended Dietary Intakes for Omega-6 and Omega-3 Fatty Acids (52) recommends a daily dose of DHA of at least 220 mg, the equivalent of about one or two of the typically available commercial capsules. Preliminary data from Martek Biosciences (Columbia, MD; unpublished observations, 1999) suggest that 800 mg per day of high-grade DHA may be enough to quadruple serum levels of DHA in humans, but the ultimate clinical usefulness of this is unclear.

In a study conducted by Stoll et al. (31), participants received the equivalent of about 3.4 g of DHA divided in twice-a-day dosing. These investigators selected their dose based on the tolerability of prior dosing for other disease states. These doses are significantly higher than those typically taken by individuals who choose to self-medicate with ω3 preparations. Therefore, lower doses of DHA may be effective for depression. More studies to test minimal effective dosing may be of value, particularly when comparing outcomes in depressed individuals who have a DHA deficiency versus depressed individuals without DHA deficiency.

SUMMARY AND FUTURE DIRECTIONS FOR RESEARCH WITH DOCOSAHEXANOIC ACID AND OMEGA-3 FATTY ACIDS

Geographic areas where consumption of DHA is higher are associated with decreased rates of depression. DHA deficiency states, such as alcoholism and the postpartum period, are also linked with depression. Individuals with major depression have marked depletions in ω3 FAs (especially DHA) in red blood cell phospholipids compared to those in controls. These data suggest that DHA may be associated with depression, and the limited data available on supplementation with DHA or other ω3 FAs appear to support the hypothesis that DHA may have psychotropic effects. Overall, the use of EFAs is promising, particularly in view of the variety of illnesses potentially treatable with these substances. However, larger, carefully designed studies are needed to establish whether DHA is an effective and safe antidepressant, mood stabilizer, or antipsychotic.

A few preliminary trials of DHA are currently in progress, but to the authors' knowledge, no studies comparing DHA against a placebo or against an established antidepressant have been carried out. Studies to address this question are currently being developed at the Massachusetts General Hospital. Studies will likely require escalating doses of DHA, eventually reaching high levels to ensure that patients avoid a potentially ineffective subclinical dose. Careful monitoring of dietary intake among subjects will also be necessary because a high intake of ω3- rich foods may potentially confound results. Finally, large-scale placebo-controlled, double-blind trials comparing the efficacy and safety of DHA against standard antidepressants will be required before psychiatrists can recommend DHA as effective and safe for depression and other mood disorders.

Based on the popularity of self-medication by patients who are already taking antidepressant medications, studies examining the use of DHA as an augmentor to standard antidepressant drugs may answer whether DHA can occupy a niche as an augmenting agent for those who have a partial response or who have not responded to conventional antidepressant drugs. Because natural medications generally seem best for mild-to-moderate illness, the role of DHA as a treatment for minor and subsyndromal depression should be considered. Studies of these types hope to help clarify some of the knowledge gaps outlined in this paper.

ACKNOWLEDGMENT

Dr. Mischoulon was supported in part by a NARSAD Young Investigator Award.

REFERENCES

1. Uauy-Dagach R, Mena P. Nutritional role of omega-3 fatty acids during the perinatal period. *Clin Perinatol* 1995;22:157–175.
2. Salem N Jr, Ward GR. Are omega 3 fatty acids essential nutrients for mammals? *World Rev Nutr Diet* 1993;72:128–147.
3. Stensby ME. Nutritional properties of fish oils. *World Rev Nutr Diet* 1968;11:46–105.
4. Hibbeln JR, Salem N Jr. Dietary polyunsaturated fatty acids and depression: when cholesterol does not satisfy. *Am J Clin Nutr* 1995;62:1–9.
5. Hibbeln JR, Salem N Jr. Risks of cholesterol-lowering therapies. *Biol Psychiatry* 1996;40:686–687.
6. Maes M, Smith R, Christophe A, et al. Fatty acid composition in major depression: decreased omega 3 fractions in cholesteryl esters and increased C20: 4 omega 6/C20:5 omega 3 ratio in cholesteryl esters and phospholipids. *J Affect Disord* 1996;38:35–46.
7. Peet M, Murphy B, Shay J, et al. Depletion of omega-3 fatty acid levels in red blood cell membranes of depressive patients. *Biol Psychiatry* 1998;43:315–319.
8. Sun GY, Sun AY. Effect of chronic ethanol administration on phospholipid acyl groups of synaptic plasma membrane fraction isolated from guinea pig brain. *Res Commun Chem Pathol Pharmacol* 1979;24:405–408.
9. Salem N Jr, Kim HY, Yergey JA. Docosahexanoic acid: membrane function and metabolism. In: Simopoulos A, Kifer RR, Martin R, eds. *Health effects of polyunsaturated fatty acids in seafoods*, Vol. 15. New York: Academic Press, 1986:263–317.
10. Bernsohn J, Stephanides LM. Aetiology of multiple sclerosis. *Nature* 1967;215:821–823.
11. Holman RT, Johnson SB, Kokman E. Deficiencies in polyunsaturated fatty acids and replacement by

nonessential fatty acids in plasma lipids in multiple sclerosis. *Proc Natl Acad Sci U S A* 1989;86: 4720–4724.

12. Nightingale S, Woo E, Smith AD, et al. Red blood cell and adipose tissue fatty acids in mild inactive multiple sclerosis. *Acta Neurol Scand* 1990;82:43–50.
13. Hibbeln JR, Linnoila M, Umhau JC, et al. Essential fatty acids predict metabolites of serotonin and dopamine in cerebrospinal fluid among healthy control subjects, and early- and late-onset alcoholics. *Biol Psychiatry* 1998;44:235–242.
14. Hibbeln JR, Umhau JC, George DT, et al. Do plasma polyunsaturates predict hostility and depression? *World Rev Nutr Dietetics* 1997;82:175–186.
15. Hibbeln JR, Umhau JC, Linnoila M, et al. A replication study of violent and nonviolent subjects: cerebrospinal fluid metabolites of serotonin and dopamine are predicted by plasma essential fatty acids. *Biol Psychiatry* 1998;44:243–249.
16. Vartialnen E, Dianjun D, Marks JS, et al. Mortality, cardiovascular risk factors, and diet in China, Finland and the United States. *Public Health Rep* 1991;106:41–46.
17. Cross National Collaborative Group. The changing rate of major depression: cross national comparisons. *JAMA* 1992;268:3098–3105.
18. Farquharson J. Infant cerebral cortex and dietary fatty acids. *Eur J Clin Nutr* 1994;48:S24–S26.
19. Farquharson J, Cockburn F, Patrick WA, et al. Infant cerebral cortex phospholipid fatty-acid composition and diet. *Lancet* 1992;340:810–813.
20. Farquharson J, Jamieson EC, Logan RW, et al. Age- and dietary-related distributions of hepatic arachidonic and docosahexaenoic acid in early infancy. *Pediatr Res* 1995;38:361–365.
21. Farquharson J, Cockburn F, Patrick WA, et al. Effect of diet on infant subcutaneous tissue triglyceride fatty acids. *Arch Dis Child* 1993;69:589–593.
22. Farquharson J, Jamieson EC, Abbasi KA, et al. Effect of diet on the fatty acid composition of the major phospholipids of infant cerebral cortex. *Arch Dis Child* 1995;72:198–203.
23. Weidner G, Connor SL, Hollis JF, et al. Improvements in hostility and depression in relation to dietary change and cholesterol lowering. The Family Heart Study. *Ann Intern Med* 1992;117:820–823.
24. Edwards R, Peet M, Shay J, et al. Omega-3 polyunsaturated fatty acid levels in the diet and in red blood cell membranes of depressed patients. *J Affect Disord* 1998;48:149–155.
25. Adams PB, Lawson S, Sanigorski A, et al. Arachidonic acid to eicosapentaenoic acid ratio in blood correlates positively with clinical symptoms of depression. *Lipids* 1996;31:S157–S161.
26. Holman RT, Johnson SB, Ogburn PL. Deficiency of essential fatty acids and membrane fluidity during pregnancy and lactation. *Proc Natl Acad Sci U S A* 1991;88:4835–4839.
27. Houwelingen AC, Honstra G. *Docosahexanoic acid, 22:6(n3), cervonic acid (CA), and hypertension in pregnancy: consequences for mother and child.* Scientific conference on omega-3 fatty acids in nutrition, vascular biology and medicine. Houston, TX: American Heart Association 17-9 (abstr 56), 1994.
28. Cohen LS, Altshuler LL. Pharmacologic management of psychiatric illness during pregnancy and the postpartum period. *Psychiatr Clin North Am Annu Drug Ther* 1997;4:21–60.
29. Salem N Jr, Ward G. The effects of ethanol on polyunsaturated fatty acid composition. In: Alling C, Diamond I, Leslie SW, et al, eds. *Alcohol, cell membranes and signal transduction in brain.* New York: Plenum Press, 1993:33–46.
30. Weissman MW. The treatment of depressive symptoms secondary to alcoholism, opiate addiction and schizophrenia: evidence for the efficacy of tricyclics. In: Clayton PJ, Barret JE, eds. *Treatment of depression: old controversies and new approaches.* New York: Raven Press, 1983:207–216.
31. Stoll A, Severus WE, Freeman MP, et al. Omega 3 fatty acids in bipolar disorder. *Arch Gen Psychiatry* 1999;56:407–412.
32. Laugharne JD, Mellor JE, Peet M. Fatty acids and schizophrenia. *Lipids* 1996;31:S163–S165.
33. Mellor JE, Laugharne JD, Peet M. Schizophrenic symptoms and dietary intake of n-3 fatty acids. *Schizophrenia Res* 1995;18:85–86.
34. Peet M, Laugharne J, Rangarajan N, et al. Depleted red cell membrane essential fatty acids in drug-treated schizophrenic patients. *J Psychiatr Res* 1995;29:227–232.
35. Peet M, Laugharne JD, Mellor J, et al. Essential fatty acid deficiency in erythrocyte membranes from chronic schizophrenic patients, and the clinical effects of dietary supplementation. *Prostaglandins Leukotr Essent Fatty Acids* 1996;55:71–75.
36. Zubenko GS, Cohen BM, Reynolds CF, et al. Platelet membrane fluidity of Alzheimer's disease and major depression. *Am J Psychiatry* 1987;144:860–868.
37. Corrigan FM, Horrobin DF, Skinner ER, et al. Abnormal content of n-6 and n-3 long-chain unsaturated fatty acids in the phosphoglycerides and cholesterol esters of parahippocampal cortex from

Alzheimer's disease patients and its relationship to acetyl CoA content. *Int J Biochem Cell Biol* 1998; 30:197–207.

38. Kalmijn S, Launer LJ, Ott A, et al. Dietary fat intake and the risk of incident dementia in the Rotterdam study. *Ann Neurol* 1997;42:776–782.

39. Peers RJ. Alzheimer's disease and omega-3 fatty acids: hypothesis. *Med J Australia* 1990;153:563–564.

40. Kaplan JR, Manuck SB, Shively C. The effects of fat and cholesterol on social behavior in monkeys. *Psychosom Med* 1991;53:634–642.

41. Slater SJ, Kelly MB, Taddeo FJ, et al. The modulation of protein kinase C activity by membrane lipid bilayer structure. *J Biol Chem* 1994;269:4866–4871.

42. Maes M, Christophe A, Delanghe J, et al. Lowered omega3 polyunsaturated fatty acids in serum phospholipids and cholesteryl esters of depressed patients. *Psychiatry Res* 1999;85:275–291.

43. Crawford MA, Gale MM, Woodford MH. The polyenoic acids and their elongation products in the muscle tissue of Phacochoerus aethiopicus: a re-evaluation of "animal fat." *Biochem J* 1969;114:68P.

44. Crawford MA, Gale MM, Woodford MH. Linoleic acid and linolenic acid elongation products in muscle tissue of Sncerus caffer and other ruminant species. *Biochem J* 1969;115:25–27.

45. Hamazaki T, Sawazaki S, Kobayashi M. The effect of docosahexanoic acid on aggression in young adults. A double-blind study. *J Clin Invest* 1996;97:1129–1134.

46. Cenacchi T, Bertoldin T, Farina C, et al. Cognitive decline in the elderly: a double-blind, placebo-controlled multicenter study on efficacy of phosphatidyl-serine administration. *Aging Clin Exp Res* 1993;5:123–133.

47. Maggioni M, Picotti GB, Bondiolotti GP, et al. Effects of phosphatidylserine therapy in geriatric patients with depressive disorders. *Acta Psychiatr Scand* 1990;81:265–270.

48. Maes M, Smith RS. Fatty acids, cytokines, and major depression. *Biol Psychiatry* 1998;43:313–314.

49. Block E, Edwards D. Effects of plasma membrane fluidity on serotonin transport by endothelial cells. *Am J Physiol* 1987;253:C672–C678.

50. Engler MB, Karanian JW, Salem N Jr. Docosahexaenoic acid (22:6n3)-induced relaxation of the rat aorta. *Eur J Pharmacol* 1990;185:223–226.

51. Lee CR, Hamm MW. Effect of dietary fat and cholesterol supplements on glucagon receptor binding and adenylate cyclase activity of rat liver plasma membrane. *J Nutr* 1989;119:539–546.

52. Simopoulos AP, Leaf A, Salem N. *Workshop on the essentiality of and recommended dietary intakes for omega-6 and omega-3 fatty acids.* The Cloisters, National Institutes of Health (NIH) in Bethesda, Maryland, April 7–9, 1999.

4

One-Carbon Metabolism and the Treatment of Depression

Roles of S-Adenosyl-L-Methionine and Folic Acid

Jonathan E. Alpert and David Mischoulon

INTRODUCTION

The putative psychotropics reviewed in the chapter include the B-vitamin folic acid and S-adenosyl-L-methionine (SAMe), a cofactor in various metabolic processes in the brain and elsewhere in the body. These substances, which are metabolically interrelated, are therefore discussed together. While deficiencies in folic acid (and vitamin B_{12}) are linked with depression and its replenishment appears to result in a greater response to antidepressant drugs, none of the B vitamins has been touted as an antidepressant agent. SAMe, on the other hand, has an extensive body of evidence supporting its use as an antidepressant agent, for which it has been marketed both in Europe and more recently in the United States.

S-ADENOSYL-L-METHIONINE

Overview

SAMe is a naturally occurring substance produced in mammals from L-methionine and adenosine triphosphate. Although it has been studied in Europe for nearly 30 years, SAMe has recently risen from relative obscurity in the United States following its release in 1998 to 1999 as an over-the-counter dietary supplement. As SAMe is claimed to improve mood and emotional well-being, it has been the subject of national media coverage and several popular books, and it has steadily attracted the attention of patients and clinicians.

Unlike St. John's wort, SAMe is not a plant extract, a vitamin, or a mineral. However, SAMe is ubiquitous among living organisms, and it plays a critical role in a broad range of metabolic reactions. It is found throughout the human body, although particularly high concentrations have been measured in the liver, adrenal glands, and the pineal gland. SAMe appears to be uniformly distributed in the brain where it serves as a major donor of the methyl groups required for key transmethylation reactions (Figs. 4.1 and 4.2).

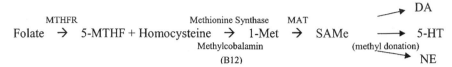

FIG. 4.1. SAMe-folate-vitamin B_{12} pathways. Abbreviations: DA, dopamine; 5-HT, serotonin (5-hydroxytryptamine); MAT, methionine adenosine transferase; I-Met, methionine; MTHF, methyl-tetrahydrofolate; MTHFR, methylene tetrahydrofolate reductase; NE, norepinephrine; SAMe, S-adenosyl-L-methionine.

SAMe is involved in the synthesis of a large number of neural messengers, including the monoamines (e.g., norepinephrine and serotonin) and melatonin, and of neuronal membrane constituents, particularly phospholipids, which play a critical role in signal transduction. It functions mainly through methyl-transferase reactions that shift the methyl group of SAMe to a wide variety of methyl acceptor molecules, such as catecholamines and other biogenic amines, proteins, and phospholipids (1).

SAMe also participates in the production of proteoglycans for cartilage and in the formation of cysteine and glutathione and of endogenous antiinflammatory and antioxidant substances and in the synthesis, repair, and recombination of DNA (2,3). In view of its widespread distribution and pervasive metabolic functions, that SAMe has been advanced—with varying degrees of empirical support—as a potential treatment for a broad range of conditions in addition to clinical depression should come as no surprise; these include dementia, Parkinson disease, cirrhosis, osteoarthritis, and fibromyalgia.

SAMe is continuously recycled in the body within a metabolic pathway referred to as the one-carbon cycle. SAMe is formed from the essential amino acid L-methionine in a reaction that requires adequate amounts of vitamin B_{12}

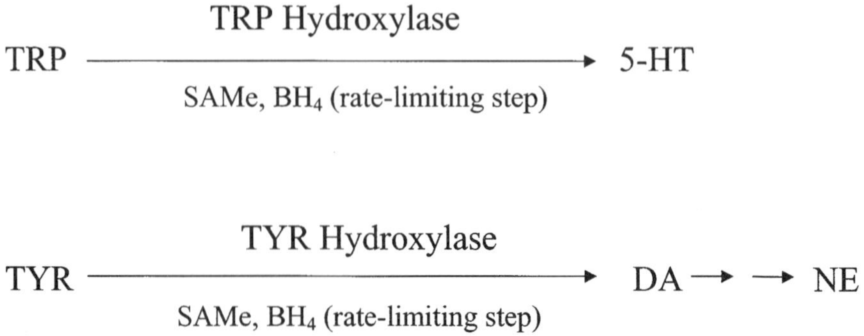

$$\text{TRP} \xrightarrow[\text{SAMe, BH}_4 \text{ (rate-limiting step)}]{\text{TRP Hydroxylase}} \text{5-HT}$$

$$\text{TYR} \xrightarrow[\text{SAMe, BH}_4 \text{ (rate-limiting step)}]{\text{TYR Hydroxylase}} \text{DA} \rightarrow \rightarrow \text{NE}$$

FIG. 4.2. SAMe and neurotransmitter synthesis. Abbreviations: BH_4, tetrahydrobiopterin; DA, dopamine; 5-HT, serotonin (5-hydroxytryptamine); NE, norepinephrine; SAMe, S-adenosyl-L-methionine; TRP, tryptophan; TYR, tyrosine.

and folic acid. Since dietary sources of L-methionine are insufficent, SAMe synthesis also depends on the endogenous formation of this amino acid from homocysteine. SAMe, in turn, is ultimately metabolized back to homocysteine, thereby replenishing the substrate needed to synthesize L-methionine and, eventually, to produce SAMe once again.

S-Adenosyl-L-Methionine and Methylation in Depression

Smythies (5) formulated the "one-carbon cycle" hypothesis that a defect in the mechanism of the one-carbon cycle causes some psychiatric illnesses. Tolbert et al. (6) observed that patients with unipolar depression had significantly lower levels of methionine adenosine transferase (MAT), which is one of the enzymes of the one-carbon cycle (Fig. 4.1). Smythies et al. (7) also reported that, following antidepressant treatment, patients with major depression displayed a significant increase in the V_{max} (the highest amount of substrate per unit time that an enzyme can process) of their MAT activity. L-Methionine is converted by MAT into SAMe, which, in turn, donates its methyl group to a variety of molecules in the brain (8). Reynolds et al. (9) hypothesized that a methylation deficit occurred in depression, based primarily on the discovery of a reduction in central nervous system (CNS) methylation in depression that was reversed with recovery. In support of this view, cerebrospinal fluid (CSF) SAMe levels were found to be significantly lower in severely depressed patients than in a neurologic control group (10).

Also of potential interest is the effect of SAMe on neuronal membranes since it increases the conversion of phosphatidylethanolamine to phosphatidylcholine, thereby increasing the fluidity of cell membranes and possibly facilitating neurotransmission by increasing the density of available receptors or the efficiency of receptor–effector coupling (11). Small alterations in membrane molecular dynamics can produce significant effects on signal transduction across cell membranes (12,13); in patients with dementia, the intravenous administration of SAMe (IV SAMe) has been reported to decrease the microviscosity of platelet membranes (14). In a study of patients with depression (15), the overall effects of oral SAMe on membrane fluidity were quite inconsistent. Nine depressed patients showed a fairly significant increase in platelet membrane fluidity after treatment with SAMe; but the membrane fluidity actually decreased in seven patients, and it was essentially unchanged in three.

Although the effects of SAMe on monoamines are not consistent, SAMe does have an impact on monoaminergic systems (1). SAMe is involved in the methylation of catecholamines, and it appears to increase the serotonin turnover (16,17), to inhibit the reuptake of norepinephrine in a temperature-dependent fashion (11), and to augment dopaminergic activity (16). Increased CSF levels of homovanillic acid (HVA) have also been correlated with increasing CSF levels of SAMe (18). One report of decreased prolactin secretion (17,19) may also be indirect evidence of an increased dopaminergic transmission. Folate levels, which some have implicated as having a role in depression, are also increased by SAMe (20).

Clinical Studies with S-Adenosyl-ʟ-Methionine in Depression

The first clinical trial of SAMe in the treatment of depression was published in 1973 (21). Since then, nearly 40 controlled and uncontrolled clinical trials have been reported; most, although not all, have shown some degree of antidepressant benefit from either oral, intravenous, or intramuscular administration of the compound.

After an initial, serendipitous observation of mood elevation in patients treated with SAMe (22), Fazio et al. (21) reported remission in 14 of 35 depressed patients in an open trial of parenteral SAMe. In 1975, Agnoli et al. (23) reported marked improvement of depression in 30 of 51 patients who were given intramuscular SAMe. Following these two reports, a large number of open studies (24–28) showed that treatment with parenteral SAMe was followed by a marked improvement in a substantial proportion of patients. Lipinski et al. (29), using IV SAMe in a single-blind study of inpatient depressives, reported improvement or remission in seven of nine subjects. The antidepressant response was rapid and was without side effects. Two other uncontrolled trials (30,31) suggested the efficacy of SAMe in depression.

Several double-blind studies showed that parenteral SAMe, when compared with a number of standard tricyclic antidepressants (TCAs), such as clomipramine, amitriptyline, and imipramine, was generally equally or more effective; and it tended to produce an earlier response (often within 3–7 days) and fewer side effects (32–40). Similarly, in studies examining the efficacy of IV SAMe compared with a placebo, the parenteral SAMe was significantly more effective (26,40), demonstrating a 56% response rate with SAMe and a 13% response rate with placebo.

Although parenteral SAMe appears to be an effective antidepressant, whether similar clinical efficacy can be achieved with its oral preparation is unclear. A highly labile compound, SAMe may be too labile and too polar to survive absorption without giving up its methyl group. On the other hand, the oral administration of SAMe is associated with a significant rise of CSF SAMe, suggesting that it crosses the blood-brain barrier in humans (10). In an open trial conducted with oral SAMe on 11 nontreatment-resistant depressed outpatients and nine treatment-resistant depressed outpatients (15), eight (73%) of the 11 nontreatment-resistant patients were considered responders. Complete response was defined as a greater than 50% reduction in the 21-item Hamilton Rating Scale for Depression (41) score from baseline, an endpoint Clinician Global Impression Severity (CGI-S) Scale (42) score of 1 or 2, and/or a CGI-S decrease greater than 2 points from baseline. The markedly significant clinical improvement found in this study following treatment with oral SAMe was also accompanied by significant neuroendocrine effects (19).

These findings, which suggest the efficacy of the oral preparation, were confirmed by the double-blind studies by Kagan et al. (43) and Salmaggi et al. (44) showing SAMe, 1,600 mg per day, to be more effective than a placebo in treating depressive symptoms among inpatients with major depression (N=18; N is the number of patients) and depressed postmenopausal women (N=80). Bell et al. (45) and De Vanna et al. (46) also showed the efficacy of oral SAMe (1,600 mg per day) to be comparable to that of desipramine and imipramine in two depressed populations (N=28 and 30, respectively).

However, when Fava et al. (47) evaluated the efficacy of oral SAMe in a double-blind, placebo-controlled study on 44 depressed outpatients, the sample as a whole improved significantly during the administration of either oral SAMe or placebo, but a significant difference between treatments was not observed. One may postulate that the failure of SAMe to produce effects significantly different from those of placebo in the double-blind study by Fava et al. might have been due to problems in the stability of the new preparation of this compound, as an analysis of the content of the 400-mg tablets of SAMe by Trapp et al. suggested (unpublished results). Ten SAMe tablets from that study, dated September 1988, were examined by compositional analysis in August 1990 (Trapp et al., unpublished results). Results from spectrophotometric and colorimetric analyses indicated that the tablets contained approximately the correct molar ratios of adenine and methionine for their labeled weight (107% and 90% of theoretical yield, respectively). However, although the molar ratios remained predominantly unaffected by prolonged storage, thin-layer chromatographic separation of compounds indicated that more than 50% of SAMe (R_f=0.36; R_f, movement of the substance relative to the solvent front) had degraded into a material (R_f=0.81) that probably contained the adenine nucleus and methionine as shown by spectrophotometric analysis (l max=260 nm) but that could not otherwise be identified. One of the inferences that can be drawn from this experience is that low doses of SAMe may have little or no discernible antidepressant benefit over a placebo.

In a 1994 formal metaanalysis by Bressa (48), 13 prospective double-blind, randomized clinical trials were selected as having met the criteria for a meaningful comparison. In six of these studies, SAMe had been compared with a placebo. In the seven remaining studies, SAMe had been compared with one of the various TCAs. SAMe was found to be significantly more effective than the placebo and equivalently effective to and typically better tolerated than the TCAs in the treatment of depression. The metaanalysis (48) of all the studies with oral and parenteral SAMe (including the authors') showed a superior response rate with SAMe when compared with the placebo, with an average global effect size of 27.5%. This effect size range is comparable to the average effect size of 25% for trazodone and two heterocyclic antidepressants (amoxapine and maprotiline) and is slightly higher than the average effect size of 19% for two standard TCAs (imipramine or amitriptyline) that was reported by Greenberg et al. (49) in their metaanalysis of 22 studies of antidepressant outcome. Further support for the comparable efficacy of SAMe when compared to TCAs is derived from the Bressa metaanalysis of all the trials comparing SAMe with other antidepressant agents (48). His analysis showed, among full responders, a global response of 61% for SAMe and of 59% for TCAs.

Of relevance to SAMe's putative antidepressant efficacy is the observation by Carney et al. (28) that three of 12 responders to IV SAMe underwent an early switch to mania or hypomania. Furthermore, in an open trial of oral SAMe, Carney reported that three of the first six patients treated with oral SAMe (500 to 1,600 mg daily for 14 to 42 days) experienced 1 to 3 days of euthymia, followed by hypomanic switches with symptoms including increased speech and activity, grandiose ideas, and, in one subject, increased libido (50). These samples included subjects with bipolar, as well as unipolar, depression, which undoubtedly contributed to the higher switch rates.

Although parenteral SAMe is an effective antidepressant, its route of administration diminishes its appeal to patients even though it is a naturally occurring compound. However, SAMe oral preparations with adequate bioavailability appear to be more acceptable with relatively few side effects. Information on the safety of oral SAMe administered for 6 weeks in the treatment of depression is available. Although no long-term safety data are available in depression, a 2-year study of the use of SAMe in hepatic cirrhosis found this compound to be safe and devoid of significant side effects (51). The encouraging results obtained in the course of four of five previously published double-blind preliminary studies support the hypothesis that this compound, even in its oral form, may have antidepressant effects.

If safe and effective, a stable oral formulation of SAMe would be a major contribution to the antidepressant pharmacopoeia for a number of reasons. Treatments that are perceived as natural currently enjoy a high degree of acceptability among patients (52). Many individuals with depression who are reluctant to take prescribed medications are nonetheless willing to try supplements such as St. John's wort, chromium picolonate, or SAMe, at least as a first step. Furthermore, in previous clinical trials, SAMe has also been well tolerated; it thus is potentially quite useful in the treatment of elderly or medically ill populations in whom depression has typically been undertreated because of concerns about the potentially serious side effects (e.g., cardiac toxicity, orthostatic hypotension, and drowsiness) of standard antidepressant drugs. Similarly, SAMe does not appear to cause sexual dysfunction, a common complaint with conventional antidepressant drugs, particularly the selective serotonin reuptake inhibitors (SSRIs); nor is it known to cause weight gain, a side effect that may cause significant distress and compliance problems. In addition, SAMe appears to be nontoxic, and therefore, it is not likely to be effective as an agent in a suicide attempt.

In addition, previous work has suggested the possibility that SAMe may be associated with a shorter latency of response than the conventional antidepressant agents, which typically require as much as 3 to 6 weeks before significant improvement in depression severity is observed (4). If so, SAMe, as monotherapy or, potentially, as an augmenting agent to other treatments, could benefit individuals with severe depression by reducing their period of functional impairment, risk of suicide, and length of stay for inpatient treatment.

Finally, in view of the prevalence of depressions that are refractory to standard treatment, much interest in the development of antidepressant agents that exploit quite different pharmacologic strategies continues to be expressed. Adequately sized double-blind studies of stable oral formulations of SAMe that are compared with current first-line pharmacotherapy (SSRIs), as well as a placebo, in depressed outpatients are clearly needed.

Recommendations in Clinical Practice

SAMe is relatively new to most patients and clinicians in the United States. However, attesting to its popularity overseas, an Italian survey over 4 years ago found that SAMe is the third most commonly administered antidepressant in and around Rome, trailing only fluoxetine and amitriptyline in the early 1990s (53). To expect that SAMe could attain comparable popularity in the United States is reasonable, particularly if further studies support its putative role as an antidepressant.

When assessing the relevance of the reviewed studies to clinical practice, one must bear in mind that, in most studies, SAMe was administered at doses that are extremely high in comparison with the doses currently recommended by distributors in the United States. The studies cited in the metaanalysis involved the administration of up to 1,600 mg per day of oral SAMe. By comparison, the suggested oral dose of SAMe recommended by distributors of the dietary supplement is generally 400 mg per day. Clinicians and patients must consider the likelihood that daily doses in excess of the 400 mg generally recommended in package inserts will be needed when treating clinical forms of depression, although 400 mg may be an acceptable starting dose.

At a cost of approximately $0.75 or more per 200-mg tablet, a daily dose of 1,600 mg, or 8 tablets per day, comparable to the doses studied in the European trials, could easily exceed $180.00 per month. What may prove to be a full therapeutic dose for most patients may therefore be difficult to swallow for many, both literally and figuratively, and the risk that patients will gravitate toward subtherapeutic doses is high.

Remembering that a majority of the controlled studies that have been reported to date have involved the administration of parenteral rather than oral preparations of SAMe is also important. In addition, these studies typically examined only short-term outcomes, and they enrolled patients with a variety of depressive disorders, including dysthymia and bipolar disorder, rather than those with major depression alone. The degree to which the studies that have been conducted on SAMe are relevant to particular clinical situations must be judged, therefore, in the context of potential differences in doses, route of administration, lengths of treatment, and the depressive disorder under treatment.

For now, the most logical applications of SAMe appear to be in the treatment of patients with mild depressions who prefer trying it over prescription agents, in patients who have proven to be intolerant of conventional antidepressant drugs, and in patients whose depression has proven refractory to a series of adequate antidepressant trials.

Several caveats, however, are necessary. Because SAMe, like most of the natural psychotropics, is marketed as a dietary supplement with no claims to treat specific disorders, it is not subject to Food and Drug Administration regulation, and manufacturers are not bound by standards that ensure consistency or equivalent bioavailability across different preparations. As an example, even when the stated dose strengths are identical, SAMe tablets from one supply may provide only 25% of the actual amount of SAMe contained in a supply coming from a different manufacturer or even a different batch. No published information exists that compares the over half-dozen different SAMe products on the market. However, one can reasonably surmise that some relapses on SAMe will occur when patients change preparations, and a patient doing well on a particular preparation of SAMe should generally be discouraged from changing brands in mid-treatment.

Although the majority of patients tolerate SAMe as well as they do the placebo, several reports of mania while on SAMe already exist in the literature (29,43,50,54,55). The relative risk of developing manic symptoms on SAMe in comparison to that of conventional antidepressants is unknown. At present, the same degree of caution that is exercised in the use of standard agents must be extended to SAMe, particularly when treating depressed patients with a personal or family history of mania. In the setting of bipolar I disorder, one can reasonably assume that SAMe should be avoided unless patients are also taking a mood stabilizer.

In addition, systematic studies of drug-drug interactions with SAMe are lacking. Although no known contraindications to combining SAMe with other medications and supplements exist, reports of drug-drug interactions may emerge as its use becomes more widespread.

Finally, because of its metabolic links with homocysteine, concern has been raised about the theoretical possibility that elevated levels of serum homocysteine will develop, which is a risk factor for occlusive vascular disorders, in some individuals receiving exogenous SAMe. To the authors' knowledge, no evidence has been found to suggest that serum homocysteine levels rise in patients receiving oral SAMe. Pending further study, however, the prudent course would be to consider monitoring homocysteine levels periodically during treatment when recommending SAMe to depressed patients who have a personal history or a particularly impressive family history of heart disease, peripheral vascular disease, or stroke or who are known to have significantly elevated homocysteine levels. In addition, some clinicians recommend folate and vitamin B_{12} supplements for such patients since these vitamins have been shown to facilitate the metabolism of homocysteine in some conditions in which elevated levels occur.

Before the medical community can incorporate SAMe with confidence into psychopharmacologic practice, a number of fundamental clinical research questions need to be answered. In particular, how does SAMe compare with newer antidepressants, particularly the SSRIs and atypical antidepressants, such as bupropion or nefazodone, in terms of safety, tolerability, drug-drug interactions, and efficacy? What are the optimal doses for oral administration? Is it safe for long-term use, and how does it compare with conventional antidepressants in the prevention of relapses and recurrences of depression? Can it be used effectively for patients with refractory depression, whether by itself or as a jumpstart to standard antidepressant drugs?

As greater clinical familiarity with SAMe is gained over the coming years and as well controlled studies on these topics get underway, the answers to many of these questions—whether these answers promote greater enthusiasm or dictate greater caution—will undoubtedly contribute to the development of innovative strategies for the treatment of the major mood disorders.

FOLIC ACID

Introduction

With the development of clinically reliable assays for folate in the 1960s, evidence began to accumulate for an association between folate-deficient states and depression (56–58), which helped to explain earlier observations on the various neuropsychiatric presentations of megaloblastic anemia (59). More recently, enhanced recognition of the relevance of folate in other medical conditions, such as neural tube defects (60) and cardiovascular disease (61), together with the increasingly avid attention to the potential antidepressant efficacy of agents marketed as dietary supplements or nutraceuticals (62,63), has generated new interest in old questions. The field has moved toward a better understanding of the impact of folate deficiency, replacement, and supplementation on the course and management of depressive disorders, particularly major depressive disorder, and the putative roles of folate in CNS function (64–66).

An association between folate deficiency and depression has been inferred from multiple disparate and imprecise, although essentially convergent, lines of evidence. Neuropsychiatric and particularly depressive symptoms, including apathy, fatigue, insomnia, irritability, and impaired concentration, have figured prominently in the clinical descriptions of folate deficiency states associated with malabsorption (67), anticonvulsant-treated epilepsy (68,69), megaloblastic anemia (70), and dietary folate restriction (56). Higher rates (up to 38%) of low serum or red blood cell folate or methyltetrahydrofolic acid (MTHF) have been reported among depressed patients than among psychiatric and non-psychiatric controls (57,58,71–74).

Bottiglieri has marshaled evidence regarding the role of folate in CNS function, including the essential role of folate in the one-carbon cycle that furnishes SAMe (64). Folate deficiency in animals and human inborn errors of folate metabolism have been associated with lower levels of SAMe (4,48,75–77), and low SAMe levels have been associated with depression. In addition, reduced red blood cell folate levels have been correlated with reduced levels of the serotonin metabolite, 5-hydroxyindoleacetic acid (5-HIAA), in the CSF (71).

Folate also appears to influence the rate of synthesis of tetrahydrobiopterin (BH_4) (71), a cofactor in the hydoxylation of phenylalanine and tryptophan, which are rate-limiting steps in the biosynthesis of dopamine, norepinephrine, and serotonin, neurotransmitters postulated to play a role in the pathogenesis of depression. In addition, MTHF has been shown to bind to presynaptic glutamate receptors (78), where it may potentially modulate the release of other neurotransmitters, including the monoamines. Finally, elevated levels of homocysteine resulting from folate deficiency may play a role in mediating some of its neuropsychiatric complications, both by generating elevated levels of S-adenosylhomocysteine, which broadly inhibits methylation reactions (79), and also possibly by exerting direct excitoxic effects via activity at the N-methyl D-aspartate glutamate receptors (80).

Low CSF levels of the serotonin metabolite 5-HIAA and the dopamine metabolite HVA have been reported in several, although not all (81), studies among folate-deficient patients with epilepsy (82), other neuropsychiatric disorders (83), and congenital folate deficiency states (84). The reciprocal tenets, however, have not been established; that is, whether folate supplementation actually enhances monoamine synthesis or release or furnishes additional SAMe has not been determined. At this time, human studies examining the impact of supraphysiologic doses of folate on CSF metabolites are lacking in the literature. Indeed, an older study in rats yielded the paradoxical finding that folate supplementation, as well as folate deficiency, lowered brain serotonin (83). The possibility of a similarly complex pattern in humans cannot be excluded.

Folate deficiency has been more closely linked to depression than vitamin B_{12} deficiency, with the former nearly twice as common as the latter among depressed patients (58). Mood disorders are more prevalent among individuals with folate deficiency (56%) than among those with vitamin B_{12} deficiency (20%) (59).

Low folate has been associated with particular depressive subtypes. Among psychiatric inpatients, low serum folate has been associated with endogenous depression (72). Among outpatients with depression, low serum folate, but not vitamin B_{12}, has been associated with melancholic depression (85), a more recent construct overlapping endogenous depression.

Folate Replenishment and the Treatment of Depression

Correlational analyses have suggested that, among individuals with major mood disorders, higher folate values predict better acute (86) and long-term outcomes (87). In the latter study of individuals with unipolar depression or bipolar disorder, folate levels were boosted with daily low-dose folate supplementation (200 µg) that was accompanied by pharmacologic prophylaxis of affective symptoms. Further demonstration of the potential antidepressant benefit of folate has come from a double-blind study of 96 nonfolate-deficient patients with senile dementia and depressive symptoms in which significant improvement of depression was reported among patients randomized to methylene tetrahydrofolate (MTHF) (50 mg), which is similar to that observed on the active antidepressant comparator, trazodone (100 mg per day) (88). In 16 elderly nondemented subjects with major depression, an open trial of MTHF (50 mg) also resulted in substantial improvement in depressive symptoms, even among the 14 subjects who had normal baseline serum folate levels (89).

Changes in folate may correlate with the response to certain antidepressant treatments. In depressed adults, responders to acute treatment with desipramine (90) or desipramine plus levothyroxine (T_4), triiodothyronine (T_3), or a placebo (91) exhibited a significant increase in red blood cell (RBC) folate in comparison to that observed in nonresponders. Reciprocally, well over 20 surveys concerning the folate status among patients with psychiatric disorders (66,92,93) revealed that as many as one-third of the patients among psychiatric cohorts, mainly from the United Kingdom, exhibited low or deficient serum folate values; generally comparable findings were observed in the few studies that assessed RBC folate as a more accurate reflection of tissue folate stores.

In the subset of surveys in which depressed patients were compared with psychiatric or nonpsychiatric controls, depressed patients were found to have serum folate (57,73), RBC folate (71), or serum MTHF (74) levels that were lower than those of all other groups except for patients with alcoholism who had a similar prevalence of low folate levels (72). Furthermore, low serum or RBC folate and serum MTHF levels were often associated with greater symptom severity among depressed patients (58,74,86,94).

In studies that failed to demonstrate this relationship between low folate and depression severity, one nevertheless found an inverse relationship between folate and the duration of the depressive episode (95), and another described an inverse relation with the length of hospitalization, thus suggesting a relationship between folate and treatment outcome (96).

Pursuing these leads regarding folate and treatment outcome, the authors assessed serum folate and response to the SSRI antidepressant fluoxetine (Prozac) among 213 adults with major depression (85). In this outpatient depressed but medically healthy study sample, the prevalence of actual folate deficiency, defined in this study as <1.5 ng per mL, was low (2%), while borderline low values (from 1.5 to 2.5 ng per mL) were more common (17%). Pretreatment folate, but not vitamin B_{12}, status was significantly related to the response. Individuals with a low or deficient serum folate exhibited a 35% rate of nonresponse to an adequate course of fluoxetine, compared with a 20% rate of nonresponse among those with values in the normal range. A similar result was reported among 22 depressed patients over the age of 60 who were treated with nortriptyline or sertraline; for these patients, an inverse relationship between RBC folate and antidepressant response existed (97).

Consistent with this, in an earlier study of 101 depressed inpatients receiving a variety of treatments, including electroconvulsive therapy (ECT), antidepressant agents, or tryptophan, outcome was significantly poorer for patients with low serum folate (58), although, in a small series of patients undergoing ECT, the serum MTHF did not appear to correlate with the response (74). Although many investigators have searched for predictors of refractoriness to antidepressant treatment, very few predictors have in fact emerged (98). From this light, the apparent relationship between low folate and nonresponse, at least to SSRI antidepressants, is particularly interesting.

If lack of folate hinders antidepressant response, furnishing folate to deficient subjects should improve treatment outcome. To test this, Godfrey et al. (99) administered MTHF, 15 mg, in an oral form of folate that is actively transported across the blood-brain barrier to 24 patients with major depression and low or deficient folate (RBC folate <200 μg/L). In this 6-month, randomized, double-blind trial, those 13 depressed patients who received MTHF were globally rated as having superior symptom improvement and social adjustment at 3 and 6 months in comparison to the 11 patients who were assigned to the placebo. Limitations of this study included the relatively small sample, nonsystematic concomitant treatments (e.g., antidepressants, lithium, or no medications), symptom improvement on some, but not all, measures, and similar, although somewhat less dramatic, response to MTHF among comparably treated patients with schizophrenia, suggesting that the positive effects of MTHF may not have been specific to depression.

Nonetheless, these findings extended to other depressed samples where folate replacement showed improved long-term neuropsychiatric outcome among folate-deficient patients with psychiatric (100) and gastrointestinal (67) disorders and in some, although not all, studies on anticonvulsant-treated patients with epilepsy (68).

Studies on folate deficiency and replacement in neuropsychiatric disorders have suggested a connection between folate and depression and have helped to delineate some of the characteristics of this relationship. The actual clinical relevance of these studies, however, may be increasingly limited. Recent work suggests that the prevalence of folate deficiency or borderline low values is lower among contemporary psychiatric cohorts than was initially suggested by studies carried out several decades ago (85) and also that Western estimates may not generalize well to other parts of the world, including Asia (101). Moreover, much of what is surmised about folate and depression is based upon data gathered prior to the implementation of folic acid fortification programs and the widespread public awareness about the possible health benefits of folate. In the United States, the Food and Drug Administration mandate requiring folic acid fortification of all enriched grain products by 1998 appears to have exerted a rapid and substantial impact on the prevalence of low and deficient folate in the community, nearly eradicating low serum folate values (<3 ng/mL) among 350 middle-aged and older adults in the Framingham Offspring Study Cohort (102). When low plasma folate is defined as less than 3 ng/mL, the prevalence of low plasma folate among the Framingham Offspring Cohort dropped from 22.0%

(1991–1994) to 1.7% (1995–1998) (N=248). Among those who also took B vitamin supplements, the prevalence of low folate was further reduced from 3.9% (1991–1994) to 0.0% (1995–1998) (N=102) (102).

Potential Role for Folate Supplementation as an Antidepressant

A comparable study on the prevalence of low folate among carefully diagnosed, depressed cohorts in this postfortification era is needed, particularly since the extent to which dietary intake contributes to low folate among depressed individuals is not well established (57,58,85,86,103,104). Nevertheless, the prevalence of low folate levels in patients with depression has likely been reduced to well below the earlier estimates. If so, the more compelling clinical focus for clinicians who treat depression shifts from the need for folate replacement to that of folate supplementation and to the question of whether supraphysiologic doses of folate, as monotherapy or augmentation of conventional agents, may confer antidepressant benefit among depressed, normofolatemic patients.

In this regard, Coppen and Bailey (105) examined whether the coadministration of folic acid would enhance the antidepressant action of fluoxetine. They treated 127 normofolatemic, depressed patients with either 500 µg of folic acid or a placebo in addition to 20 mg of fluoxetine daily for 10 weeks. This folate dose exceeds the usual amount in standard multivitamins that are marketed in the United States by only 25%. Patients receiving folate generally showed a significant increase in plasma folate; plasma homocysteine was unchanged in men, but it was significantly decreased in women by 20.6%. Subjects in the fluoxetine plus folic acid group, particularly the women, demonstrated greater improvement in depressive symptoms. Of women who received the folic acid supplement, 93.3% showed a good response (defined as >50% reduction in score) as compared with 61.1% of women who received the placebo ($P<0.005$). The authors concluded that folic acid is effective in improving the antidepressant action of fluoxetine and probably of other antidepressants, and they recommend folic acid supplementation in doses that are sufficient to decrease plasma homocysteine.

In a recent study (106), the authors examined 22 adults with major depression who had shown an inadequate antidepressant response to an initial course of treatment with an SSRI; they then had 15 to 30 mg of folinic acid (leucovorin) added to their antidepressant over an 8-week open trial (106). These individuals had serum folate values greater than 6 ng per mL. No individuals in this sample were folate deficient; in fact, most had pretreatment serum values in the moderate-to-high range, which apparently reflected the nutrition consciousness of this group. A modest open trial response rate was observed, based upon a conservative estimate from the intent-to-treat sample (ranging from 18% with stringent remission criteria to 41% for global ratings of improvement) and a more liberal estimate from among the completer sample (ranging from 19% to 44%). One quarter of those who completed the study showed an improvement greater than

50%. Leucovorin appeared to be well tolerated; dropouts were due to lack of efficacy or noncompliance. Limitations of the study included the lack of placebo control, and the potential ceiling effects from subjects with a baseline high serum folate. Among individuals who do not exhibit low or deficient serum folate—as is likely to be increasingly typical of most outpatient samples since 1996—the true response rate to leucovorin among SSRI refractory adults appears to be modest, although it is probably comparable to some conventional antidepressant adjuncts. Double-blind studies involving cohorts with a wider range of folate values and of comorbid conditions would be useful for further clarifying the potential utility of folate or leucovorin as adjunctive strategies among certain patient populations with treatment-refractory depression.

More rigorous, double-blind studies are needed to address important clinical questions regarding the magnitude of these effects compared with standard therapies and compared across different forms of oral folate, including folic acid, MTHF, and folinic acid, and folate doses; possible predictors of response that would help identify the patients most likely to benefit from folate supplementation; and the potential long-term consequences of high folate in this population. Nevertheless, these preliminary studies support the proposal that the relevance of folate to depression treatment may extend beyond its more obvious role in reversing the sequelae of folate deficiency.

Conclusions and Recommendations

Studies of low folate and its relationship to the expression, course, and treatment of neuropsychiatric disorders have provided intriguing clues about the apparent links between folate and depression. These studies clearly suggest that assessment of folate status ought to be included in any comprehensive medical workup for refractoriness to antidepressant treatment and that folate replacement among individuals with conditions leading to folate deficiency states, such as alcoholism, inborn errors of metabolism, and malabsorption, may well reduce the risk or severity of depressive symptoms.

Determination of serum or RBC folate levels alone may be an overly simplistic probe of overall folate status. Steady advances in knowledge about the interaction among genes, folate, and other key participants in one-carbon metabolism, including homocysteine and SAMe, seem likely to yield important insights in this respect. Thus, for example, individuals homozygous for the common mutant form of MTHFR are at significantly higher risk for elevated plasma homocysteine if they have lower plasma folate levels (107–109). Quite speculatively, perhaps folate plays a similar protective effect against depression among individuals with this or similar genetic polymorphisms. At this point, clinicians clearly need to know much more about the clinical and neurobiologic consequences of folate supplementation before informed decisions can be made about the circumstances under which high doses of folate (i.e., exceeding the equivalent of 400 µg of folic acid) should be recommended to depressed individuals, as well as in what form and for how long.

The combination of well designed clinical trials, epidemiologic and genetic analyses, and increasingly refined brain imaging techniques that provide an unprecedented window on receptor physiology and CNS metabolism will surely help pave the way.

ACKNOWLEDGMENT

Drs. Alpert and Mischoulon were supported in part by NARSAD Young Investigator Awards.

REFERENCES

1. Baldessarini RJ. The neuropharmacology of S-adenosyl-L-methionine. *Am J Med* 1987;83:95–103.
2. Shane B, Stokstad ELB. Vitamin B_{12}-folate interrelationships. *Annu Rev Nutr* 1985;5:115–141.
3. Young SN, Ghadirian M. Folic acid and psychopathology. *Prog Neuropsychopharmacol Biol Psychiatry* 1989;13:841–863.
4. Spillman M, Fava M. S-Adenosyl-methionine (ademethionine) in psychiatric disorders. *CNS Drugs* 1996;6:416–425.
5. Smythies JR. Biochemistry of schizophrenia. *Postgrad Med J* 1963;39:16–33.
6. Tolbert LC, Monti JA, O'Shields H, et al. Defects in transmethylation and membrane lipids in schizophrenia. *Psychopharm Bull* 1983;19:594–599.
7. Smythies JR, Alarcon RD, Bancroft AJ, et al. Role of the one-carbon cycle in neuropsychiatry. In: Borchardt RT, Creveling CR, Ueland PM, eds. *Biological methylation and drug design*. Clifton, NJ: Humana Press, 1986;351–362.
8. Cantoni GL. S-adenosylmethionine: a new intermediate formed enzymatically from L-methionine and adenosine triphosphate. *J Biol Chem* 1953;204:403–416.
9. Reynolds EH, Carney MWP, Toone BK. Methylation and mood. *Lancet* 1984;ii:196–198.
10. Bottiglieri T, Godfrey P, Flynn T, et al. Cerebrospinal fluid s-adenosylmethionine in depression and dementia: effects of treatment with parenteral and oral S-adenosylmethionine. *J Neurol Neurosurg Psychiatry* 1990;53:1096–1098.
11. Cimino M, Vantini G, Algeri S, et al. Age-related modification of dopaminergic and β-adrenergic receptor system: restoration to normal activity by modifying membrane fluidity with S-adenosyl-methionine. *Life Sci* 1984;34:2029–2039.
12. Zubenko GS, Cohen BM, Reynolds CF, et al. Platelet membrane fluidity of Alzheimer's disease and major depression. *Am J Psychiatry* 1987;144:860–868.
13. Zubenko GS, Cohen BM. Effects of phenothiazine treatment on the physical properties of platelet membranes from psychiatric patients. *Biol Psychiatry* 1985;20:384–396.
14. Cohen BM, Satlin A, Zubenko GS. S-Adenosyl-L-methionine in the treatment of Alzheimer's disease. *J Clin Psychopharmacol* 1987;7:254–257.
15. Rosenbaum JF, Fava M, Falk WE, et al. The antidepressant potential of oral S-adenosyl-L-methionine. *Acta Psychiatr Scand* 1990;81:432–436.
16. Agnoli A, Ruggieri S, Cerone G, et al. The dopamine hypothesis of depression: results of treatment with dopaminergic drugs. In: Garattini S, ed. *Depressive disorders*. Stuttgard: Schattauer, 1977: 447–458.
17. Bottiglieri T, Carney MWP, Edeh J. A biochemical study of depressed patients receiving S-adenosyl-L-methionine (SAM). In: Borchardt RT, Creveling CR, Ueland PM, eds. *Biological methylation and drug design*. Clifton, NJ: Humana Press, 1986;327–338.
18. Carney MW, Edeh J, Bottiglieri T, et al. Affective illness and S-adenosyl methionine: a preliminary report. *Clin Neuropharmacol* 1986;9:379–385.
19. Fava M, Rosenbaum JF, MacLaughlin R, et al. Neuroendocrine effects of S-adenosyl-L-methionine, a novel putative antidepressant. *J Psychiatr Res* 1990;24:177–184.
20. Reynolds EH, Stramentinoli G. Folic acid, S-adenosyl-L-methionine and affective disorder. *Psychol Med* 1983;13:705–710.
21. Fazio C, Andreoli V, Agnoli A, et al. Effetti terapeutici e meccanismo d'azione della S-adenosil-L-metionina (SAMe) nelle sindromi depressive. *Minerva Med* 1973;64:1515–1529.
22. Pinzello A, Andreoli V. Le transmetilazioni SAM-dipendenti nelle sindromi depressive: valutazione

dell-effetto terapeutico della S-adenosilmetionina con la scala di Hamilton. *Quad Ter Sper Suppl Bioch Biol Sper* 1972;X/2:3–11.

23. Agnoli A, Fazio C, Andreoli V. Disturbi neuropsichiatrici e transmetilazioni: effetti terapeutici della S-adenosil-L-metionina. *La Clin Ter* 1975;75:567–579.

24. Mantero M, Pastorino P. Sindromi depressive, malattie cutanee e transmetilazioni. Effetti terapeutici della S-adenosyl-L-metionina. *Gazzetta Med Ital* 1976;135:707–716.

25. Andreoli V, Campedelli A, Maffei F. La S-adenosil-L-metionina (SAMe) in geropsichiatria: uno studio clinico controllato "in aperto" nelle sindromi depressive dell'eta' senile. *G Gerontol* 1977;25:172–180.

26. Barberi A, Pusateri C. Sugli effetti clinici della S-adenosil-L-metionina (SAMe) nelle sindromi depressive. *Min Psichiatr* 1978;19:235–243.

27. Salvadorini F, Galeone F, Saba P, et al. Evaluation of S-adenosylmethionine (SAMe) effectiveness on depression. *Curr Ther Res* 1980;27:908–918.

28. Carney MWP, Martin G, Bottiglieri T, et al. Switch mechanism in affective illness and S-adenosyl-methionine. *Lancet* 1983;i:820–821.

29. Lipinski JF, Cohen BM, Frankenburg F, et al. An open trial of S-adenosylmethionine for treatment of depression. *Am J Psychiatry* 1984;141:448–450.

30. Labriola FR, Kalina E, Glina H, et al. *Accion de la SAMe en depresiones endogenas.* Paper presented at the V Congreso Nacional de la Sociedad Mexicana de Psiquiatria Biologica y II Symposium de la Federacion Latinoamericana de Psiquiatria Biologica. Cd. de Pueble, Mexico, 1986.

31. Antun F. *Open study of SAMe in depression.* Symposium on Transmethylations, Trieste, Italy, 1987.

32. Mantero M, Pastorino P, Carolei A, Agnoli A. Studio controllato in doppio cieco (SAMe-imipramina) nelle sindromi depressive. *Minerva Med* 1975;66:4098–4101.

33. Scarzella R, Appiotti A. *A double clinical comparison of SAMe versus chlorimipramine in depressive syndromes.* Paper presented at the VI World Congress of Psychiatry, Honolulu, 1977.

34. Miccoli L, Porro V, Bertolino A. Comparison between the antidepressant activity of S-adenosyl-L-methionine (SAMe) and that of some tricyclic drugs. *Acta Neurol* 1978;33:243–255.

35. Del Vecchio M, Iorio G, Cocorullo M, et al. Has SAMe (Ado-Met) an antidepressant effect? A preliminary trial versus chlorimipramine. *Riv Sper Freniatria* 1978;102:344–358.

36. Monaco P, Quattrocchi F. Studio degli effetti antidepressivi di un transmetilante biologico (S-adenosil-metionina-SAMe). *Riv Neurol* 1979;49:417–439.

37. Calandra C, Roxas M, Rapisarda V. Azione antidepressiva della SAMe a paragone della clorimipramina. Ipotesi interpretative del meccanismo d'azione. *Minerva Psichiatr* 1979;20:147–152.

38. Kufferle B, Grunberger J. Early clinical double-blind study with S-adenosyl-L-methionine: a new potential antidepressant. In: Costa E, Racagni G, eds. *Typical and atypical antidepressants.* New York: Raven Press, 1982:175–180.

39. Bell KM, Plon L, Bunney WE Jr, Potkin SG. S-adenosylmethionine treatment of depression: a controlled clinical trial. *Am J Psychiatry* 1988;145:1110–1114.

40. Janicak PG, Lipinski J, Davis JM, et al. S-adenosylmethionine in depression: a literature review and preliminary report. *Ala J Med Sci* 1988;25:306–313.

41. Hamilton M. A rating scale for depression. *J Neurol Neurosurg Psychiatry* 1960;23:56–62.

42. Guy W, ed. *ECDEU assessment manual for psychopharmacology,* revised. DHEW Pub. No. (ADM)76-338. Rockville, MD: National Institute of Mental Health, 1976.

43. Kagan BL, Sultzer DL, Rosenlicht N, Gerner RH. Oral S-adenosylmethionine in depression: a randomized, double-blind, placebo-controlled trial. *Am J Psychiatry* 1990;147:591–595.

44. Salmaggi P, Bressa GM, Nicchia G, et al. Double-blind, placebo-controlled study of S-adenosyl-L-methionine in depressed post-menopausal women. *Psychother Psychosom* 1993;59:34–40.

45. Bell MB, Carreon D, Plon L, et al. *Oral S-adenosylmethionine in the treatment of depression: a double-blind comparison with desipramine.* Study Report. BioResearch file, 1990.

46. De Vanna M, Rigamonti R. Oral S-adenosyl-L-methionine in depression. *Curr Ther Res* 1992;52:478–485.

47. Fava M, Rosenbaum JF, Birnbaum R, Kelly K, et al. The thyrotropin response to TRH as a predictor of response to treatment in depressed outpatients. *Acta Psychiatr Scand* 1992;86:42–45.

48. Bressa GM. S-Adenosyl-L-Methionine (SAMe) as antidepressant: meta-analysis of clinical studies. *Acta Neurol Scand Suppl* 1994;154:7–14.

49. Greenberg RP, Bornstein RF, Greenberg MD, Fisher S. A meta-analysis of antidepressant outcome under "blinder" conditions. *J Consult Clin Psychol* 1992;5:664–669.

50. Carney MWP, Chary TNK, Bottiglieri T. Switch mechanism in affective illness and oral S-adenosylmethionine (SAM). *Br J Psychiatry* 1987;150:724–725.

51. Mato JM, Camara J, Fernandez de Paz J, et al. S-adenosylmethionine in alcoholic liver cirrhosis: a randomized, placebo-controlled, double-blind, multicenter clinical trial. *J Hepatol* 1999;30:1081–1089.
52. Mischoulon D, Rosenbaum JF. The use of natural medications in psychiatry. A commentary. *Harv Rev Psychiatry* 1999;6:279–283.
53. Arpino C, Da Cas R, Donini G, et al. Use and misuse of antidepressant drugs in a random sample of the population of Rome, Italy. *Acta Psychiatr Scand* 1995;92:7–9.
54. Carney MW, Chary TK, Bottiglieri T, Reynolds EH. The switch mechanism and the bipolar/unipolar dichotomy. *Br J Psychiatry* 1989;154:48–51.
55. Carney MW, Chary TK, Bottiglieri T, Reynolds EH. Switch and S-adenosylmethionine. *Ala J Med Sci* 1988;25:316–319.
56. Herbert V. Experimental nutritional folate defiency in man. *Trans Assoc Am Physicians* 1961;75: 307–320.
57. Carney MWP. Serum folate values in 423 psychiatric patients. *BMJ* 1967;4:512–516.
58. Reynolds EH, Preece JM, Bailey J, Coppen A. Folate deficiency in depressive illness. *Br J Psychiatry* 1970;117:287–292.
59. Shorvon SD, Carney MWP, Chanarin I, Reynolds EH. The neuropsychiatry of megaloblastic anaemia. *Br Med J* 1980;281:1036–1038.
60. MRC Vitamin Study Research Group. Prevention of neural tube defects: results of the Medical Research Council Vitamin Study. *Lancet* 1991;338:131–137.
61. Rimm EB, Willett WC, Hu FB, et al. Folate and vitamin B_6 from diet and supplements in relation to risk of coronary heart disease among women. *JAMA* 1998;279:359–364.
62. Mischoulon D. Herbal remedies for mental illness. *Psychiatr Clin North Am Ann Drug Ther* 1999;6:1–20.
63. Fugh-Berman A, Cott JM. Dietary supplements and natural products as psychotherapeutic agents. *Psychosom Med* 1999;61:712–728.
64. Bottiglieri T. Folate, vitamin B_{12}, and neuropsychiatric disorders. *Nutr Rev* 1997;54:382–390.
65. Alpert JE, Fava M. Nutrition and depression: the role of folate. *Nutr Rev* 1997;55:145–149.
66. Hutto BR. Folate and cobalamin in psychiatric illness. *Compr Psychiatry* 1997;38:305–314.
67. Botez MI, Botez T, Leveille J, et al. Neurological correlates of folic acid deficiency: facts and hypotheses. In: Botez MI, Reynolds EH, eds. *Folic acid in neurology, psychiatry and internal medicine.* New York: Raven Press, 1979:435–461.
68. Reynolds EH. Anticonvulsant drugs, folate metabolism and mental symptoms. In: Dam M, Gram L, Penry JK, eds. *Advances in epileptology.* XIIth Epilepsy International Symposium. New York: Raven Press, 1981:621–625.
69. Edeh J, Toone BK. Antiepileptic therapy, folate deficiency, and psychiatric morbidity: a general practice survey. *Epilepsia* 1985;26:434–440.
70. Shorvon SD, Carney MWP, Chanarin I, Reynolds EH. The neuropsychiatry of megaloblastic anemia. *Br Med J* 1980;281:1036–1038.
71. Bottiglieri T, Hyland K, Laundy M, et al. Folate deficiency, biopterin and monoamine metabolism in depression. *Psychol Med* 1992;22:871–876.
72. Carney MWP, Chary TKN, Laundy M, et al. Red cell folate concentrations in psychiatric patients. *J Affect Dis* 1990;19:207–213.
73. Ghadirian AM, Anath J, Engelsmann F. Folic acid deficiency in depression. *Psychosomatics* 1980; 21:926–929.
74. Wilkinson A, Anderson D, Abou-Saleh M, et al. 5-Methyltetrahydrofolate level in the serum of depressed subjects and its relationship to the outcome of ECT. *J Affect Disord* 1994;32:163–168.
75. Ordonez LA, Wurtman RJ. Folic acid deficiency and methyl group metabolism in rat brain: effects of L-dopa. *Arch Biochem Biophys* 1974;160:372–376.
76. Bottiglieri T, Hyland K, Reynolds EH. The clinical potential of ademetionine (S-adenosylmethionine) in neurological disorders. *Drugs* 1994;48:137–152.
77. Bottiglieri T, Hyland K. S-adenosylmethionine levels in psychiatric and neurological disorders: a review. *Acta Neurol Scand Suppl* 1994;154:19–26.
78. Ruck A, Kramer S, Metz J, Brennan M. Methyltetrahydrofolate is a potent and selective agonist for kainic acid receptors. *Nature* 1980;287:852–853.
79. Schatz RA, Wilens TE, Sellinger OZ. Decreased in vivo protein and phospholipid methylation after in vivo elevation of brain S-adenosylhomocysteine. *Biochem Biophys Res Commun* 1981;98:1097.
80. Shaw PJ. Excitatory amino acid receptors, excitotoxicity and the human nervous system. *Curr Opin Neurol Neurosurg* 1993;6:414.

81. Bowers MB Jr, Reynolds EH. Cerebrospinal fluid folate and acid monoamine metabolites. *Lancet* 1972;2:137.

82. Botez MI, Young SN. Effects of anticonvulsants and low levels of folate and thiamine on amine metabolites in cerebrospinal fluid. *Brain* 1991;114:333–348.

83. Botez MI, Young SN, Bachevalier J, Gauthier S. Folate deficiency and decreased brain 5-hydroxy-tryptamine synthesis in man and rat. *Nature* 1979;278:182–183.

84. Surtees R, Heales S, Bowron A. Association of cerebrospinal fluid deficiency of 5-methyltetrahy-drofolate, but not S-adenosylmethionine, with reduced concentrations of the acid metabolites of 5-hydroxytryptamine and dopamine. *Clin Sci* 1994;986:697–702.

85. Fava M, Borus JS, Alpert JE, et al. Folate, B_{12}, and homocysteine in major depressive disorder. *Am J Psychiatry* 1997;154:426–428.

86. Wesson VA, Levitt AJ, Joffe RT. Change in folate status with antidepressant treatment. *Psychiatry Res* 1994;53:313–322.

87. Coppen A, Chaudry S, Swade C. Folic acid enhances lithium prophylaxis. *J Affect Disord* 1986;10:9–13.

89. Guaraldi G, Fava M, Mazzi F, LaGreca P. An open trial of methyltetrahydrofolate (MTHF) in elderly depressed patients. *Ann Clin Psychiatry* 1993;5:101–106.

90. Wesson VA, Levitt AJ, Joffe RT. Change in folate status with antidepressant treatment. *Psychiatry Res* 1994;53:313–322.

91. Levitt AJ, Wesson VA, Joffe RT. Impact of suppression of thyroxine on folate status during acute antidepressant therapy. *Psychiatry Res* 1998;79:123–129.

92. Young SN, Ghadirian M. Folic acid and psychopathology. *Prog Neuropsychopharm Biol Psychiatry* 1989;13:841–863.

93. Crellin R, Bottiglieri T, Reynolds EH. Folates and psychiatric disorders: clinical potential. *Drugs* 1993;45:623–636.

88. Passeri M, Ventura S, Abate G, Cucinotta D, LaGreca P. Oral 5-methyltetrahydrofolate (MTHF) in depression association with senile organic mental disorders (OMDs): a double-blind, multicenter study vs. trazodone (TRZ). *Eur J Clin Invest* 1993;21:24.

94. Abou-Saleh MT, Coppen A. Serum and red blood cell folate in depression. *Acta Psychiatry Scand* 1989;80:78–82.

95. Levitt A, Joffee R. Folate, B_{12}, and life course of depressive illness. *Biol Psychiatry* 1989;25:867–872.

96. Bell IR, Edman JS, Marby DW, et al. Vitamin B_{12} and folate status in acute geropsychiatric inpatients: affective and cognitive characteristics of a vitamin nondeficient population. *Biol Psychiatry* 1990;27:125–137.

97. Alpert M, Silva R, Pouget E. *Folate as a predictor of response to sertraline or nortriptyline in geriatric depression.* Presented at the 36th Annual Meeting of the NCDEU, Boca Raton, FL, May 28–31, 1996.

98. Fava M, Davidson KG. Definition and epidemiology of treatment-resistant depression. *Psychiatr Clin North Am* 1996;119:176–200.

99. Godfrey PSA, Toone BK, Carney MWP, et al. Enhancement of recovery from psychiatric illness by methylfolate. *Lancet* 1990;336:392–395.

100. Carney MWP, Sheffield BF. Associations of subnormal serum folate and vitamin B_{12} values and effects of replacement therapy. *J Nerv Ment Dis* 1970;150:404–412.

101. Lee S, Wing YK, Fong S. A controlled study of folate levels in Chinese inpatients with major depression in Hong Kong. *J Affect Disord* 1998;49:73–77.

102. Jacques PF, Selhub J, Bostom AG, et al. The effect of folic acid fortification on plasma folate and total homocysteine concentrations. *New Engl J Med* 1999;340:1449–1454.

103. Abou-Saleh MT, Coppen A. The biology of folate in depression: implications for nutritional hypotheses of psychoses. *J Psychiatr Res* 1986;20:91–101.

104. Thorton WE, Thornton BP. Folic acid, mental function and dietary habits. *J Clin Psychiatry* 1978; 39:315–322.

105. Coppen A, Bailey J. Enhancement of the antidepressant action of fluoxetine by folic acid: a randomised, placebo controlled trial. *J Affect Disord* 2000;60:121–130.

106. Alpert JE, Pingol MG, Rankin MA, et al. *Methylfolate as an adjunct in SSRI refractory depression.* Presented at the 152nd Annual Meeting of the American Psychiatric Association, Washington, D.C., 1999.

107. Kang SS, Wong PW, Bock HG, et al. Intermediate hyperhomocysteinemia resulting from compound heterozygosity of methylenetetrahydrofolate reductase mutations. *Am J Hum Genet* 1991;48:546–551.

108. Jacques PF, Bostom AG, Williams RR, et al. Relation between folate status, a common mutation in methylenetetrahydrofolate reductase, and plasma homocysteine concentrations. *Circulation* 1996; 93:7–9.
109. Lee BH, Cheong HI, Shin YS, et al. The effect of C677T mutation of methylene tetrahydrofolate reductase gene and plasma folate level on hyperhomocysteinemia in patients with meningomyelocele. *Childs Nerv Syst* 2000;16:559–563.

5

Dehydroepiandrosterone as a Neurohormone in the Treatment of Depression and Dementia

Owen M. Wolkowitz and Victor I. Reus

"Whether diandrone [dehydroepiandrosterone] turns out to be of therapeutic value in psychiatric practice remains to be seen.... However, we appear to have at our disposal a chemical agent that can exert a direct and prolonged action on the mental state." (1)

INTRODUCTION

Dehydroepiandrosterone (DHEA) has been evaluated in the treatment of psychiatric disorders almost from the time of its initial discovery and synthesis, with published reports appearing as early as 1952 (2,3). Several uncontrolled positive reports were subsequently published in the 1950s, but large-scale enthusiasm for this potential therapy languished until the late 1980s through the mid-1990s. At that time, an expanding body of preclinical data, plus the first adequately controlled clinical trial (4), fostered hope that DHEA might, conservatively, increase well-being and, hopefully, extend life, protect the brain, and retard the ravages of aging. A citation count of the number of published articles in the MedLine database containing the key words, dehydroepiandrosterone, DHEA, or DHEA-S (sulfate), confirms the exponential rise in scientific interest in this hormone since approximately 1990 (Fig. 5.1).

Coinciding with this burst of scientific activity, consumer interest in DHEA was enlivened by the passage of the 1994 Dietary Supplement Health and Education Act, which allowed the marketing and sale of DHEA as a food supplement (these are not subject to usual Food and Drug Administration regulation) rather than as a hormonal medication. Shortly thereafter, popular mass-market books began promoting the substance, as the following titles illustrate: *The DHEA breakthrough: look younger, live longer, feel better* (5) and *DHEA: the miracle hormone that can help you boost immunity, increase energy, lighten your mood, improve your sex drive and lengthen your lifespan* (6). Such claims, as well as the widespread unreg-

Portions of this chapter are adapted from Wolkowitz OM, Kroboth P, Reus VI, Fabian TJ. Dehydroepiandrosterone in aging and mental health. In: Morrison M, ed. *Hormones, gender and the aging brain: the endocrine basis of geriatric psychiatry.* Oxford: Cambridge University Press, 2000:144–167.

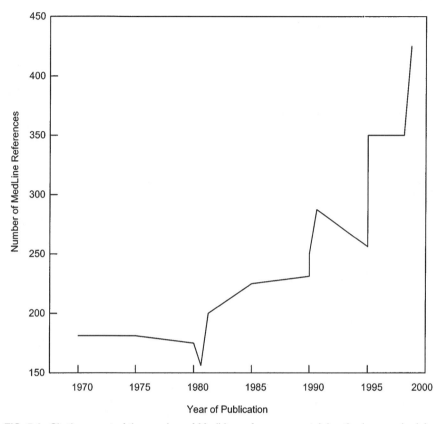

FIG. 5.1. Citation count of the number of MedLine references containing the key words dehydroepiandrosterone, DHEA, or DHEA-S by year of publication.

ulated use of DHEA, have concerned many medical investigators and practitioners because preclinical data may not readily extrapolate to clinical situations, much of the clinical data that exist have been derived from uncontrolled studies, and the full risk-to-benefit ratio of long-term DHEA use remains unknown (7,8).

This chapter seeks to put the possible role of DHEA as a psychotropic agent into scientific context and to review clinical data regarding its use in neuropsychiatric illnesses. The main focus will be on clinical efficacy, feasibility, and safety; more extensive reviews of pertinent preclinical studies are available elsewhere (9–20).

DEHYDROEPIANDROSTERONE AS A NEUROHORMONE

DHEA and its sulfated metabolite, DHEA-S (together abbreviated DHEA-(S)), are the most plentiful adrenal corticosteroids in humans, yet their physiologic roles remain uncertain. Important actions in the central nervous system, however, have been inferred from the fact that DHEA-S is synthesized *in situ* in brain; indeed, it has been termed a neurosteroid for this reason (19,21). Highlighting the potential importance of DHEA-S for brain functioning, the accumulation of DHEA-S in rat brain is largely independent of adrenal and gonadal synthesis, remaining constant after orchiectomy, adrenalectomy, and dexamethasone administration and increasing in response to acute stress independent of changes in plasma levels (22,23).

DEHYDROEPIANDROSTERONE(S) LEVELS DECREASE AS A FUNCTION OF AGING, CHRONIC STRESS, AND ILLNESS

Perhaps the most remarkable and well replicated observation about DHEA-S in humans is that its circulating levels (in both the plasma and CSF) peak in the mid-20s and then progressively decline with age, approaching a nadir (approximately 20% of peak levels) at approximately 65 to 70 years, the age at which the incidence of many age-related illnesses steeply increases (13,24,25). Levels of DHEA-S also decrease with chronic stress and medical illness (26–29). Glucocorticoids fail to show a similar pattern of decrease with age, illness, or stress. Indeed, cortisol levels typically rise or do not change in these conditions, and a highly significant decrease is observed in plasma ratios of DHEA-S–to–cortisol with age and chronic stress (24,27–38). Since DHEA-S may physiologically "buffer" the deleterious effects of excessive glucocorticoid exposure (see below), decreasing DHEA-S–to–cortisol ratios may prove especially problematic in hypercortisolemic states, including aging, depression, and other conditions (34,39,40). Indeed, Lupien et al. (41) noted greater cognitive deterioration in elderly men and women who showed larger decreases in DHEA-S–to–cortisol ratios over a 2-year period; changes in DHEA-S levels alone, however, were not significantly correlated with cognitive change.

BEHAVIORAL EFFECTS OF DEHYDROEPIANDROSTERONE(S) IN ANIMALS

By necessity, much of the data about the effects of DHEA-S derive from animal or tissue culture–based studies. Species typically studied, such as rats and mice, have significant concentrations of brain DHEA-S but minimal peripheral (adrenally derived) levels, challenging the relevance of such preclinical data to effects in humans. Nonetheless, such studies have provided valuable leads for designing clinical trials and have suggested possible mechanisms of the behavioral effects of DHEA-S.

DHEA and DHEA-S generally have memory-enhancing effects in animals, restoring the memory of old male mice and rats to the levels seen in young animals (42,43) and reversing pharmacologically induced amnesia in mice (14,44,45). Of particular clinical significance is the fact that DHEA-S reverses scopolamine amnesia in mice (14,45); scopolamine, an anticholinergic agent, has been proposed as a pharmacologic model of Alzheimer disease in healthy humans.

DHEA-S also has antidepressant-like effects in mice tested in the Porsolt forced swim test, significantly decreasing immobility time (46). The nonsulfated parent compound, DHEA, also displays antidepressant effects in this test but, interestingly, only in high-anxiety rats (47). Antianxiety effects of DHEA and DHEA-S have also been demonstrated in mice using the elevated plus maze test (48). However, while DHEA augments the anxiolytic effect of ethanol in this model, DHEA-S blocks it (48). Consistent with the possible difference in effects of DHEA and DHEA-S in animal models of anxiety, DHEA-S has been found to be anxiogenic in the mirrored chamber test, another test of anxiety in mice (49). DHEA, but not DHEA-S, administration also decreases mouse aggressive behavior in certain paradigms (e.g., the attack by group-housed triads of castrated male mice on lactating female mouse intruders) (22). The specificity of DHEA versus DHEA-S in these models of depression, anxiety, and aggression may be related to the differential effects of the two hormones at the brain γ-aminobutyric acid (GABA)-A receptors (22,50,51), although, physiologically, DHEA and DHEA-S are readily interconvertible in the circulation.

DHEA-S also affects eating behavior, producing hypophagia in food-deprived male mice (52). This effect may, at least partly, involve a N-methyl-D-aspartic acid (NMDA) receptor mechanism, since it is blocked by dizocilpine, a NMDA receptor antagonist (52). DHEA also decreases feeding in obese Zucker rats; this effect may be related to DHEA-induced increases in hypothalamic serotonin or dopamine activity (53,54).

NEUROTROPHIC POTENTIAL OF DEHYDROEPIANDROSTERONE(S)

Several studies also suggest that DHEA-S has neurotrophic potential. DHEA and DHEA-S, for example, enhance neuronal and glial survival and differentiation in dissociated cultures of the mouse embryo brain (15,55) and induce the formation of hypertrophic cells in hippocampal section culture specimens derived from orchiectomized adult male rats (56). These hypertrophic cells appear similar to the reactive astroglia that may be involved in restorative events following brain injury (56). DHEA-S has also been shown to prevent or to reduce the hippocampal neurotoxicity induced by the glutamate agonist, NMDA (57), as well as by corticosterone (58). Because glutamate release has been implicated in the neural damage resulting from cerebral ischemia and other neuronal insults and because excessive corticosterone exposure has been linked to hippocampal atrophy, these data raise the possibility that decreased DHEA-S levels may contribute to the increased vulnerability of the aging or stressed human brain to neurotoxic damage (30,33,34,39,57–60).

DEHYDROEPIANDROSTERONE(S) LEVELS CORRELATE WITH MOOD, MEMORY, AND FUNCTIONAL ABILITIES IN HUMANS

Correlational studies have provided indirect evidence of an effect of DHEA on mood, memory, and functional abilities in humans, but numerous caveats, which are outlined elsewhere (9), are important to consider before ascribing causality in these relationships.

Many, but not all, studies have reported lowered levels of DHEA-S in patients with depression, poor life satisfaction, psychosocial stress, and functional limitations (61–64). Osran et al. (65) and Ferrari et al. (66) found that DHEA-to-cortisol ratios more accurately discriminated depressed from nondepressed individuals than the levels of either hormone alone did, with lower morning ratios being seen in the depressed individuals (65). Low DHEA levels have also been reported in child and adolescent patients with depression. Goodyer et al. (67) found that morning DHEA hyposecretion, as well as evening cortisol hypersecretion, were significantly and independently associated with major depression in children from the ages of 8 to 16 years and that patients who remained depressed 36 weeks after initial assessment had baseline evening DHEA-to-cortisol ratios lower than the median group value (68). The authors speculated that, in the presence of adequate DHEA concentrations, high cortisol concentrations alone may not inhibit recovery (68).

Low levels of DHEA-S have also been associated with higher ratings of perceived stress (69), trait anxiety (70), Type A behavior, cynicism, and hostility (71–74), while higher levels of DHEA-S have been associated with greater amount, frequency, and enjoyment of leisure activities (71); sexual gratification and frequency of masturbation (in women) (75–76); healthier psychological profiles (71); more expansive personality ratings (characterized by self-centeredness, high activity drive, and high capacity for work) (77); and greater sensation-seeking and monotony avoidance attributes (78).

In a recently published study, Buckwalter et al. (79) examined hormonal correlates of mood and cognitive function in pregnancy and in the postpartum period. They reported a very consistent pattern of associations of higher plasma DHEA levels with better mood and memory. During pregnancy and following delivery, higher DHEA levels were correlated with lower ratings of depression, interpersonal sensitivity or tension, and anxiety and with better executive control processes and free recall. The authors proposed that DHEA endogenously regulates mood and cognitive function during pregnancy and that postpartum depression may be exacerbated by declines in DHEA. Therefore, they suggested that DHEA supplementation, in theory, might be a viable option for treating postpartum mood disturbances (79).

The remaining literature examining endogenous serum or urinary DHEA-S levels in depression is inconsistent, with reports of increased (80–83), decreased (84), or unaltered (32,38,85) levels. In one of the studies showing high DHEA-S levels in depressed patients, the levels were positively correlated with depression severity ratings (80); however, hormone levels tended to be inversely correlated with depression severity ratings ($P<0.10$) in another report (83).

DHEA-S levels have also been examined in other psychiatric illnesses. Increased, rather than decreased, DHEA-S-to–cortisol ratios have been reported in patients with panic disorder (38). Perhaps consistent with this, Herbert et al., who reported the low morning DHEA levels in depressed adolescents (67), found that depressed adolescents with comorbid panic or phobic disorder did not show low morning DHEA levels (86).

Patients with anorexia nervosa reportedly have low DHEA-S levels (87,88), as well as extremely low DHEA–to–cortisol ratios (89). These abnormalities revert to normal with partial clinical recovery (89). Gordon et al. (88) recently treated young anorexic women with oral DHEA (50 to 200 mg per day) and noted significant improvement in bone turnover markers (88) without any significant effects on weight or psychological measures.

Two recent studies have also demonstrated low DHEA-S levels in patients with chronic fatigue syndrome (CFS) (90,91). The latter authors speculated that this decrease in DHEA-S levels is directly responsible for the neuropsychiatric aspects of this condition (91). Such a hypothesis would be consistent with reports that exogenous DHEA administration alleviates fatigue in normal patients (4), as well as in medically ill patients (92). To the authors' knowledge, DHEA has not been formally tested as a treatment for CFS, although infusions of DHEA plus high-dose vitamin C have been reported to alleviate CFS in a series of uncontrolled studies in Japan (93,94).

A large number of studies has also assessed the relationship of DHEA-S levels to overall well-being and cognitive and general functioning. In many population-based studies in the elderly, cognitive and general functional abilities are positively correlated with DHEA-S levels (32,61,95–102), but, in some studies, the relationships were gender specific. Based on such data, investigators have proposed that DHEA-S plays a role in successful aging (100,101).

Other studies, however, have reported that higher DHEA levels are associated with poorer performance on cognitive tests in men and women with Alzheimer disease (103) and in women (but not men) who are nursing home residents (97). The latter authors concluded that contradictory relationships exist between DHEA-S levels and neuropsychiatric function and that these relationships may be gender specific. Adding to the uncertain nature of the relationship of DHEA-S to cognitive function, patients with Alzheimer disease have been reported to exhibit both decreased (104–107) and increased or unchanged (61,63,108–111) DHEA-S levels. Studies have also evaluated whether low DHEA-S levels at an index time point predict the subsequent development or progression of dementia or cognitive decline (62,103,112). Such studies, although sometimes suffering from methodologic flaws (103,112,cf. [9] for discussion), failed to ascertain a significant predictive relationship.

Cumulatively, then, the descriptive and epidemiologic data in humans raise the possibility of a direct relationship between DHEA-S levels and functional abilities, memory, mood, and sense of well-being, although many inconsistencies exist in the literature and abnormalities in patients with depression and dementia have not been uniformly replicated. Nonetheless, even if endogenous DHEA-S levels are not decreased in depression and dementia, the pharmacologic increases in their levels may possibly have mood-enhancing and memory-enhancing effects. This possibility is reviewed in the following section.

DEHYDROEPIANDROSTERONE TREATMENT EFFECTS ON WELL-BEING, MOOD, AND MEMORY IN HUMANS

Discrepancies among the treatment studies may relate to several factors, including the age and gender of the subjects treated, the formulation (e.g., powder, cream, micronized) and the dose and route (e.g., oral, sublingual, transdermal, intramuscular) of DHEA-S administration, the duration of treatment, and the sensitivity and appropriateness of the dependent variables. The potential importance of dose is highlighted by preclinical and clinical studies in which intermediate doses or serum levels of DHEA-S were more effective than lower or higher doses or levels (14,45,55,113,114).

In the first published clinical trials of DHEA, Strauss and Sands et al. (1–3, 115) reported that patients with schizophrenia, inadequate personality, or emotional immaturity showed rapid and impressive improvements in energy, insight, self-confidence, emotionality, vitality, adjustment to the environment, and school and occupational performance and decreases in anxiety, depression, apathy, and withdrawal. Although these studies were largely uncontrolled, in several cases the improvements dissipated following single-blind crossover to the placebo and returned with single-blind crossover back to DHEA. Similar beneficial results, seen in open-label trials, were reported in patients with phobic-obsessive psychoneuroses, neuropsychasthenia, psychopathic personality, involutive syndromes, and depressive psychoses by early Italian investigators (116,117). Based on these studies and others (118,119), DHEA, also referred to in Europe as prasterone, was approved under the trade name Astenile for prescription in Italy for indications such as nervousness, mild depression (especially when associated with the climacteric period), asthenia, insufficient personality, psychophysical stress, and psychosomatic disturbances associated with senescence and menopause (120). However, it was subsequently withdrawn from the market due to the lack of double-blind trials addressing these indications.

In the first double-blind, placebo-controlled clinical trial of DHEA, Forrest et al. (121) treated eight patients who had depression, anxiety, social phobia, shyness, lack of confidence, hyposexuality, and so on (classified by the authors as having vulnerable personalities) with DHEA (5 to 20 mg per day) or a placebo for 3 weeks each in a within-subject crossover design that had a 1-week washout between treatment arms. DHEA treatment was associated with slightly more global positive assessments and with fewer negative global assessments than the placebo, but this was not interpreted as significant by the authors. Unfortunately, the sample size was small, the doses were low, the trial was short, and it used nonstandardized ratings and did not present statistical analyses of these effects.

After a 30-year to 40-year hiatus, clinical trials with DHEA resumed. Patients with multiple sclerosis and systemic lupus erythematosus, for example, showed increased energy, libido, and sense of well-being in open-label trials (92,122,123). More recently, DHEA was administered to healthy, normal middle-aged and elderly subjects in a randomized, placebo-controlled, double-blind, crossover study (4). Subjects, aged from 40 to 70 years old, received DHEA (50 mg) or the placebo every evening for 3 months. This dosing schedule restored DHEA-S levels to youthful levels within 2 weeks, and levels were sustained for the entire 3-month period. DHEA-treated subjects showed significant increases in perceived physical and psychological well-being with no change in libido. Reported improvements included increased energy, deeper sleep, improved mood, a more relaxed feeling, and having an enhanced ability to handle stressful events. These results generated considerable interest in the possibility of significant behavioral effects of DHEA, but the global subjective measure used to assess behavioral change (a single visual analog scale measuring sense of well-being) was relatively crude.

Labrie and Diamond et al. both treated 60-year-old to 70-year-old women with single daily percutaneous applications of a 10% DHEA cream for 12 months (124,125). This was preceded or was followed by 6 months of placebo cream, although the study does not state if this was open-label, single-blind, or double-blind. They noted, as did Morales et al. (4), that 80% of the women reported well-being and an increase in energy during DHEA treatment. Unfortunately, these behavioral changes were also assessed via nonstandardized daily diaries. Vogiatzi et al. (126) administered micronized DHEA, 40 mg twice daily sublingually, versus the placebo in a double-blind manner to 13 morbidly obese adolescents. They reported no change in the sense of well-being in these subjects; but their assessment method was not specified, and the sample size was too small to gauge this effect meaningfully. An additional double-blind study recently examined the effects of 2 weeks of treatment with DHEA, 50 mg per day, compared to 2 weeks of placebo in healthy elderly men and women (127,128). Only women tended to report an increase in well-being ($P=0.11$) and mood ($P=0.10$), as assessed with questionnaires. They also showed better performance in one of six cognitive tests (picture memory) after DHEA treatment. However, after post-hoc correction for multiple comparisons, this difference was no longer significant. No such trends were observed in the male subjects ($P>0.20$). This study used reliable neuropsychological test instruments and had an adequate sample size, but the duration of treatment may have been too short for behavioral changes to become manifest (129).

Other studies have specifically assessed the effect of DHEA on mood in depressed or dysthymic subjects. In an initial small-scale (N=6; N, number of patients studied), open-label pilot study, Wolkowitz et al. (130) reported antidepressant effects of DHEA in middle-aged to elderly patients with major depression. The doses of DHEA were individually adjusted between 30 and 90 mg per day for 4 weeks to achieve circulating DHEA-S levels in the mid-to-high normal range for healthy young adults. Subjects demonstrated highly significant improvements in the Hamilton Depression Ratings and Symptom Checklist-90 ratings and showed a significant improvement in automatic cognitive processing at week 3 of DHEA treatment. Mood improvements were significantly related to increases in the circulating levels of DHEA and DHEA-S and to their ratios with cortisol; changes in cortisol concentrations alone were not correlated with behavioral changes. One subject from this study, a previously treatment-resistant elderly depressed woman, received extended open-label treatment with DHEA (60 mg per day for 4 months, followed by 90 mg per day for an additional 2 months). Her depression ratings improved approximately 50%, and her access to semantic memory improved 63% during DHEA treatment and returned to pre-treatment levels after DHEA discontinuation. Increases in DHEA-S levels over time were also directly correlated in this patient with improvements in depression ratings and recognition memory.

These open-label studies were followed by a double-blind, placebo-controlled trial in which 22 depressed patients received either DHEA (60 to 90 mg per day) or a placebo for 6 weeks (131). Some patients were medication free at the time of entering the study; others remained depressed despite being on prestabilized (>6 weeks) antidepressant medication. In the former group, DHEA or the placebo was used alone; in the latter group, DHEA or the placebo was added to the stabilized antidepressant regimen. DHEA, compared to the placebo, was associated with significant antidepressant responses; five of 11 DHEA-treated patients showed greater than 50% improvement in depression ratings and had endpoint Hamilton Depression Rating Scale ratings of less than 10. These were seen in none of the 11 placebo-treated patients. These results have not yet been replicated in larger studies, but they raise the possibility that DHEA, used alone or as an antidepressant adjunct in refractory patients, has significant antidepressant effects in some patients.

Bloch et al. (132) recently concluded a 12-week, double-blind, placebo-controlled study in unmedicated patients with mid-life dysthymia (one patient had concurrent major depression). Subjects received, in randomized order, DHEA (90 mg per day for 3 weeks, followed by 450 mg per day for 3 weeks) or the placebo for 6 weeks. DHEA, compared to the placebo, produced a robust antidepressant response at both doses. No changes in cognitive function were noted.

Gordon et al. (88) recently treated young women with anorexia nervosa with DHEA (50, 100, or 200 mg per day for 3 months). Although the specific DHEA dosage group assignment was double blind, no placebo control group was used. They noted that, despite having patients with significant levels of depression and anxiety at baseline, DHEA treatment had no significant effects on the self-ratings of either symptom. This study should be interpreted cautiously since no placebo control group was used, the sample size was small, the subjects may have been sporadically noncompliant with the study drug regimens (per the authors' estimation), and the psychological measures were all self-ratings. Self-ratings in patients with anorexia nervosa may be less reliable than corresponding observer ratings (133,134).

Another important area of clinical investigation has been the possible cognition-enhancing effects of DHEA. In 1990, a single case was reported of a 47-year-old woman with low serum DHEA-S levels and a 20-year history of treatment-refractory learning and memory dysfunction. She was treated openly with high daily doses of DHEA ranging from 12.5 to 37 mg per kg for 2 years; she demonstrated improved verbal recall and recognition along with a normalization in electroencephalography (EEG) and P300 brain electrophysiology (135).

Recent studies by Wolf and others in Germany (127,128,136–138) have failed to detect major cognitive effects of short-term DHEA administration in normal volunteers, although these conclusions are limited by the short duration of DHEA administration used in those studies (129). Single-dose DHEA administration (300 mg dissolved in 5 mL of ethanol) to healthy young adults failed to alter memory performance, despite significantly lowering cortisol levels (136). In another study that was previously described (127), 2 weeks of double-blind DHEA administration to healthy elderly controls produced only a trend toward improvement in picture memory in women, but this was not significant after adjusting for the number of tests administered. Event-related potentials (ERPs) were assessed in the men, but not the women, in this treatment paradigm (137). Certain significant ERP changes were induced by DHEA treatment, indicating changes in central nervous system stimulus processing, but these changes were apparently insufficient to alter memory performance significantly in these men (137). If DHEA exerts memory-enhancing effects via antiglucocorticoid actions, such benefits might only be apparent under conditions of hypercortisolemia or stress. To test this hypothesis, the same group of investigators tested cognitive performance before and after a laboratory stressor in DHEA-treated versus placebo-treated subjects. DHEA treatment yielded opposing effects on memory performance as follows: it decreased the post-stress recall of visual material learned prior to the stressor, but it enhanced post-stress attentional performance (138).

Most recently, DHEA has been studied as a possible memory enhancer in patients with Alzheimer disease. A great deal of excitement followed the initial reports of low serum DHEA-S levels in patients with Alzheimer disease (104). Although these reports were only inconsistently replicated, as was previously reviewed, they raised the possibility that increasing DHEA-S levels in these patients to the physiologic levels seen in healthy young adults might have salutary cognitive effects. An initial small-scale study addressing this possibility yielded negative findings (139). Dukoff et al. (139) reported that DHEA, 1,600 mg orally daily for 4 weeks, had no significant cognitive or mood effects in demented or nondemented elderly individuals. This negative report should be interpreted cautiously, however, since the sample size was small, the demented population was heterogeneous, and the trial duration may have been too short to see cognitive change in this population. Furthermore, very high (pharmacologic, as opposed to physiologic) doses of DHEA were used; these may have exceeded a therapeutic window, as prior preclinical and clinical data have suggested (15, 16,55,113,122).

Wolkowitz et al. (140) recently treated 58 patients with Alzheimer disease with either DHEA (NPI-34133), 50 mg orally twice daily, or a placebo for 6 months in a between-groups design. At these doses, DHEA treatment restored serum DHEA-S levels to, or slightly above, those seen in healthy young adults. DHEA treatment, relative to the placebo, was associated with a significant improvement in cognitive performance at month 3 ($P<0.02$) and a non-significant trend toward significant improvement at month 6 ($P=0.010$). Although cognitive performance improved with DHEA at month 3 but not at month 6, no significant difference between treatments was seen on a global rating measure that assessed overall clinical impressions of change at either month 3 or month 6.

Review of the DHEA treatment literature cumulatively suggests that, in certain situations, DHEA administration enhances mood, energy, sleep, sense of well-being, functional capabilities, and memory. Such effects may be more likely in elderly, depressed, or infirm patients than in young, healthy individuals. They may also be more likely to emerge after 1 or more months of treatment, and they may continue to evolve over 6 months or longer (140,141). Cognitive and mood effects in normal subjects following short duration treatment (2 weeks or less) seem unlikely or else are quite mild.

NOTE ON POSSIBLE MECHANISMS OF NEUROPSYCHIATRIC EFFECTS OF DEHYDROEPIANDROSTERONE

A full review of the postulated mechanisms underlying the neuropsychiatric effects of DHEA is beyond the scope of this chapter, but the most relevant references are cited for the interested reader. Although DHEA-S or its metabolites may regulate gene transcription (142–144), most research has focused on its nongenomic, membrane receptor–based effects. Electrophysiologic and neurochemical data suggest that DHEA and DHEA-S have GABA-antagonistic (10,145–148) and NMDA-potentiating and sigma-receptor–potentiating (149–151) properties. DHEA-S also increases the hippocampal primed burst potentiation (152) and reduces the amplitude of inhibitory postsynaptic potentials, thereby enhancing neuronal depolarization and excitation (145,153). It also facilitates the activation of CA1 neurons in hippocampal slices (154) and, perhaps most importantly, increases hippocampal cholinergic function (155,156).

DHEA-S could have antidepressant effects by increasing brain serotonin and dopamine activity (53,54,157), as well as by potentiating NMDA-induced hippocampal norepinephrine release (11,149), but direct effects of DHEA administration on biogenic amine levels in humans have yet to be assessed. Actions on the hypothalamic-pituitary-adrenal axis are also likely to be involved in the mood and other neuropsychiatric effects of DHEA (30,33,40,59,60,130,158,159). Antagonism of glucocorticoid effects by DHEA or its metabolites has been demonstrated in multiple model systems in peripheral tissue (159–168) and in the brain (58). Antiglucocorticoid effects could, in theory, account for both the antidepressant (34,36,40,59,169,170) and neuroprotective (30,33,39,171) effects of DHEA.

Other miscellaneous mechanisms that could contribute to the neuropsychiatric effects of DHEA include increased serum insulin-like growth factor-1 levels and bioavailability (4), as well as inhibition of proinflammatory brain cytokines (e.g., interleukin-1 [IL-1], IL-6, and tumor necrosis factor-α) and of free radical formation, both of which have been implicated in neurodegeneration (107,172–178). Of relevance to aging and dementia, the serum amyloid component in aged rats is also decreased by DHEA administration (179), and DHEA *in vitro* augments amyloid precursor protein secretion following cholinergic stimulation of desensitized M1-muscarinic receptors in PC12M1 cells (180,181).

TREATMENT GUIDELINES

Due to the paucity of adequately controlled and powered studies of DHEA administration, DHEA cannot be recommended for clinical use at this time (7,8,17,182). This may change, however, as new studies emerge in the near future. For patients who are interested in trying DHEA despite these caveats, the following recommendations for physicians (as well as the recommendations outlined by van Vollenhoven [8]) seem prudent, although most are derived from clinical intuition and informed reading of the extant literature rather than from empirical evidence:

1. The current state of knowledge about the effects and potential side effects of DHEA should be reviewed with patients, placing particular emphasis on diminishing any unrealistic expectations about its antiaging effects.

2. Patients should be monitored for the occasional development of hypomanic, aggressive, psychotic, or disinhibited behavior (1,3,140,183,184).

3. Patients at increased risk for hormonally sensitive tumors (e.g., cancer of the breast, ovary, uterus, cervix, or prostate or malignant melanoma) should be advised not to take DHEA, although antitumor, as well as protumor, effects have been reported (182,185–189). For other patients, baseline and follow-up assessments, such as prostate-specific antigen measurements (182), mammograms, uterine ultrasounds, Pap smears, and so on, may be prudent (8). For non-hysterectomized women contemplating long-term DHEA treatment (e.g., >3 months), periodic progesterone treatment aimed at shedding the uterine lining (which may hypertrophy under DHEA's estrogenic influence) may also be prudent.

4. Baseline serum levels of DHEA-S should be measured to assess the relative appropriateness of DHEA replacement and to establish a baseline against which the treatment-induced increases can be compared.

5. Although no clear relationships have yet been demonstrated between serum DHEA-S levels and therapeutic outcome (8,140), assaying serum DHEA-S levels after each dosage adjustment to guide the achievement of levels in the high-normal range for young adults seems reasonable (although, for some conditions, supraphysiologic levels may be more efficacious [190]).

6. Periodic assays of serum testosterone (in particular, bioavailable testosterone) and estradiol levels should be performed to preclude excessive increases in the levels of either hormone.

7. Appropriate dosing for most of the neuropsychiatric conditions reviewed here seems to be in the range of 25 to 100 mg per day, although few studies have systematically compared the efficacy and tolerability of different doses. Indeed, clinical trials have used doses as low as 5 mg per day to as high as several grams per day (16). Due to the relatively short half-lives of DHEA-S and, especially, DHEA, the authors have generally divided the total daily doses into twice-daily or thrice-daily dosing in their studies, with the larger portion of the dose given in the morning to mimic the endogenous circadian rhythm (17). Doses late in the evening (e.g., after 6:00 or 8:00 PM) may be overly activating, causing insomnia in some patients.

8. If no benefit is observed after approximately 3 months, any additional benefit appears unlikely to accrue, and discontinuation of DHEA may be appropriate.

9. As noted, DHEA can be widely procured without prescription in the United States. No federal regulatory control exists over the purity and bioavailability of these uncontrolled commercial preparations, and the actual content of over-the-counter preparations varies from 0% to 150% of the claimed DHEA content (191). Nonetheless, the products of the larger, reputable manufacturers (especially those assaying hormone content by high-performance liquid chromatography) may be suitable. However, preparations advertising natural DHEA derived from Mexican wild mountain yams should be avoided since they contain diosgenin, a manufacturing source of steroid products that is itself ineffective *in vivo*. Patients wishing to try DHEA ideally should procure it from a compounding pharmacy, which requires a physician's prescription.

SUMMARY

Despite the meteoric rise in research in DHEA-S in recent years, its role in human neuropsychiatric diseases and its possible place in clinical therapeutics remain uncertain. This situation will hopefully be remedied in coming years. The provocative clinical and preclinical leads reviewed in this chapter should bolster enthusiasm for exploring the neuropsychotropic properties of DHEA-S.

In the authors' opinion, DHEA supplementation is not yet ready for unsupervised clinical use because its benefits and safety with long-term use have yet to be clearly established. Individuals wishing to undertake DHEA supplementation should obtain DHEA from a reputable source and should take it under medical supervision with appropriate laboratory and clinical monitoring.

ACKNOWLEDGMENTS

The authors gratefully acknowledge the following individuals who provided stimulating discussions and ideas about the role of DHEA in human illness:

Louann Brizendine, M.D.; Eugene Roberts, PH.D.; William Regelson, M.D.; Joe Herbert, M.D.; David Rubinow, M.D.; and Steven Paul, M.D.

This research was partially funded by grants to Owen M. Wolkowitz from the National Alliance for Research in Schizophrenia and Affective Disorders, the Stanley Foundation, the Alzheimer's Association, and the National Institute on Aging.

REFERENCES

1. Strauss EB, Stevenson WAH. Use of dehydroisoandrosterone in psychiatric practice. *J Neurol Neurosurg Psychiatr* 1955;18:137–144.
2. Sands DE, Chamberlain GHA. Treatment of inadequate personality in juveniles by dehydroisoandrosterone. *Br Med J* 1952;2:66.
3. Strauss EB, Sands DE, Robinson AM, Tindall WJ, Stevenson WAH. Use of dehydroisoandrosterone in psychiatric treatment: a preliminary survey. *Br Med J* 1952;2:64–66.
4. Morales AJ, Nolan JJ, Nelson JC, Yen SS. Effects of replacement dose of dehydroepiandrosterone in men and women of advancing age [published erratum appears in *J Clin Endocrinol Metab* 1995;80: 2799]. *J Clin Endocrinol Metab* 1994;78:1360–1367.
5. Cherniske S. *The DHEA breakthrough*. New York: Ballantine Books, 1998.
6. Callahan M. *DHEA: the miracle hormone that can help you boost immunity, increase energy, lighten your mood, improve your sex drive and lengthen your lifespan.* New York: Signet, 1997.
7. Katz S, Morales AJ. Dehydroepiandrosterone (DHEA) and DHEA-sulfate (DS) as therapeutic options in menopause. *Semin Reprod Endocrinol* 1998;16:161–170.
8. van Vollenhoven RF. Dehydroepiandrosterone: uses and abuses. In: Kelley WN, Harris ED Jr, Sledge CB, eds. *Textbook of rheumatology*. Update Series, Vol. 25. Philadelphia: WB Saunders, 1997:1–25.
9. Wolkowitz OM, Kroboth P, Reus VI, Fabian TJ. Dehydroepiandrosterone in aging and mental health. In: Morrison M, ed. *Hormones, gender and the aging brain: the endocrine basis of geriatric psychiatry*. Oxford: Cambridge University Press, 2000:144–167.
10. Majewska MD. Neurosteroids: endogenous bimodal modulators of the GABAA receptor. Mechanism of action and physiological significance. *Prog Neurobiol* 1992;38:379–395.
11. Majewska MD. Neuronal actions of dehydroepiandrosterone. Possible roles in brain development, aging, memory, and affect. *Ann N Y Acad Sci* 1995;774:111–120.
12. Regelson W, Kalimi M, Loria R. DHEA: Some thoughts as to its biologic and clinical action. In: Kalimi M, Regelson W, eds. *The biologic role of dehydroepiandrosterone (DHEA).* Berlin: de Gruyter, 1990:405–445.
13. Regelson W, Kalimi M. Dehydroepiandrosterone (DHEA)—the multifunctional steroid. II. Effects on the CNS, cell proliferation, metabolic and vascular, clinical and other effects. Mechanism of action? *Ann N Y Acad Sci* 1994;719:564–575.
14. Roberts E. Dehydroepiandrosterone (DHEA) and its sulfate (DHEAS) as neural facilitators: effects on brain tissue in culture and on memory in young and old mice. A cyclic GMP hypothesis of action of DHEA and DHEAS in nervous system and other tissues. In: Kalimi M, Regelson W, eds. *The biologic role of dehydroepiandrosterone (DHEA).* Berlin: de Gruyter, 1990:13–42.
15. Roberts E, Bologa L, Flood JF, Smith GE. Effects of dehydroepiandrosterone and its sulfate on brain tissue in culture and on memory in mice. *Brain Res* 1987;406:357–362.
16. Svec F, Porter JR. The actions of exogenous dehydroepiandrosterone in experimental animals and humans. *PSEBM* 1998;218:174–191.
17. Svec F. Ageing and adrenal cortical function. *Baill Clin Endocrinol Metab* 1997;11:271–287.
18. Baulieu EE, Robel P. Dehydroepiandrosterone (DHEA) and dehydroepiandrosterone sulfate (DHEAS) as neuroactive neurosteroids [comment]. *Proc Natl Acad Sci U S A* 1998;95:4089–4091.
19. Baulieu EE. Neurosteroids: of the nervous system, by the nervous system, for the nervous system. *Recent Prog Horm Res* 1997;52:1–32.
20. Baulieu EE, Robel P. Dehydroepiandrosterone and dehydroepiandrosterone sulfate as neuroactive neurosteroids. *J Endocrinol* 1996;150:S221–S239.
21. Zwain IH, Yen SS. Dehydroepiandrosterone: biosynthesis and metabolism in the brain. *Endocrinology* 1999;140:880–887.
22. Robel P, Baulieu EE. Dehydroepiandrosterone (DHEA) is a neuroactive neurosteroid. *Ann N Y Acad Sci* 1995;774:82–110.

23. Corpechot C, Robel P, Axelson M, et al. Characterization and measurement of dehydroepiandros-terone sulfate in rat brain. *Proc Natl Acad Sci U S A* 1981;78:4704–4707.
24. Guazzo EP, Kirkpatrick PJ, Goodyer IM, et al. Cortisol, dehydroepiandrosterone (DHEA), and DHEA sulfate in the cerebrospinal fluid of man: relation to blood levels and the effects of age. *J Clin Endocrinol Metab* 1996;81:3951–3960.
25. Azuma T, Matsubara T, Shima Y, et al. Neurosteroids in cerebrospinal fluid in neurologic disorders. *J Neurol Sci* 1993;120:87–92.
26. Spratt DI, Longcope C, Cox PM, Bigos ST, Wilbur-Welling C. Differential changes in serum con-centrations of androgens and estrogens (in relation with cortisol) in postmenopausal women with acute illness. *J Clin Endocrinol Metab* 1993;76:1542–1547.
27. Parker LN, Levin ER, Lifrak ET. Evidence for adrenocortical adaptation to severe illness. *J Clin Endocrinol Metab* 1985;60:947–952.
28. Nishikaze O. [17-KS sulfate as a biomarker in health and disease]. *Rinsho Byori* 1998;46:520–528.
29. Ozasa H, Kita M, Inoue T, Mori T. Plasma dehydroepiandrosterone-to-cortisol ratios as an indicator of stress in gynecologic patients. *Gynecol Oncol* 1990;37:178–182.
30. Leblhuber F, Windhager E, Neubauer C, et al. Antiglucocorticoid effects of DHEA-S in Alzheimer's disease [letter] [published erratum appears in *Am J Psychiatry* 1992;149:1622]. *Am J Psychiatry* 1992;149:1125–1126.
31. Leblhuber F, Neubauer C, Peichl M, et al. Age and sex differences of dehydroepiandrosterone sul-fate (DHEAS) and cortisol (CRT) plasma levels in normal controls and Alzheimer's disease (AD). *Psychopharmacology* 1993;111:23–26.
32. Reus VI, Wolkowitz OM, Roberts E, et al. Dehydroepiandrosterone (DHEA) and memory in depressed patients. *Neuropsychopharmacology* 1993;9:66S.
33. Wolkowitz OM, Reus VI, Manfredi F, Roberts E. Antiglucocorticoid effects of DHEA-S in Alzheimer's disease [reply]. *Am J Psychiatry* 1992;149:1126.
34. Hechter O, Grossman A, Chatterton RT Jr. Relationship of dehydroepiandrosterone and cortisol in disease. *Med Hypotheses* 1997;49:85–91.
35. McKenna TJ, Fearon U, Clarke D, Cunningham SK. A critical review of the origin and control of adrenal androgens. *Baillieres Clin Obstet Gynaecol* 1997;11:229–248.
36. Goodyer IM, Herbert J, Altham PM. Adrenal steroid secretion and major depression in 8- to 16-year-olds, III. Influence of cortisol/DHEA ratio at presentation on subsequent rates of disappointing life events and persistent major depression. *Psychol Med* 1998;28:265–273.
37. Oberbeck R, Benschop RJ, Jacobs R, et al. Endocrine mechanisms of stress-induced DHEA-secretion. *J Endocrinol Invest* 1998;21:148–153.
38. Fava M, Rosenbaum JF, MacLaughlin RA, et al. Dehydroepiandrosterone-sulfate/cortisol ratio in panic disorder. *Psychiatry Res* 1989;28:345–350.
39. Herbert J. Neurosteroids, brain damage, and mental illness. *Exp Gerontol* 1998;33:713–727.
40. Dubrovsky B. Natural steroids counteracting some actions of putative depressogenic steroids on the central nervous system: potential therapeutic benefits. *Med Hypotheses* 1997;49:51–55.
41. Lupien S, Sharma S, Arcand JF, et al. Dehydroepiandrosterone-sulfate (DHEA-S) levels, cortisol levels and cognitive function in elderly human subjects. In: *International society of psychoneuroen-docrinology.* Munich: International Society of Psychoneuroendocrinology, 1995:24.
42. Flood JF, Roberts E. Dehydroepiandrosterone sulfate improves memory in aging mice. *Brain Research* 1988;448:178–181.
43. Tejkalova H, Beneova O, Kritofikova Z, et al. Neuro-behavioral effects of dehydroepiandrosterone in model experiments with old rats. In: *XXIst collegium internationale neuro-psychopharmacolog-icum congress.* Glasgow: XXIst Collegium Internationale Neuropsychopharmacologicum Congress, 1998:Abstract #PW11027.
44. Melchior CL, Ritzmann RF. Neurosteroids block the memory-impairing effects of ethanol in mice. *Pharmacol Biochem Behav* 1996;53:51–56.
45. Flood JF, Smith GE, Roberts E. Dehydroepiandrosterone and its sulfate enhance memory retention in mice. *Brain Res* 1988;447:269–278.
46. Reddy DS, Kaur G, Kulkarni SK. Sigma (sigma1) receptor mediated anti-depressant-like effects of neurosteroids in the Porsolt forced swim test. *Neuroreport* 1998;9:3069–3073.
47. Prasad A, Imamura M, Prasad C. Dehydroepiandrosterone decreases behavioral despair in high- but not low-anxiety rats. *Physiol Behav* 1997;62:1053–1057.
48. Melchior CL, Ritzmann RF. Dehydroepiandrosterone is an anxiolytic in mice on the plus maze. *Pharmacol Biochem Behav* 1994;47:437–441.
49. Reddy DS, Kulkarni SK. Differential anxiolytic effects of neurosteroids in the mirrored chamber behavior test in mice. *Brain Res* 1997;752:61–71.

50. Demirgoren S, Majewska MD, Spivak CE, London ED. Receptor binding and electrophysiological effects of dehydroepiandrosterone sulfate, an antagonist of the GABAA receptor. *Neuroscience* 1991;45:127–135.
51. Corpechot C, Robel P, Lachapelle N, et al. Dehydroepiandrosterone libre et sulfo-conjugee dans le cerveau du Souris dysmyeliniques. *CR Acad Sci Paris* 1981;292:231–234.
52. Reddy DS, Kulkarni SK. The role of GABA-A and mitochondrial diazepam-binding inhibitor receptors on the effects of neurosteroids on food intake in mice. *Psychopharmacology* 1998;137: 391–400.
53. Abadie JM, Wright B, Correa G, et al. Effect of dehydroepiandrosterone on neurotransmitter levels and appetite regulation of the obese Zucker rat. The obesity research program. *Diabetes* 1993;42:662–669.
54. Porter JR, Abadie JM, Wright BE, et al. The effect of discontinuing dehydroepiandrosterone supplementation on Zucker rat food intake and hypothalamic neurotransmitters. *Int J Obes Relat Metab Disord* 1995;19:480–488.
55. Bologa L, Sharma J, Roberts E. Dehydroepiandrosterone and its sulfate derivative reduce neuronal death and enhance astrocytic differentiation in brain cell cultures. *J Neurosci Res* 1987;17:225–234.
56. Del Cerro S, Garcia-Estrada J, Garcia-Segura LM. Neuroactive steroids regulate astroglia morphology in hippocampal cultures from adult rats. *Glia* 1995;14:65–71.
57. Kimonides VG, Khatibi NH, Svendsen CN, et al. Dehydroepiandrosterone (DHEA) and DHEA-sulfate (DHEAS) protect hippocampal neurons against excitatory amino acid-induced neurotoxicity. *Proc Natl Acad Sci U S A* 1998;95:1852–1857.
58. Kimonides VG, Spillantini MG, Sofroniew MV, et al. Dehydroepiandrosterone antagonizes the neurotoxic effects of corticosterone and translocation of stress-activated protein kinase 3 in hippocampal primary cultures. *Neuroscience* 1999;89:429–436.
59. Herbert J. Fortnightly review. Stress, the brain, and mental illness. *BMJ* 1997;315:530–535.
60. Herbert J. Stress, the brain, and mental illness. *BMJ* 1997;315:530–535.
61. Berr C, Lafont S, Debuire B, et al. Relationships of dehydroepiandrosterone sulfate in the elderly with functional, psychological, and mental status, and short-term mortality: a French community-based study. *Proc Natl Acad Sci U S A* 1996;93:13410–13415.
62. Yaffe K, Ettinger B, Pressman A, et al. Neuropsychiatric function and dehydroepiandrosterone sulfate in elderly women: a prospective study. *Biol Psychiatry* 1998;43:694–700.
63. Legrain S, Berr C, Frenoy N, et al. Dehydroepiandrosterone sulfate in a long-term care aged population. *Gerontology* 1995;41:343–351.
64. Furuya E, Maezawa M, Nishikaze O. [17-KS sulfate as a biomarker in psychosocial stress]. *Rinsho Byori* 1998;46:529–537.
65. Osran H, Reist C, Chen CC, et al. Adrenal androgens and cortisol in major depression. *Am J Psychiatry* 1993;150:806–809.
66. Ferrari E, Borri R, Casarotti D, et al. Major depression in elderly patients: a chrono-neuroendocrine study. *Aging Clin. Exp Res* 1997;9:83.
67. Goodyer IM, Herbert J, Altham PM, et al. Adrenal secretion during major depression in 8- to 16-year-olds, I. Altered diurnal rhythms in salivary cortisol and dehydroepiandrosterone (DHEA) at presentation. *Psychol Med* 1996;26:245–256.
68. Goodyer IM, Herbert J, Altham PME. Adrenal steroid secretion and major depression in 8- to-16-year olds, III. Influence of cortisol/DHEA ratio at presentation on subsequent rates of disappointing life events and persistent major depression. *Psychol Med* 1998;28:265–273.
69. Labbate LA, Fava M, Oleshansky M, et al. Physical fitness and perceived stress. Relationships with coronary artery disease risk factors. *Psychosomatics* 1995;36:555–560.
70. Diamond P, Brisson GR, Candas B, Peronnet F. Trait anxiety, submaximal physical exercise and blood androgens. *Eur J Appl Physiol* 1989;58:699–704.
71. Fava M, Littman A, Lamon-Fava S, et al. Psychological, behavioral and biochemical risk factors for coronary artery disease among American and Italian male corporate managers. *Am J Cardiol* 1992; 70:1412–1416.
72. Fava M, Littman A, Halperin P. Neuroendocrine correlates of the type A behavior pattern: a review and new hypothesis. *Int J Psychiatry Med* 1987;17:289–307.
73. Littman AB, Fava M, Halperin P, et al. Psychologic benefits of a stress reduction program for healthy middle-aged army officers. *J Psychosom Res* 1993;37:345–354.
74. Schneider RH, Mills PJ, Schramm W, et al. Dehydroepiandrosterone sulfate (DHEAS) levels in type A behavior and the transcendental meditation program. *Psychosom Med* 1989;51:256.
75. van Goozen SH, Wiegant VM, Endert E, et al. Psychoendocrinological assessment of the menstrual cycle: the relationship between hormones, sexuality, and mood. *Arch Sexual Behav* 1997;26:359–382.
76. Persky H, Dreisbach L, Miller WR, et al. The relation of plasma androgen levels to sexual behaviors and attitudes of women. *Psychosom Med* 1982;44:305–319.

77. Hermida RC, Halberg F, del Pozo F. Chronobiologic pattern discrimination of plasma hormones, notably DHEA-S and TSH, classifies an expansive personality. *Chronobiologia* 1985;12:105–136.
78. Klinteberg B, Hallman J, Oreland L, et al. Exploring the connections between platelet monoamine oxidase activity and behavior. II. Impulsive personality without neuropsychological signs of disinhibition in air force pilot recruits. *Neuropsychobiology* 1992;26:136–145.
79. Buckwalter JG, Stanczyc FZ, McCleary CA, et al. Pregnancy, the postpartum, and steroid hormones: effects on cognition and mood. *Psychoneuroendocrinology* 1999;24:69–84.
80. Tollefson GD, Haus E, Garvey MJ, et al. 24 hour urinary dehydroepiandrosterone sulfate in unipolar depression treated with cognitive and/or pharmacotherapy. *Ann Clin Psychiatry* 1990;2:39–45.
81. Hansen CR Jr, Kroll J, Mackenzie TB. Dehydroepiandrosterone and affective disorders [letter]. *Am J Psychiatry* 1982;139:386–387.
82. Heuser I, Deuschle M, Luppa P, et al. Increased diurnal plasma concentrations of dehydroepiandrosterone in depressed patients. *J Clin Endocrinol Metab* 1998;83:3130–3133.
83. Takebayashi M, Kagaya A, Uchitomi Y, et al. Plasma dehydroepiandrosterone sulfate in unipolar major depression. Short communication. *J Neural Transm* 1998;105:537–542.
84. Ferguson HC, Bartram ACG, Fowlie HC, et al. A preliminary investigation of steroid excretion in depressed patients before and after electroconvulsive therapy. *Acta Endocrinol* 1964;47:58–66.
85. Shulman LH, DeRogatis L, Spielvogel R, et al. Serum androgens and depression in women with facial hirsutism. *J Am Acad Dermatol* 1992;27:178–181.
86. Herbert J, Goodyer IM, Altham PME, et al. Adrenal secretion and major depression in 8- to 16-year-olds, II. Influence of co-morbidity at presentation. *Psychol Med* 1996;26:257–263.
87. Winterer J, Gwirtsman HE, George DT, et al. Adrenocorticotropin-stimulated adrenal androgen secretion in anorexia nervosa: impaired secretion at low weight with normalization after long-term weight recovery. *J Clin Endocrinol Metab* 1985;61:693–697.
88. Gordon CM, Grace E, Jean Emans S, et al. Changes in bone turnover markers and menstrual function after short-term oral DHEA in young women with anorexia nervosa. *J Bone Miner Res* 1999;14:136–145.
89. Zumoff B, Walsh BT, Katz JL, et al. Subnormal plasma dehydroepiandrosterone to cortisol ratio in anorexia nervosa: a second hormonal parameter of ontogenic regression. *J Clin Endocrinol Metab* 1983;56:668–672.
90. Salahuddin F, Svec F, Dinan TG. Low DHEA and DHEA-S levels in patients with chronic fatigue syndrome. *J Invest Med* 1997;45:56A.
91. Kuratsune H, Yamaguti K, Sawada M, et al. Dehydroepiandrosterone sulfate deficiency in chronic fatigue syndrome. *Int J Mol Med* 1998;1:143–146.
92. Calabrese VP, Isaacs ER, Regelson W. Dehydroepiandosterone in multiple sclerosis: positive effects on the fatigue syndrome in a non-randomized study. In: Kalimi M, Regelson W, eds. *The biologic role of dehydroepiandrosterone (DHEA)*. Berlin: de Gruyter, 1990:95–100.
93. Kodama M, Kodama T, Murakami M. The value of the dehydroepiandrosterone-annexed vitamin C infusion treatment in the clinical control of chronic fatigue syndrome (CFS). II. Characterization of CFS patients with special reference to their response to a new vitamin C infusion treatment. *In Vivo* 1996;10:585–596.
94. Kodama M, Kodama T, Murakami M. The value of the dehydroepiandrosterone-annexed vitamin C infusion treatment in the clinical control of chronic fatigue syndrome (CFS). I. A Pilot study of the new vitamin C infusion treatment with a volunteer CFS patient. *In Vivo* 1996;10:575–584.
95. Berkman LF, Seeman TE, Albert M, et al. High, usual and impaired functioning in community-dwelling older men and women: findings from the MacArthur foundation research network on successful aging. *J Clin Epidemiol* 1993;46:1129–1140.
96. Abbasi A, Duthie EH Jr, Sheldahl L, et al. Association of dehydroepiandrosterone sulfate, body composition, and physical fitness in independent community-dwelling older men and women [see comments]. *J Am Geriatr Soc* 1998;46:263–273.
97. Morrison MF, Katz IR, Parmelee P, et al. Dehydroepiandrosterone sulfate (DHEA-S) and psychiatric and laboratory measures of frailty in a residential care population. *Am J Geriatr Psychiatry* 1998;6: 277–284.
98. Cawood EH, Bancroft J. Steroid hormones, the menopause, sexuality and well-being of women. *Psychol Med* 1996;26:925–936.
99. Rudman D, Shetty KR, Mattson DE. Plasma dehydroepiandrosterone sulfate in nursing home men. *J Am Geriatr Soc* 1990;38:421–427.
100. Ravaglia G, Forti P, Maioli F, et al. Determinants of functional status in healthy Italian nonagenari-

ans and centenarians: a comprehensive functional assessment by the instruments of geriatric practice. *J Am Geriatr Soc* 1997;45:1196–1202.

101. Ravaglia G, Forti P, Maioli F, et al. The relationship of dehydroepiandrosterone sulfate (DHEAS) to endocrine-metabolic parameters and functional status in the oldest-old. Results from an Italian study on healthy free-living over-ninety-year-olds. *J Clin Endocrinol Metab* 1996;81:1173–1178.

102. Kalmijn S, Launer LJ, Stolk RP, et al. A prospective study on cortisol, dehydroepiandrosterone sulfate, and cognitive function in the elderly. *J Clin Endocrinol Metab* 1998;83:3487–3492.

103. Miller TP, Taylor J, Rogerson S, et al. Cognitive and noncognitive symptoms in dementia patients: relationship to cortisol and dehydroepiandrosterone. *Int Psychogeriatr* 1998;10:85–96.

104. Sunderland T, Merril CR, Harrington M, et al. Reduced plasma dehydroepiandrosterone concentrations in Alzheimer's disease. *Lancet* 1989;2:570.

105. Nasman B, Olsson T, Beckstrom T, et al. Serum dehydroepiandrosterone sulfate in Alzheimer's disease and in multi-infarct dementia. *Biol Psychiatry* 1991;30:684–690.

106. Yanase T, Fukahori M, Taniguchi S, et al. Serum dehydroepiandrosterone (DHEA) and DHEA-sulfate (DHEA-S) in Alzheimer's disease and in cerebrovascular dementia. *Endocrine J* 1996;43:119–123.

107. Solerte SB, Fioravanti M, Schifino N, et al. Dehydroepiandrosterone sulfate decreases the interleukin-2-mediated overactivity of the natural killer cell compartment in senile dementia of the Alzheimer type. *Dement Geriatr Cogn Disord* 1999;10:21–27.

108. Cuckle H, Stone R, Smith D, et al. Dehydroepiandrosterone sulphate in Alzheimer's disease. *Lancet* 1990;2:449–450.

109. Spath-Schwalbe E, Dodt C, Dittmann J, et al. Dehydroepiandrosterone sulfate in Alzheimer's disease. *Lancet* 1990;335:1412.

110. Schneider LS, Hinsey M, Lyness S. Plasma dehydroepiandrosterone sulfate in Alzheimer's disease. *Biol Psychiatry* 1992;31:205–208.

111. Birkenhager-Gillesse EG, Derksen J, Lagaay AM. Dehydroepiandrosterone sulphate (DHEAS) in the oldest old, aged 85 and over. *Ann N Y Acad Sci* 1994;719:543–552.

112. Barrett-Connor E, Edelstein SL. A prospective study of dehydroepiandrosterone sulfate and cognitive function in an older population: the Rancho Bernardo Study. *J Am Geriatr Soc* 1994;42:420–423.

113. Lynda Lee YS, Kohlmeier L, van Vollenhoven RF, et al. The effcts of dehydroepiandrosterone (DHEA) on bone metabolism in healthy post-menopausal women. *Arthritis Rheum* 1994;37:S182.

114. Kroboth PD, Salek FS, Stone RA, et al. Alprazolam increases dehydroepiandrosterone concentrations. *J Clin Psychopharmacol* 1999;19:114–124.

115. Sands D. Further studies on endocrine treatment in adolescence and early adult life. *J Ment Sci* 1954;100:211–219.

116. Serra C. *Minerva Med* 1953;44:1731.

117. Zubiani A, Laricchia R. *Minerva Med* 1953;44:344–000.

118. Pelliccioni E, Nonis E, Ronchini P, et al. Impiego del deidroandrosterone nelle forme neuroasteniche e depressive in geriatria. *G Gerontol* 1981;29:602–603.

119. Scali G, Nonis E, Petronio G, Casa B. Impiego del dinistile e dell'astenile nelle forme neurastheiche e depressive in geriatria. *G Ital Richerche Clin Ter* 1980;85:85–87.

120. Recordati Industria Chimica e Farmaceutica SpA: Astenile. Milan, Italy, Recordati Industria Chimica e Farmaceutica S.p.A., 1995.

121. Forrest AD, Drewery J, Fotherby K, Laverty SG. A clinical trial of dehydroepiandrosterone (Diandrone). *J Neurol Neurosurg Psychiatry* 1960;23:52–55.

122. Roberts E, Fauble T. Oral dehydroepiandrosterone in multiple sclerosis. Results of a phase one, open study. In: Kalimi M, Regelson W, eds. *The biologic role of dehydroepiandrosterone (DHEA)*. Berlin: de Gruyter, 1990:81–94.

123. van Vollenhoven RF, Engleman EG, McGuire J. An open study of dehydroepiandrosterone in systemic lupus erythematosus. *Arthritis Rheum* 1994;37:1305–1310.

124. Diamond P, Cusan L, Gomez JL, et al. Metabolic effects of 12-month percutaneous dehydroepiandrosterone replacement therapy in postmenopausal women. *J Endocrinol* 1996;150:S43–S50.

125. Labrie F, Diamond P, Cusan L, et al. Effect of 12-month dehydroepiandrosterone replacement therapy on bone, vagina, and endometrium in postmenopausal women. *J Clin Endocrinol Metab* 1997; 82:3498–3505.

126. Vogiatzi MG, Boeck MA, Vlachopapadopoulou E, et al. Dehydroepiandrosterone in morbidly obese adolescents: effects on weight, body composition, lipids, and insulin resistance. *Metabolism* 1996; 45:1011–1015.

127. Wolf OT, Neumann O, Hellhammer DH, et al. Effects of a two-week physiological dehydroepiandro-sterone substitution on cognitive performance and well-being in healthy elderly women and men. *J Clin Endocrinol Metab* 1997;82:2363–2367.
128. Kudielka BM, Hellhammer J, Hellhammer DH, et al. Sex differences in endocrine and psychologi-cal responses to psychosocial stress in healthy elderly subjects and the impact of a 2-week dehy-droepiandrosterone treatment. *J Clin Endocrinol Metab* 1998;83:1756–1761.
129. Polleri A, Gianelli MV, Murialdo G. Dehydroepiandrosterone: dream or nightmare? *J Endocrinol Invest* 1998;21:544.
130. Wolkowitz OM, Reus VI, Roberts E, et al. Dehydroepiandrosterone (DHEA) treatment of depres-sion. *Biol Psychiatry* 1997;41:311–318.
131. Wolkowitz OM, Reus VI, Keebler A, et al. Double-blind treatment of major depression with dehy-droepiandrosterone (DHEA). *Am J Psychiatry* 1999;156:646–649.
132. Bloch M, Schmidt PJ, Danaceau MA, et al. Dehydroepiandrosterone treatment of mid-life dys-thymia. *Biol Psychiatry* 1999;45:1533–1541.
133. Johnson-Sabine EC, Wood KH, Wakeling A. Mood changes in bulimia nervosa. *Br J Psychiatry* 1984;145:512–516.
134. Kennedy SH, McVey G, Katz R. Personality disorders in anorexia nervosa and bulimia nervosa. *J Psychiatr Res* 1990;24:259–269.
135. Bonnet KA, Brown RP. Cognitive effects of DHEA replacement therapy. In: Kalimi M, Regelson W, eds. *The biologic role of dehydroepiandrosterone (DHEA)*. New York: de Gruyter, 1990:65–79.
136. Wolf OT, Koster B, Kirschbaum C, et al. A single administration of dehydroepiandrosterone does not enhance memory performance in young healthy adults, but immediately reduces cortisol levels. *Biol Psychiatry* 1997;42:845–848.
137. Wolf OT, Naumann E, Hellhammer DH, Kirschbaum C. Effects of dehydroepiandrosterone replace-ment in elderly men on event-related potentials, memory, and well-being. *J Gerontol Med Sci* 1998;53A:M385–M390.
138. Wolf OT, Kudielka BM, Hellhammer DH, et al. Opposing effects of DHEA replacement in elderly subjects on declarative memory and attention after exposure to a laboratory stressor. *Psychoneuroendocrinology* 1998;23:617–629.
139. Dukoff R, Molchan S, Putnam K, Lai J, Sunderland T. Dehydroepiandrosterone administration in demented patients and non-demented elderly volunteers (abstract). *Biol Psychiatry* 1998;43:55S.
140. Wolkowitz OM, Kramer JH, Reus VI, et al. Dehydroepiandrosterone (NPI-34133) treatment of Alzheimer's disease: a randomized, double-blind, placebo-controlled, parallel group study. *In review* (*Neurology*).
141. van Vollenhoven RF, Morabito LM, Engleman EG, McGuire JL. Treatment of systemic lupus erythema-tosus with dehydroepiandrosterone: 50 patients treated up to 12 months. *J Rheumatol* 1998;25:285–289.
142. Rupprecht R. The neuropsychopharmacological potential of neuroactive steroids. *J Psychiatr Res* 1997;31:297–314.
143. Bruder JM, Sobek L, Oettel M. Dehydroepiandrosterone stimulates the estrogen response element. *J Steroid Biochem Mol Biol* 1997;62:461–466.
144. Nephew KP, Sheeler CQ, Dudley MD, et al. Studies of dehydroepiandrosterone (DHEA) with the human estrogen receptor in yeast. *Mol Cell Endocrinol* 1998;143:133–142.
145. Spivak CE. Desensitization and noncompetitive blockade of GABAA receptors in ventral midbrain neurons by a neurosteroid dehydroepiandrosterone sulfate. *Synapse* 1994;16:113–122.
146. Steffensen SC. Dehydroepiandrosterone sulfate suppresses hippocampal recurrent inhibition and synchronizes neuronal activity to theta rhythm. *Hippocampus* 1995;5:320–328.
147. Friess E, Trachsel L, Guldner J, et al. DHEA administration increases rapid eye movement sleep and EEG power in the sigma frequency range. *Am J Physiol* 1995;268:E107–E113.
148. Yoo A, Harris J, Dubrovsky B. Dose-response study of dehydroepiandrosterone sulfate on dentate gyrus long-term potentiation. *Exp Neurol* 1996;137:151–156.
149. Monnet FP, Mahe V, Robel P, Baulieu EE. Neurosteroids, via sigma receptors, modulate the [3H] norepinephrine release evoked by N-methyl-D-aspartate in the rat hippocampus. *Proc Natl Acad Sci U S A* 1995;92:3774–3778.
150. Bergeron R, de Montigny C, Debonnel G. Potentiation of neuronal NMDA response induced by dehydroepiandrosterone and its suppression by progesterone: effects mediated via sigma receptors. *J Neurosci* 1996;16:1193–1202.
151. Urani A, Privat A, Maurice T. The modulation by neurosteroids of the scopolamine-induced learn-

ing impairment in mice involves an interaction with sigma1 (sigma1) receptors. *Brain Res* 1998; 799:64–77.

152. Diamond DM, Branch BJ, Fleshner M, Rose GM. Effects of dehydroepiandrosterone sulfate and stress on hippocampal electrophysiological plasticity. *Ann N Y Acad Sci* 1995;774:304–307.

153. Carette B, Poulain P. Excitatory effect of dehydroepiandrosterone, its sulphate ester and pregnenolone sulphate, applied by iontophoresis and pressure, on single neurones in the septo-preoptic area of the guinea pig. *Neurosci Lett* 1984;45:205–210.

154. Meyer JH, Gruol DL. Dehydroepiandrosterone sulfate alters synaptic potentials in area CA1 of the hippocampal slice. *Brain Res* 1994;633:253–261.

155. Rhodes ME, Li PK, Flood JF, Johnson DA. Enhancement of hippocampal acetylcholine release by the neurosteroid dehydroepiandrosterone sulfate: an in vivo microdialysis study. *Brain Res* 1996; 733:284–286.

156. Rhodes ME, Li PK, Burke AM, Johnson DA. Enhanced plasma DHEAS, brain acetylcholine and memory mediated by steroid sulfatase inhibition. *Brain Res* 1997;773:28–32.

157. Murray HE, Gillies GE. Differential effects of neuroactive steroids on somatostatin and dopamine secretion from primary hypothalamic cell cultures. *J Neuroendocrinol* 1997;9:287–295.

158. Holsboer F, Grasser A, Friess E, Wiedemann K. Steroid effects on central neurons and implications for psychiatric and neurological disorders. *Ann N Y Acad Sci* 1994;746:345–361.

159. Svec F, Lopez A. Antiglucocorticoid actions of dehydroepiandrosterone and low concentrations in Alzheimer's disease [letter]. *Lancet* 1989;2:1335–1336.

160. Riley V, Fitzmaurice MA, Regelson W. DHEA and thymus integrity in the mouse. In: Kalimi M, Regelson W, eds. *The biologic role of dehydroepiandrosterone (DHEA).* Berlin: de Gruyter, 1990; 131–155.

161. Blauer KL, Poth M, Rogers WM, Bernton EW. Dehydroepiandrosterone antagonizes the suppressive effects of dexamethasone on lymphocyte proliferation. *Endocrinology* 1991;129:3174–-3179.

162. Ben-Nathan D, Feuerstein G. The influence of cold or isolation stress on resistance of mice to West Nile virus encephalitis. *Experientia* 1990;46:285–290.

163. Browne ES, Wright BE, Porter JR, Svec F. Dehydroepiandrosterone: antiglucocorticoid action in mice. *Am J Med Sci* 1992;303:366–371.

164. Fleshner M, Pugh CR, Tremblay D, Rudy JW. DHEA-S selectively impairs contextual-fear conditioning: support for the antiglucocorticoid hypothesis. *Behav Neurosci* 1997;111:512–517.

165. Attal-Khemis S, Dalmeyda V, Morfin R. Change of 7 alpha-hydroxy-dehydroepiandrosterone levels in serum of mice treated by cytochrome P450-modifying agents. *Life Sci* 1998;63:1543–1553.

166. Loria RM. Antiglucocorticoid function of androstenetriol. *Psychoneuroendocrinology* 1997;22: S103–S108.

167. Morfin R, Chmielewski V. Antiglucocorticoid and immune-promoting effect of 7-alpha-hydroxylated steroids. In: *2nd international conference on cortisol and anti-cortisols.* Las Vegas, NV, 1997:38.

168. Padgett DA, Loria RM, Sheridan JF. Androstenediol, a metabolite of dehydroepiandrosterone, counter-regulates the influence of corticosterone on immune function. In: *2nd international conference on cortisol and anti-cortisols.* Las Vegas, NV, 1997:44.

169. Reus VI, Wolkowitz OM, Frederick S. Antiglucocorticoid treatments in psychiatry. 1997;22: S121–S124.

170. Murphy BEP, Wolkowitz OM. The pathophysiologic significance of hyperadrenocorticism: antiglucocorticoid strategies. *Psychiatr Ann* 1993;23:682–690.

171. Sapolsky RM. The neuroendocrinology of stress and aging: the glucocorticoid cascade hypothesis. *Endocr Rev* 1986;7:284–301.

172. Griffin WS, Stanley LC, Ling C, et al. Brain interleukin 1 and S-100 immunoreactivity are elevated in Down syndrome and Alzheimer disease. *Proc Natl Acad Sci U S A* 1989;86:7611–7615.

173. Danenberg HD, Alpen G, Lustig S, Ben-Nathan D. Dehydroepiandrosterone protects mice from endotoxin toxicity and reduces tumor necrosis factor production. *Antimicrob Agents Chemother* 1992;36:2275–2279.

174. Daynes RA, Araneo BA, Ershler WB, et al. Altered regulation of IL-6 production with normal aging. *J Immunol* 1993;150:5219–5230.

175. Straub RH, Konecna L, Hrach S, et al. Serum dehydroepiandrosterone (DHEA) and DHEA sulfate are negatively correlated with serum interleukin-6 (IL-6), and DHEA inhibits IL-6 secretion from mononuclear cells in man in vitro: possible link between endocrinosenescence and immunosenescence. *J Clin Endocrinol Metab* 1998;83:2012–2017.

176. Tamagno E, Aragno M, Boccuzzi G, et al. Oxygen free radical scavenger properties of dehydroepiandrosterone. *Cell Biochem Funct* 1998;16:57–63.
177. Aragno M, Brignardello E, Tamagno E, et al. Dehydroepiandrosterone administration prevents the oxidative damage induced by acute hyperglycemia in rats. *J Endocrinol* 1997;155:233–240.
178. Khalil A, Lehoux JG, Wagner RJ, et al. Dehydroepiandrosterone protects low density lipoproteins against peroxidation by free radicals produced by gamma-radiolysis of ethanol-water mixtures. *Atherosclerosis* 1998;136:99–107.
179. Hashimoto S, Migita S. Serum amyloid P component regulation by sex steroids in rats. *Nippon Ketsueki Gakkai Zasshi* 1990;53:89–97.
180. Danenberg HD, Haring R, Heldman E, et al. Dehydroepiandrosterone augments M1-muscarinic receptor-stimulated amyloid precursor protein secretion in desensitized PC12M1 cells. *Ann NY Acad Sci* 1995;774:300–303.
181. Danenberg HD, Haring R, Fisher A, Pittel Z, Gurwitz D, Heldman E. Dehydroepiandrosterone (DHEA) increases production and release of Alzheimer's amyloid precursor protein. *Life Sci* 1996; 59:1651–1657.
182. Goldberg M. Dehydroepiandrosterone, insulin-like growth factor-I, and prostate cancer [letter]. *Ann Intern Med* 1998;129:587–588.
183. Markowitz JS, Carson WH, Jackson CW. Possible dehydroepiandrosterone-induced mania. *Biol Psychiatry* 1999;45:241–242.
184. Howard JS III. Severe psychosis and the adrenal androgens. *Integr Physiol Behav Sci* 1992;27: 209–215.
185. Schwartz AG, Pashko L, Whitcomb JM. Inhibition of tumor development by dehydroepiandrosterone and related steroids. *Toxicol Pathol* 1986;14:357–362.
186. Comstock GW, Gordon GB, Hsing AW. The relationship of serum dehydroepiandrostreone and its sulfate to subsequent cancer of the prostate. *Cancer Epidemiol Biomarkers Prev* 1993;2:219–221.
187. Dorgan JF, Stanczyk FZ, Longcope C, et al. Relationship of serum dehydroepiandrosterone (DHEA), DHEA sulfate, and 5-androstene-3 beta, 17 beta-diol to risk of breast cancer in postmenopausal women. *Cancer Epidemiol Biomarkers Prevent* 1997;6:177–181.
188. Jones JA, Nguyen A, Straub M, et al. Use of DHEA in a patient with advanced prostate cancer: a case report and review. *Urology* 1997;50:784–788.
189. McNeil C. Potential drug DHEA hits snags on way to clinic [news]. *J Natl Cancer Inst* 1997;89: 681–683.
190. Barry NN, McGuire JL, Watts J, et al. Treatment of systemic lupus erythematosus with dehydroepiandrosterone (DHEA): optimum of clinical responses at DHEA-sulfate serum level of 1,700-2,000 µg/ml [abstract]. *Arthritis Rheum* 1995;38:S302.
191. Parasrampuria J, Schwartz K, Petesch R. Quality control of dehydroepiandrosterone dietary supplement products. *JAMA* 1998;280:1565.

6

Phenylethylamine Deficit and Replacement in Depressive Illness

Hector Sabelli

INTRODUCTION

Phenylethylamine as the Chemical Messenger for Psychological Energy

Thyroid hormones sustain bodily energy; their deficit produces a characteristic syndrome that includes depression in the adult and mental retardation in the child. Similarly, the brain neurohormone 2-phenylethylamine (PEA) sustains psychological energy, and its deficit produces depression. This is the PEA hypothesis of depression as originally proposed by my mentor, pharmacologist and psychiatrist Dr. Edmund Fischer (1,2), to whom I dedicate this chapter.

This PEA hypothesis (1–6) has led to the development of a physiologic approach to the diagnosis and treatment of depressive illnesses. Physiologic diagnosis means the demonstration of metabolic abnormalities, such as the deficit of a mood-elevating neurohormone, by objective biochemical tests. Physiologic treatment implies the replacement of the neurohormone demonstrated to be in deficit. However, physiology should not be reduced to biology. Physiology, signifying the study of nature, is an integral science of both physical and psychological processes. Biologic treatments complement, but do not replace, family and individual psychotherapy.

PEA is the only endogenous amine that produces behavioral effects when systemically administered. Its amphetamine-like effects include sympathomimetic effects, increases in nonspecific motor activity, increases in specific exploratory behavior (Fig. 6.1), stereotypic behaviors, electrophysiologic alerting, reinforcement of complex sequences behavior, and anorectic effects (6,7). Because of its high sensitivity to monoamine oxidase (MAO), PEA induces pharmacologic effects only at high doses or following pretreatment with MAO inhibitors (MAOI).

PEA meets all the criteria required to demonstrate that it is a chemical mediator sustaining energy and mood as follows:

1. PEA is present in brain tissue and is distributed nonuniformly.
2. PEA is produced and metabolized by brain tissue.
3. PEA is pharmacologically active, and it produces behavioral stimulation when administered.

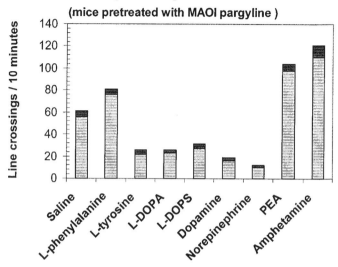

FIG. 6.1. Amphetamine-like stimulant effect of phenylethylamine (PEA) and its precursor L-phenyl-alanine, in contrast to the sedative effect of catecholamines and their amino acid precursors. Abbreviations: DOPA, 3,4-dihydroxyphenylalanine; MAOI, monoamine oxidase inhibitor.

4. Drugs that increase or reduce PEA turnover produce behavioral changes in the expected direction.
5. PEA's main metabolite, phenylacetic acid (PAA), is reduced in the biologic tissues and/or fluids of depressed subjects, indicating a decrease in PEA turnover.
6. PEA replacement relieves depression in a significant number of subjects.

The PEA hypothesis originates with the observation that amphetamine increases energy and mood in normal subjects and in a large subgroup of depressed patients. Amphetamine is a phenylethylamine with a methyl group in the alpha carbon that renders it insensitive to MAO (Fig. 6.2). These stimulant effects have been attributed to catecholamine release, and they are, in fact, the origin of the catecholamine-deficit hypothesis of depression. However, neither catecholamines nor their precursors tyrosine, 3,4-dihydroxyphenylalanine (DOPA), and DOPS, produce the behavioral stimulant effects of amphetamine—instead, they depress motor activity and exploratory behavior (1) (Fig. 6.1). The behavioral depressant effects of administered catecholamines have been attributed to their peripheral effects, because these amines do not readily cross the blood-brain barrier. However, the catecholamine precursors DOPA and DOPS produce central depressant effects. Dopamine, norepinephrine, and their amino acid precursors DOPA and DOPS induce sleep in newly hatched chicks, which lack a blood-brain barrier (Table 6.1). DOPA does not relieve depression; in fact, some patients with Parkinson disease become more depressed when they receive

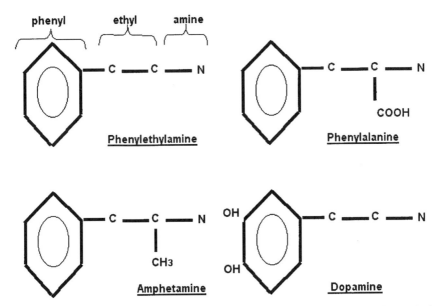

FIG. 6.2. Chemical structure of 2-phenylethylamine, its precursor L-phenylalanine, its synthetic analog amphetamine, and the related synaptic transmitter dopamine.

DOPA, despite the obvious neurologic improvement. These discrepancies between experimental data and the purported stimulant role of brain catecholamines suggested to the authors that a different endogenous amphetamine-like substance probably mediated the energizing and mood-elevating functions attributed to brain catecholamines (1). Fischer suggested PEA because (a) the

TABLE 6.1. *Phenylethylamine promotes alertness, and catecholamines induce sleep in animals without a blood-brain barrier*

Treatment	Sleep	Excitement
None (saline)	0	0
Amphetamine	0	100
L-phenylalanine (PEA precursor)	0	20
PEA	0	100
Tyrosine (tyramine precursor)	70	0
Tyramine	85	0
DOPA (dopamine precursor)	100	0
Dopamine	100	0
DOPS (norepinephrine precursor)	100	0
Norepinephrine	100	0
Epinephrine	100	0

Percentage of newly hatched chicks asleep or excited within 5 to 15 minutes after treatment.

Abbreviations: DOPA, 3,4-dihydroxyphenylalanine; PEA, phenyl-ethylamine.

administration of PEA induces amphetamine-like effects (Fig. 6.1); (b) amphetamine is chemically and pharmacologically more similar to PEA than to the catecholamines (Fig. 6.2); (c) PEA could be readily formed from phenylalanine; and (d) PEA had been found in the brain of mice treated with a MAOI (8).

Phenylethylamine Synthesis and Metabolism

The author's research group identified endogenous PEA in the human brain and biologic fluids (9–11), as well as in animal brain and peripheral tissues (12). PEA is selectively found in specific areas of the rat brain (13–15).

Endogenous PEA originates from the decarboxylation of the essential amino acid L-phenylalanine, a reaction catalyzed by L-aromatic amino acid decarboxylase (L-AAAD) (Fig. 6.3 (16). PEA can thus be formed in all tissues capable of taking up L-phenylalanine and containing L-AAAD, such as catecholaminergic neurons. L-phenylalanine is a poorer substrate for L-AAAD than DOPA, but its tissue levels are much higher. Similarly, PEA turnover rate is extremely fast (half-life of 5 to 10 minutes, as contrasted to the much slower catecholamine turnover [2 to 14 hours]) (17). These fast dynamics suggest that PEA plays a major role in brain function. PEA is metabolized by all MAOs, and it is the natural substrate for MAO type B (18,19). This metabolic pathway terminates in PAA (20,21). MAO-A and MAO-B are key isoenzymes. MAO-A preferentially oxidizes serotonin and norepinephrine, whereas MAO-B preferentially oxidizes PEA. Both forms can oxidize dopamine, but, after genetic deletion of MAO-B, only PEA is increased in the brain (22). Thus, PEA probably is the physiologic substrate for MAO-B. Given the rapid turnover, the levels of PEA in tissues are low (less than 10 ng per g of brain tissue compared to other biogenic amines, which range from 100 to 5,000 ng per g). Correspondingly, PEA levels in biologic fluids are low and variable, and hence they are a poor indication of PEA metabolism. PAA levels presumably are a better indication of PEA turnover (see later).

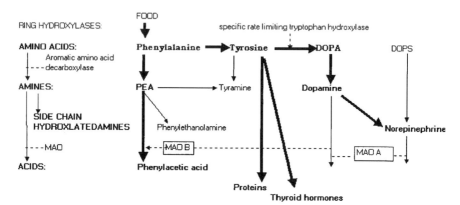

FIG. 6.3. Phenylethylamine (PEA) synthesis and metabolism. Abbreviations: DOPA, 3,4-dihydroxyphenylalanine; MAO, monoamine oxidase.

Approximately 10% of brain PEA is metabolized to phenylethanolamine (23) by dopamine β-hydroxylase. Phenylethanolamine is present in the human (9) and animal (24) brain, and it may function as a cotransmitter in norepinephrine synapses. Experiments with enzyme inhibitors indicate that the stimulant, electrophysiologic, and neurologic effects of PEA are not mediated by phenylethanolamine (25).

PHENYLETHYLAMINE AS A NEUROMODULATOR OF CATECHOLAMINE SYNAPSES

PEA is formed in catecholamine neurons. The administration of PEA releases dopamine and norepinephrine, but it also produce effects opposite to those of catecholamines. Notably, PEA and its precursor phenylalanine antagonize the sedative effects of catecholamines and of their precursor DOPA on exploratory behavior; in turn, catecholamines and DOPA reduce the stimulant effect of PEA (Tables 6.1 and 6.2).

The autonomic effects of PEA and amphetamines are largely mediated by catecholamine release from sympathetic nerve endings. In the central nervous system, PEA effects may be mediated in part by specific PEA receptors (4) and in part by the release of catecholamines and serotonin (6,7,26,27). At low doses, PEA does not release brain catecholamines (28). In the author's view, the behavioral stimulant effects of PEA are not mediated by catecholamines. Thus, the following are true: (a) the administration of either PEA or amphetamine as alerting stimuli reduces the amplitude of the visual-evoked potentials, whereas the catecholamine precursor DOPA increases their amplitude (Table 6.3); (b) the central stimulant effects of PEA and amphetamines are not prevented by either catecholamine depletion by reserpine (Table 6.4) or by blockade of the amine pump (norepinephrine reuptake) in catecholaminergic neurons by imipramine (In contrast, reserpine, as well as imipramine, prevents the peripheral sympathomimetic effects of PEA, as well as those of amphetamine [6].); and (c) using multiple-

TABLE 6.2. *Phenylethylamine and catecholamine antagonism on exploratory behavior*

| | Motor activity (6 mice per group) | | | |
	None	PEA (2.5 mg/kg)	PEA (5 mg/kg)	Phenylalanine (25 mg/kg)
None	48 ± 4	87 ± 13*	95 ± 20*	93 ± 14*
Adrenaline (1 mg/kg)	17 ± 4*	56 ± 8	98 ± 8*	39 ± 8
DOPA (100 mg/kg)	12 ± 2*	37 ± 12	84 ± 12*	31 ± 7

Method: Quantification of locomotor activity of a mouse placed alone on a novel environment using an actophotometer; all mice pretreated 1 day earlier with the monoamine oxidase inhibitor iproniazid (200 mg/kg).
*$P < 0.05$.
Abbreviation: PEA, phenylethylamine.
From Fischer E, Ludmer RI, Sabelli HC. The antagonism of phenylethylamine to catecholamines on mouse motor actvity. *Acta Fisiol Latino Am* 1967;17:15–21, with permission.

TABLE 6.3. *Opposite effects of PEA and catecholamines on visual-evoked cortical responses*

Pretreatment	Treatment	Effect on main slow negative response
Saline	Alerting stimuli (air puff)	Decrease
	Amphetamine, 1 to 10 mg/kg	Decrease
Nialamide	Alerting stimuli (air puff)	Decrease
(100 mg/kg	PEA, 1 to 10 mg/kg	Decrease
for 2 days)	Phenylalanine, 25 to 200 mg/kg	Decrease
	DOPA, 25 to 200 mg/kg	Increase

Method: Recording of averaged cortical potentials evoked by stimulated repetitive flashes from the visual cortex of the rabbit; animals pretreated with the monoamine oxidase inhibitor nialamide.
Abbreviation: PEA, phenylethylamine.
(Data from Sabelli HC, Giardina WJ, Mosnaim AD, Sabelli NH. A comparison of the functional roles of norepinephrine, dopamine and phenylethylamine in the central nervous system. *Acta Physiol Pol* 1973;24:33–40, with permission.)

TABLE 6.4. *Catecholamine depletion by reserpine prevents the cardiovascular effects of PEA but not its central nervous system effects*

A: Behavior of groups of mice, and recording of their tonic seizure response to maximal electroshock; animals pretreated 1 day earlier with the monoamine oxidase inhibitor pargyline (100 mg/kg)

Pretreatment	Treatment	Behavior	Percentage of tonic seizures after maximal electroshock
Saline	Saline	Normal	100
Saline	PEA, 50 mg/kg	Excitement	10
Reserpine, 10 mg/kg	Saline	Markedly sedated	100
Reserpine, 10 mg/kg	PEA, 50 mg/kg	Mildly sedated	25

B: Recording of blood pressure, electroencephalogram, and visual-evoked responses in rabbits pretreated 1 day earlier with the monoamine oxidase inhibitor pargyline (100 mg/kg for 2 days)

Pretreatment	Treatment	Electroencephalographic activation (sec)	Visual-evoked response	Blood pressure increase
Saline	Saline	<10	Unchanged	0
Saline	PEA, 2.5 mg/kg	350–500	Reduced	105–200 mm Hg
Reserpine, 10 mg/kg	Saline	<10	Unchanged	0
Reserpine, 10 mg/kg	PEA, 2.5 mg/kg	300–450	Reduced	0

Abbreviation: PEA, phenylethylamine.

TABLE 6.5. *PEA and dopamine exert different effects on cortical neurons*

Agent	Excitation	No effect	Inhibition
PEA	50%	50%	—
Dopamine	—	20%	80%

Rate of firing of single neurons in the brain cortex of paralyzed rabbits using microelectrode recording and microiontophoretic drug administration.
Abbreviation: PEA, phenylethylamine.
(Data from Sabelli HC, Mosnaim AD, Vazquez AJ, et al. Biochemical plasticity of synaptic transmission: a critical review of Dale's principle. *Biol Psychiatry* 1976;11:481–524, with permission.)

barreled microelectrodes for iontophoretic drug administration and single-unit recording (Table 6.5), PEA, dopamine, and norepinephrine have been found to produce opposite effects upon cortical neurons of nonanesthetized rabbits (29,30), suggesting the existence of different receptors. PEA and catecholamines exert similar effects in some, but not all, brain neurons of anesthetized rats (31). PEA reduces the density of dopamine-1 (D1)-like dopamine receptors in the rat striatum and the density of β_1-adrenoceptors, but not that of β_2-adrenoceptors, in the cerebral cortex and the cerebellum (32). Obviously, the relationship between PEA and catecholamines is extremely complex (33). In addition, PEA interacts with brain serotonin (34). Glutaminergic mechanisms may also be involved in the central actions of phenylethylamines (35).

Based on these and other experiments, Sabelli et al. (3,4,36) and others (7,13,37) proposed that PEA is a modulator of catecholaminergic activities. Whereas the catecholamine transmitter acts in a phasic manner as it is released by nerve impulses, PEA would be constantly released, modulating transmission in a tonic manner. PEA may modulate catecholamine transmission also at the peripheral synapses. Jackson and Temple (38) proposed that cardiac PEA may function as a natural cardiotonic. As yet no study of PEA metabolism in patients with heart failure exists.

While PEA is formed at synaptic endings, it may also be synthesized and metabolized at other sites. PEA is formed by the gut flora; antibiotics decrease energy and reduce PAA excretion (39). Brain PEA originates in part from peripheral sources. As a highly lipid-soluble substance, PEA readily crosses the blood-brain barrier. Furthermore, an active mechanism accumulates blood-borne PEA in the brain against a concentration gradient (40). Drugs, such as carbidopa, that inhibit decarboxylase only in the peripheral tissues because they do not cross the blood-brain barrier markedly reduce the brain levels of PEA (41) and exert antipsychotic effects in some patients with atypical bipolar disorder (42, 43), lowering their mood and reducing PAA excretion (Table 6.6). MAOIs that do not cross the blood-brain barrier markedly affect the brain levels of PEA (44). These are agents that do not affect brain catecholamines. Because central and peripheral pools of PEA are in dynamic equilibrium, PEA and PAA levels in the blood and urine reflect brain PEA turnover (6).

TABLE 6.6. *Amelioration of psychosis with carbidopa (200 mg/d)*

Patient	Before treatment	Carbidopa on psychosis	Carbidopa on mood	PAA before treatment	PAA during treatment
54-year-old man, schizoaffective	Psychotic, unresponsive to neuroleptics	4-month remission	None	223	57
56-year-old man, schizoaffective	Psychotic, manic	Improvement, then relapse	Switch to depression	210	30
24-year-old man, schizoaffective	Psychotic, unresponsive to neuroleptics	Some improvement	Depressed	—	—
26-year-old man, schizoaffective	Acutely psychotic	Some improvement	Depressed	203	23
23-year-old man, schizoaffective	Acutely psychotic	None	Depressed	150	8
25-year-old man, schizoaffective	Psychotic, depressed, unresponsive to neuroleptics	Some improvement	More depressed	120	50
51-year-old man, bipolar	Psychotic and manic, unresponsive to lithium and to carbamazepine	3-weeks remission, then relapse	Switch to mixed affect	205	30
39-year-old woman, bipolar	Acutely psychotic	8-month remission	None	167	72
30-year-old woman, atypical bipolar	Anxious and depressed, with occasional psychotic symptoms	Some improvement	Remains anxious and depressed	190	73

Acutely psychotic subjects with a history of responsiveness to lithium and/or carbamazepine.
Abbreviation: PAA, phenylacetic acid.

DIAGNOSTICS

Phenylethylamine Turnover is Reduced in 60% of Depressed Patients

Fischer et al. (45,46) noted that depressed patients excrete lower levels of a PEA-like substance than normal controls and that manic patients excrete higher amounts. These studies were promptly replicated by Boulton in Canada (47) and by Mosnaim in the United States (48). However, the methods that were used were later determined to be nonspecific. When more specific methods became available, PEA was found to be excreted in very low amounts. Furthermore, the blood and urinary levels of PEA are not only low, but they are also highly variable. Almost all PEA is rapidly metabolized to PAA. Thus, measuring urinary PAA as an indicator of PEA turnover seems more useful (49–52). This has been contested, with some claiming that PAA is derived from phenylpyruvic acid because PAA urinary excretion is not reduced after the administration of either carbidopa or an MAOI (53). In actuality, carbidopa does reduce PAA urinary excretion in humans at higher doses (Table 6.6). MAOIs cannot be expected to produce measurable changes in urinary PAA even at doses that induce a hundredfold increase in PEA excretion because PEA is excreted in microgram amounts (10^{-6} g), while urinary PAA content is one million times greater (10^{-1} g) (6). Only a negligible amount of PAA can derive from phenylalanine via phenylpyruvic acid because this acid is present only in trace amounts in bodily fluids, except in phenylketonuria. In any case, PAA levels and PEA turnover are likely to vary together because both compounds are phenylalanine metabolites. Moreover, a reduction in PAA excretion in some forms of depression is meaningful regardless of its metabolic origin.

The cerebrospinal fluid (CSF) levels of PAA are lower in depressed patients (20.8±1.95 ng/mL) than in age-matched and sex-matched controls (28.7±2.91 ng/mL) (54). In patients with Parkinson disease who experience depressive symptoms, low CSF levels of PEA are found (55).

Depressed patients also have lower plasma PAA than normal controls (Table 6.7), as the author found in three different studies (56–58) and as others replicated (59). In the author's view, urinary determinations are more useful. Single CSF, blood, or urine sampling can be misleading because of marked circadian and ultradian variations. The timing of variation differs (e.g., night versus morning persons), so averaging observations from several individuals may create the false impression that no circadian rhythms exist, as has been claimed.

The daily urinary excretion of PAA is reduced in approximately 60% of acutely depressed patients (49–52), as Fig. 6.4 illustrates. Inpatients with unipolar major depressive disorder (MDD) excreted less PAA (68.7±7.0 mg per 24 hours, N=31; N, number of patients) than healthy volunteers (141.1±10.2 mg per 24 hours, N=48). The PAA excretion was reduced to a lesser extent (86.3±11.8 mg per 24 hours) in 35 less severely depressed outpatients who met the criteria for MDD. Likewise, PAA excretion was reduced in bipolar depressed inpatients (67.9±15.3 mg per 24 hours, N=8), as well as in outpatients (89.9±14.1 mg per 24 hours, N=11). These studies have been replicated in several groups. Gonzalez-Sastre et al. (60) found that urinary PAA was significantly lower in major depression. Also in agreement with this, DeLisi et al. (61) reported that PAA excretion was reduced in acutely depressed inpatients (84.5±46 mg per 24 hours, N=10) in comparison to controls (166.8±81 mg per 24 hours, N=10).

TABLE 6.7. *Plasma phenylacetic acid (ng/mL) in depression*

Healthy controls	N	Depressed patients	N	Reference*
536 ± 55 (80% above 400 ng/mL)	10	327 ± 45 (70% below 400 ng/mL)	10	56
596 ± 55	13	274 ± 38	17	57
638 ± 543	6	266 ± 218	17	58
530 ± 130		310 ± 96		59

*See chapter references for reference information.

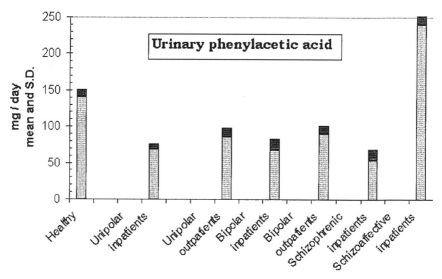

FIG. 6.4. Daily urinary excretion of phenylacetic acid in psychiatric patients. Abbreviation: S.D., standard deviation.

These same investigators (61) found no reduction in PAA in chronically depressed subjects who do not respond to tricyclic treatment; the chronic character of the depression and the lack of response to antidepressant drugs indicate that these subjects do not suffer from the same biologic illness as patients with typical MDD and that they may in fact represent a group of persons with psychologically induced depressions rather than with biologic disorders. The same consideration also applies to the group of subjects studied by Karoum et al. (53).

PAA levels are decreased only in some types of chronic depression (Table 6.8). Braun et al. (58) found that the daily urinary excretion (83±57 mg per 24 hours) and the plasma levels (266±218 ng per mL) of PAA were reduced in subjects with MDD, as well as in those with atypical depression (plasma, 104±51 ng per mL; urine, 59±37.5 mg per day) in comparison to healthy controls (plasma, 638±543 ng per mL; urine, 132±72 mg per day). In contrast, no abnormalities

TABLE 6.8. Phenylacetic acid reduction in major and atypical depression but not in dysthymic disorder

Diagnosis	N	Urine PAA (mg/d)	N	Plasma PAA (ng/mL)
Healthy	6	132 ± 72	6	638 ± 543
Major depression	20	83 ± 57	17	266 ± 218
Atypical depression	6	59 ± 37	5	104 ± 51
Dysthymic disorder	9	139 ± 42	6	638 ± 247

Abbreviations: N, number of subjects, PAA, phenylacetic acid.

were observed in patients with dysthymia (plasma, 638±247 ng per mL; urine, 139 mg±42 mg per day).

Phenylethylamine and Violence: The Levy Study

Levy's study of PAA excretion and psychologic symptoms in a prison population (62,63) is the largest study carried out in this field. It confirmed the association between PAA reduction and depression—PAA excretion was lower in 59 subjects with depressive symptoms according to the Minnesota Multiphasic Personality Inventory and Beck and Hamilton scales than in 49 subjects who were not depressed by any criterion (Table 6.9). Intermediate levels of PAA were observed in persons who showed symptoms of depression in one scale only. Analysis of variance demonstrated that this difference was significant regardless of age and history of violence.

Anger, anxiety, and depression vary largely together in both normal and depressed persons (63). This was also observed in the incarcerated population. Daily subjective reports of emotions (e.g., subjective energy, joy, anger, fear, depression, and sexual drive in a 0 to 9 scale) were obtained for 35 days or longer. In persons with low PAA excretion, reports of joy, sexual feelings, restful sleep, and positive feelings toward others were also low. The joint trajectories of anger, anxiety, and depression (Fig. 6.5) were chaotic-like, as has been previously noted in depressed outpatients (63). In contrast, in subjects with high PAA excretion, significantly higher levels of joy, sexual feelings, and positive feelings toward others were seen, with no expressions of negative feelings, except for short outbursts that were followed by a rapid return to equilibrium. One should note that this pattern that was common (67%) among violent criminals has not been observed in other individuals (63).

PAA excretion was higher for depressed and nondepressed jail inmates than for other depressed and nondepressed persons. Furthermore, persons who had committed violent crimes (e.g., homicide and other crimes of bodily injury, aggravated arson, and burglaries with a weapon) tended to excrete larger amounts of PAA than nonviolent persons, regardless of the level of depression (two-way factorial analysis of variance, $P < 0.01$).

TABLE 6.9. *Phenylacetic acid urinary excretion in criminals*

Subjects	N	Phenylacetic acid excretion (mg/d)
Not depressed*	49	180 ± 22
Moderately depressed[†]	29	143 ± 22
Severely depressed[‡]	59	116 ± 11[§]

*No symptoms.
[†]Depressed according to only one of the three scales.
[‡]Beck Depression Inventory score >20; Depression scale of the Minnesota Multiphasic Personality Inventory score >70; and Hamilton Depression Scale score >19.
[§]Analysis of variance: $P < 0.05$.
Abbreviation: N, number of subjects.

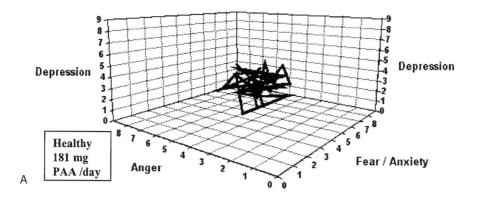

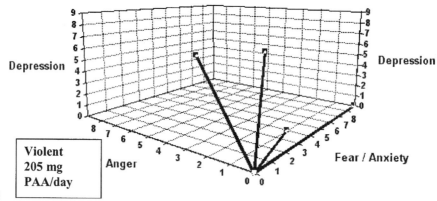

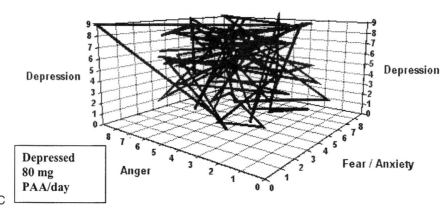

FIG. 6.5. Thirty-five–day trajectory of daily feelings of anger, fear, and depression as reported by three jail inmates. This tridimensional representation of changes is a standard method to detect pattern. **A:** The small variations of mood observed in a normal person. **B:** An equilibrium pattern, observed in 67% of violent criminals, associated with high phenylacetic acid (PAA) excretion. **C:** A chaotic-like pattern observed in 90% of depressed individuals, associated with low PAA excretion.

These results support Sandler's proposal (64) that PEA plays a role in socio-pathic behavior. Sandler found abnormally high plasma PAA levels in ten aggressive psychopaths but not in ten nonviolent control prisoners. At variance, Boulton et al. (65) found that incarcerated violent offenders had lower plasma PAA levels than nonviolent prisoners. These differences may be due to different degrees of depression in these two populations. In the author's study, the major-ity of jail inmates were depressed, and they showed low PAA excretion. These observations cast an interesting light on the relationships among depression, aggression, and crime. Crime is more often associated with failure and depres-sion than with aggression, but a distinct group of violent criminals has high PEA turnover, whether genetic or drug induced.

Further illuminating the anger–depression opposition, amphetamine increases violent behavior in humans; marijuana plus an MAOI increase fighting in mice (while neither agent does so separately) (66,67); and phenylalanine can produce irritability in euthymic persons. Animal experiments, as well as observations in human subjects, suggest that PEA may play a role in aggressive behavior (6). However, MAO-B knocked-out mice do not exhibit aggression, while deletion of MAO-A (which elevates catecholamine and serotonin levels) increases aggres-sion in both mice and humans (68).

Phenylethylamine and Laboratory Psychiatry: Differentiating Schizoaffective Illness from Schizophrenia and Panic Disorder from Depression with Panic Attacks

Although these studies are suggestive, they are extremely incomplete. Can clinicians clinically distinguish PEA deficit from serotonin-deficit types of depressions? Are PEA deficits genetically determined causes, or are they the metabolic consequences of depression? What are the alterations of PEA metab-olism in mania? Is PAA excretion a good indicator of PEA turnover?

The authors have observed both marked increases and decreases in urinary samples obtained from manic patients. Twenty-four hour urine samples are dif-ficult to obtain in these patients, but these data suggest that manic subjects excrete highly variable amounts of PAA.

Some patients with atypical bipolar affective disorders, characterized by psy-chotic manias and depressions, have fluctuating and episodic high urinary PEA excretion (69). In schizoaffective disorder with manic features, PAA excretion is elevated (70). A practical application of these observations is the use of car-bidopa as an adjunct in the treatment of atypical bipolar affective disorders (42) and of affective psychoses (43) (Table 6.6).

In contrast, PAA excretion is decreased in schizophrenia, another illness characterized by low psychological energy (70). This is at variance with the hypothesis that PEA excess contributes to the pathogenesis of schizophrenia. The biochemical difference between schizoaffective and schizophrenic patients illustrates the usefulness of biologic testing to differentiate entities that, on the

TABLE 6.10. *Urinary phenylacetic acid in panic disorders and in panic attacks associated with depression*

Diagnosis	Number of patients	Phenylacetic acid urinary excretion (mg/d)	Patients successfully treated with alprazolam (%)
Panic disorder	30	105 ± 23	70
Depression with panic attacks	9	66 ± 23	0

basis of symptoms alone, have been confused for a long time. A great need for laboratory tests in psychiatry exists. Depression, like fever, is a nonspecific symptom. In all fields of medicine, diagnosis is based on the identification of anatomic or metabolic changes and of causal factors, such as infection or intoxication. Lacking effective laboratory tests, early 20th-century psychiatrists adopted a symptomatologic definition of psychiatric syndromes, which has more recently become the organizing factor of official diagnosis. Yet only metabolic changes can define a specific illness, as the same syndrome can be produced by many different illnesses. Just as the Wassermann reaction defined syphilis, differentiating it from other venereal illnesses, so the identification of PEA deficit, if confirmed, will define an illness that is different from other illnesses that produce depressive symptoms.

Further illustrating the practical application of the PAA test, PAA excretion is decreased in patients with depression and panic attacks but not in patients with panic attacks alone (71) (Table 6.10). Alprazolam is useful for controlling panic attacks only in patients with normal PAA excretion, while imipramine is useful in patients with panic attacks and depression who show low PAA excretion (72).

PHARMACOLOGY

Pharmacologic observations in animals and humans support the role of PEA as a mediator of psychological energy. Amphetamines release and enhance the synthesis of PEA (41,73). Tetrahydrocannabinol (the main component of marijuana) inhibits PEA disposition and increases its brain levels (66,67). MAOIs increase PEA levels to a larger extent than those of any other neuroamine. Tricyclic antidepressants inhibit MAO-B (74) and reduce PEA disposition (75,76). PAA excretion is increased by imipramine, desipramine, amitriptyline, and fluoxetine (Sabelli H, unpublished, 1990–1995). PAA urinary excretion increases with effective antidepressant treatment but not with ineffective treatment (57) (Table 6.11). Lithium decreases PEA synthesis and reduces the stimulant effect of amphetamine (77). In clinical work with alcoholics and users of opiate analgesics, the authors found that these euphoriants markedly increase PAA excretion.

TABLE 6.11. *Phenylacetic acid urinary excretion (mg/d) in untreated and treated depression*

Diagnosis	Status	Treatment	N	PAA (% <70 mg/d)	PAA (mg/d)
Healthy			48	15	141 ± 10
Major depression	Inpatient	None	13	62*	69 ± 7*
Major depression	Inpatient at discharge	Effective	13	15	119 ± 17
Major depression	Outpatient	None	35	54*	86 ± 12*
Major depression	Outpatient	Effective	7	14	121 ± 27
Bipolar depression	Inpatient	Ineffective	8	71*	68 ± 15*
Bipolar depression	Outpatient	None	11	36*	90 ± 14*
Bipolar depression	Outpatient	Ineffective	5	60*	64 ± 19*

*P <0.05.
Abbreviations: N, number of patients; PAA, phenylacetic acid.

THERAPEUTICS

Phenylalanine Supplements in Depression

Attempting to test and apply these concepts, Fischer et al. (78), Beckman (79), and the author's group (57,80) explored the antidepressant effect of increasing PEA levels by the administration of its amino acid precursor, phenylalanine. Suprisingly, both Fischer and the author's group independently found that D-phenylalanine, a synthetic compound, was more effective than the actual precursor, L-phenylalanine, in increasing brain PEA in animals. These observations led to the use of the D isomer as an antidepressant in Argentina and to the sale of D-L-phenylalanine in health-food stores in the United States.

L-Phenylalanine (1 to 10 g, with pyridoxine 200 mg per day to facilitate decarboxylation) is a weak mood elevator. This combination can induce remission from depression, but only in subjects with bipolar disorder (Table 6.12). A positive response to methylphenidate predicts mood elevation by phenylalanine (Table 6.13).

The antidepressant effect of L-phenylalanine is mild, but it is useful for potentiating MAOI antidepressants. Low doses of selegiline (5 to 10 mg per day) enhance the mood-elevating effect of L-phenylalanine (1 to 6 g per day). At these low doses, selegiline selectively inhibits MAO-B, so tyramine is metabolized normally, and a low tyramine diet is not required. The antidepressant effect of L-phenylalanine in combination with selegiline is still mild, yet it is capable of eliciting remission in some treatment-resistant depressions (82).

The author views the selegiline–phenylalanine combination as an excellent treatment for mild depressions in the elderly because of its lack of cardiovascular effects. Depressed patients treated with standard antidepressants show a reduction in heart rate variation, whereas those treated with L-phenylalanine do not (Table 6.14); this is significant, as low heart rate variation is a predictor of increased mortality (83).

In summary, phenylalanine supplements (in combination with selegiline) produce a mood elevation that is useful in mild depressions, particularly in elderly

TABLE 6.12. *Phenylalanine supplements effective in bipolar depression*

Diagnosis	N	A. Full remission	B. Partial mood elevation	A + B	No effect of dysphoria
Bipolar I	8	3	4	7	1
Bipolar II*	21	8	12	20	1
All bipolars	29	11	16	27	2
Unipolars	11	0	4	4	7
All depressed	40	11	20	31	9

Method: Open study of the effects of L-phenylalanine (0.5 to 14 g/d), plus pyridoxine (200 mg/d), in 40 patients with bipolar disorder (depressed phase) or major depressive disorder (DSM-III).

*History of hypomania or soft signs of bipolarity, such as impulsivity rating >8 in the Kupfer test (81); hypersomnia instead of insomnia in present or past episode of depression; or family history of bipolar disorder.

Abbreviations: DSM-III, *Diagnostic and statistical manual of mental disorders*, 3rd edition; N, number of patients.

(Data from Sabelli HC, Fawcett J, Gusovsky F, et al. Clinical studies on the phenylethylamine hypothesis of affective disorder: urine and blood phenylacetic acid and phenylalanine dietary supplements. *J Clin Psychiatr* 1986;47:66–70; and Kravitz HM, Sabelli HC, Fawcett J. Dietary supplements of phenylalanine and other amino acid precursors of brain neuroamines in the treatment of depressive disorders. *J Am Osteopath Assoc* 1984;8:119–123, with permission.)

patients (because of low side effects). They are useful in bipolar patients, and they may be of great value in some treatment-resistant depressions.

Phenyethylamine Rapidly Relieves Depression in 60% of Patients

PEA is a much stronger antidepressant than L-phenylalanine, but only after inhibiting MAO. In patients treated with MAOIs, the addition of PEA can be extremely useful (85). Treatment of depression by PEA replacement became much more practical with the introduction of selective inhibitors of MAO-B. In an open study conducted at the University of Buenos Aires (86), six of ten out-

TABLE 6.13. *Methylphenidate test predicts phenylalanine antidepressant effect*

Response to methylphenidate	Number of patients responding with mood elevation to phenylalanine and to methylphenidate	
	Mood elevation with L-phenylalanine treatment	L-phenylalanine ineffective
Mood elevation	26	2
None or dysphoric	5	7

Method: Open study, 40 patients with bipolar disorder (depressed phase) or major depressive disorder (*Diagnostic and statistical manual of mental disorders*, 3rd edition [DSM-III]), treated with L-phenylalanine, 0.5 to 14 g/d, and pyridoxine, 200 mg/d. Stimulant challenge test with methylphenidate (Ritalin): day 1, give 5 mg in AM and 5 mg at 1 PM; subsequent days, increase 5 mg per dose up to mood elevation or anxiety or to a total of 60 mg/d.

Analysis of variance: $P < 0.001$.

(Data from Sabelli HC, Fawcett J, Javaid JI, Bagri S. The methylphenidate test to differentiate between desipramine-responsive (type I) and nortriptyline-responsive (type II) depressions. *Am J Psychiatry* 1983;140:212–219, with permission.)

TABLE 6.14. ʟ-*Phenylalanine does not reduce heart rate variation as standard antidepressants do*

Parameter	Healthy controls	Major depressive disorder	
Treatment	None	Treated with standard antidepressants	Treated with ʟ-phenylalanine
Number of subjects	10	17	3
SD of RRI (normalized)	105 ± 9	63 ± 23	114 ± 54
Median embedding dimension	59 ± 7	37 ± 5	52 ± 25

Method: 24-hour Holter monitoring. R-to-R intervals (RRI) measured with a precision of 1/128th sec. Three samples of 3500 RRI per patient obtained during wakefulness. Median embedding dimension calculated with the recurrence method. Median embedding dimension is a measure of complexity of pattern that indicates health. Low heart rate variation (small standard deviation) predicts cardiac illness; after infarction, low heart rate variation predicts death within 24 hr.

Abbreviation: SD, standard deviation.

(Data from Sabelli HC, Carlson-Sabelli L, Patel M, et al. Psycho-cardiological portraits: a clinical application of process theory. In: Abraham FD, Gilgen AR, eds. *Chaos theory in psychology.* Westport, CT: Greenwood Publishing Group, Inc., 1995;107–125, with permission.)

patients with MDD recovered within 2 weeks with PEA (15 to 60 mg per day); these subjects had been pretreated with low doses (10 mg) of selegiline to prevent rapid PEA metabolism.

In another study at Rush-Presbyterian-St.Luke's Medical Center (Table 6.15), the authors found that PEA replacement (10 to 60 mg per day) with selegiline (5 mg twice daily) rapidly induced remission in 60% of patients who were previously resistant to a wide variety of treatments, including MAOIs and selective serotonin reuptake inhibitors (87,88). These patients experienced mood elevation within a day or two of starting treatment, but remission usually required 2 weeks. Therapeutic effects included a restoration of energy, concentration, motivation, and sexual drive. Although the administration of PEA increases alertness in humans and experimental animals, PEA treatment significantly improved sleep. No side effects of nausea or fatigue, no inhibition of sexual function, no

TABLE 6.15. *Phenylethylamine treatment of depressed patients pretreated with selegiline*

Subjects	N	Responders	Nonresponders	Responders who relapsed within 3–5 wk	Relapse at follow-up	Premature terminations (<2 wk)
All	22	14 (64%)	2	2	2	4
Unipolars	13	10 (77%)		2	1	1
Bipolars	9	4 (44%)	2		1	3
Women	12	8 (67%)		2	1	2
Men	10	6 (60%)	2		1	2

Abbreviation: N, number of patients.

increases or decreases in blood pressure, no significant tachycardia, and no excitement or euphoria were observed.

PEA can be effective in patients who have not responded to standard antidepressive drugs, and likewise other antidepressant agents can be effective in patients for whom PEA is not. A predictor of response to PEA was transient mood elevation in the stimulant challenge test, which consists in the evaluation of the mood response to the intake of a dose of amphetamine or methylphenidate (81,89). However, a substantial difference exists between PEA and stimulant drugs. Patients treated with PEA experience none of the sensations of excitement, tension, euphoria, or artificial stimulation that are often associated with the intake of amphetamine.

Twelve of 14 successfully treated subjects continued to be euthymic when reexamined 20 to 50 weeks later, and none of the subjects had required an increase in dosage. In the author's view, PEA replacement maintained remission in part because the study also concomitantly addressed personal and interpersonal conflicts. Yet, prior to the use of PEA, psychologic treatment had not succeeded. In turn, PEA, as any other biologic intervention, should be a component of an integral approach to patient care. Biologic and psychologic treatments are indissolubly connected because both biologic and psychologic phenomena are physical processes.

PSYCHODYNAMICS

Phenylethylamine as Mediator for Psychological Energy, Love, and Self-Love

Freud inaugurated psychodynamics with the following concept of psychological energy: (a) psychobiologic energy is a physical energy; (b) a single psychobiologic energy exists, which includes emotional, sexual, and mental energy as its manifestations, just as multiple forms of physical energy are observed; and (c) psychobiologic energy also is interpersonal energy, meaning that warmth, affection, sexuality, and attention can be self-directed if and only if they are also other-directed. According to Freud, psychologic energy was best exemplified by sexual libido, but it has many other manifestations, such as courage, anger, and aggressiveness. Just as testosterone may increase sexual libido and mood, as well as aggressiveness, PEA may elevate mood and enhance aggressiveness by enhancing psychic energy.

Freud assumed, based on the closed system's model of nineteenth century thermodynamics, that psychic energy is constant. Energy could only be displaced, so symptoms of increased or decreased energy could not reflect actual changes in energy. For the same reason, love and self-love compete with each other, as one can grow only at the expense of the other. That energy can increase or decrease in open systems, such as biologic organisms, is now known. Furthermore, energy incessantly flows; changes in energy are associated with changes in time. This conjoint variation of energy and time is called action. Affective disorders illustrate this conjoint variation well, as feelings of low energy combine with slowness and even retardation of thinking and behavior in depression, while feelings of increased energy accompany acceleration in mania.

Depression is a shortage of psychologic action (energy flow), and mania is an overabundance (90,91). Diminished interest, attention, concentration, pleasure, self-love, self-esteem, affection, and sexuality; fatigue; helplessness; and retardation indicate a lowering of psychologic energy in depression, whereas the increased goal-directed activity, excessive involvement in pleasurable activities, increased sexuality, decreased need for sleep, talkativeness, flight of ideas, distractibility, and inflated self-esteem that define mania point to an excess of psychologic activity. Corresponding to the interpersonal dimension of psychological energy, *affective illnesses are dysfunctions of interpersonal affection and love, not only of personal mood and energy.* In depression, reductions not only in mood and self-esteem, but also in affection, sexuality, and solidarity, occur. In mania, increased affection, sexuality, and solidarity is observed. Disregarding interpersonal affect and defining depression as a mood disorder leaves something out. For example, clinically the author has observed a number of Caucasians who love African Americans while manic and who express racist notions when depressed. Love and self-love are both increased in mania and reduced in depression. This corresponds to the notion of love and self-love as complementary, each feeding on the other, as proposed by Antonio Sabelli, my father (92,93).

These changes in psychologic energy must be embodied in metabolic changes in the central nervous system. The demonstration that psychologic processes and illnesses actually are physical processes and are modifiable by drugs is perhaps the most important philosophical discovery of the twentieth century. The central tenet of biologic psychiatry is that behavior, emotion, and cognition are three aspects of complex processes in genetically determined pathways. Specific anatomic and metabolic pathways serve specific behavioral pathways. Emotional life is written in a simple alphabet of genetically determined patterns of behavior (instincts) that are coded by specific brain chemicals, a concept that has guided the development of psychopharmacology in terms of synaptic theory. Hess proposed the existence of an ergotropic system (alerting, activity, sympathetic predominance) and a trophotropic system (sleep, nutrition, parasympathetic predominance). Adrenergic neuroamines, such as noradrenaline and dopamine, undoubtedly play a role in the ergotropic system, as Brodie suggested. The data previously discussed suggested that endogenous PEA sustains attention and affect. In psychodynamic terms, *PEA is the neuromodulator of libido; that is, of psychological energy (attention, motivation, self-love) and interpersonal energy (affection and aggression).*

Klein further connected PEA with affect, suggesting that PEA deficit induces a specific type of atypical depression—women who crave relationships, feel elated in them, and fall into despair when rejected (94). However, the existence of this disease entity is questionable. As was discussed earlier, PAA excretion is reduced in atypical depression and in other types of unipolar and bipolar depression. This actually reinforces the conjecture, because sexuality is characteristically decreased in all types of depression. In further support for a role of PEA in libido, sexuality and affection are increased in mania, aphrodisiac effects are noted with agents that enhance PEA turnover (e.g., tetrahydrocannabinol, amphetamine), and chronic selegiline administration increases sexual behavior in rats. What changes, if any, in PEA metabolism occur in the process of falling in love has not been studied, but the authors did observe a decrease in PAA excretion in 50% of 16 divorcing subjects that were studied (6).

These ideas have been translated into the popular notion that PEA may be the hormone of love, leading to some fanciful speculations about romance and chocolate. Of course, a hormone of love cannot exist. Love is a complex process that includes, but is not reducible to, simpler processes such as sexuality and affection. Many neurohormones modulate sexuality. On the other hand, the author's clinical experience indicates that the administration of PEA or phenylalanine can enhance sexual arousal and thus can promote erection. PEA releases dopamine, and another dopamine releaser, apomorphine, is known to improve erection. Tetrahydrocannabinols, which increase brain PEA levels, are also known to promote sexual arousal. In contrast, serotonin is a specific inhibitor of sexual function, so serotonin reuptake inhibitors by necessity reduce sexuality, a major drawback regarding their use as antidepressants (95). Thus, the opposite effects of PEA and serotonin on sexuality may be of practical relevance in the treatment of depression.

The effects of amphetamine and of tetrahydrocannabinol, two drugs that increase PEA turnover, suggest that *PEA increases emotional warmth, intellectual attention, affection, sexuality, and feelings of physical energy when a person is in intrapsychic and interpersonal harmony.*

Clinical studies of depressed, aggressive, and anxious subjects suggest that, *when a person is involved in conflict, PEA inhibits depression and favors hostile behavior.* This is to be expected from a neuromodulator that promotes courage. PEA has little, if any, influence on fear and anxiety (Table 6.16). To restate the PEA hypothesis of affect, *depression can result from a metabolic PEA deficit or from interpersonal conflict, loss, and defeat.*

TABLE 6.16. *Plasma and urine phenylacetic acid levels are not a function of anxiety*

Diagnosis	Urine PAA (mg/d)	N	Plasma PAA (ng/mL)	N
Control	132 ± 72	6	638 ± 543	6
Generalized anxiety	123 ± 49	4	240 ± 175	2
Panic attacks and depression	56 ± 37	6	207 ± 122	3

Abbreviations: N, number of patients; PAA, phenylacetic acid.

Phenylethylamine and the Conflict Theory of Depression

Fischer postulated the existence of a specific illness, PEA deficit (2), genetically different from other types of depression. Klein et al. (94) proposed that PEA deficit was the cause of atypical depression. The data show that PAA excretion is reduced in a number of different depressive syndromes—unipolar and bipolar, typical and atypical—as well as in schizophrenia, indicating that PEA turnover is decreased in more than one specific illness. Furthermore, emotions are capable of altering PEA metabolism; for instance, the authors observed remarkably parallel changes in PAA excretion in a divorcing couple—low levels both before and after the divorce, but a large peak the day of the divorce (90). Metabolic changes obviously can be psychologically determined.

In the author's view, PEA deficit may be a component of a number of illnesses, and it represents an exaggerated expression of the genetically encoded behavioral pathway for surrender (96). The traditional fight-or-flight dichotomy proposed by Cannon and modeled by catastrophe theory ignores the third pathway of behavior commonly adopted by mammals to end conflict—surrender. This behavioral trifurcation of fight, flight, or surrender reflects the empirically demonstrated coexistence of the complementary opposite emotions of anger, fear, and grief (63). These conflict emotions are the physiologic bases for rage, anxiety, or depression. Conflict and defeat constitute the physiologic trigger for discouragement and grief. When they occur in pathologic proportions or circumstances, they constitute depression. Conflict may trigger depression, and depression often induces conflicts. Thus, anger and fear coexist and alternate with depression in depressive illness (63,91). Whereas conflict triggers all three negative emotions (anger, fear, and grief), behavior depends on both personal energy and social circumstances. Low energy promotes depression, while high energy supports courage and allows for struggle. (The original relation between courage and anger is evident in the use of the same term *coraje* for both in Mexican-Spanish.) Even when biologic and psychologic energy are adequate, however, struggling may be inhibited because of overwhelming differences in power or by love. In these cases, psychobiologic energy, which is initially high, becomes inhibited in the process of surrendering. Concomitantly, pleasure-seeking, self-love, and love for others become inhibited. If, in fact, PEA is a mediator of psychobiologic energy and interpersonal bonding, a decrease in PEA turnover would thus be the cause or the consequence of depression.

Conversely, an increase in PEA production may occur as a homeostatic compensation against depressogenic stimuli or metabolic dysfunctions; in like manner, insulin levels are often increased in adult onset diabetes, an illness clearly due to a relative insulin deficit. The lack of effect of PEA in at least 40% of depressed patients, the differential results obtained in the stimulant challenge test (89), and the selective effectiveness of particular antidepressants in a given patient prove that several different illnesses can cause similar depressive syndromes. Furthermore, inhibitors of MAO-A, but not of MAO-B, produce significant antidepressant effects, indicating a role for catecholamines or serotonin in depression.

TABLE 6.17. *Three views on phenylethylamine deficit in depression*

A. Fischer: PEA deficit as a specific illness.
B. Klein: PEA deficit as the cause of atypical depression.
C. Sabelli: PEA as mediator for psychological energy and interpersonal energy (Freud's libido), including both affection and aggression. Excessive energy underlies mania. Low energy promotes depression. Conflict induces anger, fear, and depression. Affective disorders are dysfunctions of affection, not just of affect and self-esteem.

Abbreviation: PEA, phenylethylamine.

In the author's view, PEA is not a specific mediator for a particular neuronal pathway but rather a nonspecific modulator of psychological energy (Table 6.17). According to ethological theory, behavior is organized in action pathways, which are sequences of appetitive interactions leading to consummatory behavior. Pleasurable consummation acts as a positive reinforcer and strengthens social bonding; learning thus modulates genetically determined patterns of behavior. These behavioral pathways that have been transmitted genetically are encoded anatomically and metabolically in the central nervous system. Presumably, every behavior is triggered by one (or more) neurohormone and is inhibited by one (or more) neurohormone, although evidence shows that emotions often involve multiple neuronal pathways with different neurotransmitters and, even further, that each synapse involves not only a main transmitter but also modulators. Of the conflict pathways, fear and anxiety may be triggered by norepinephrine and inhibited by γ-aminobutyric acid (anxiolytic effect of beta-blockers and of benzodiazepines). Hostility is inhibited by serotonin (97), while acetylcholine may be the trigger for anger, as the abilities of cholinergic drugs to elicit rage in cats (96) and of cholinergic blockers to decrease marital conflict illustrate (98). Anger and depression (Freud's anger turned inward) may share the same chemical modulation. Clinical observations with tryptophan and with serotonin reuptake inhibitors suggest that serotonin may inhibit depression. The *neurohormonal trigger for depression is as yet unknown* (a significant research project to be pursued), although some data suggest a role for acetylcholine. Thus, depression and anger might be both triggered by acetylcholine and inhibited by serotonin, with PEA tipping the balance between one and the other emotional response to conflict.

PHENYLETHYLAMINE IN THE CONTEXT OF AN INTEGRAL PHYSIOLOGY

PEA empirical research and theoretical hypotheses have evolved in the evolving context of modern physiology. Similar to Greek physiology, the first science, modern physiology is an integrative discipline that investigates material and psychological processes as manifestations of physical energy. Metabolic dysfunctions induce psychologic symptoms, and psychologic processes alter brain metabolism.

A specific metabolic dysfunction determines specific psychologic symptoms, and, conversely, psychodynamic processes determine specific metabolic changes. Thus, PEA deficit is associated with the inhibition of behavior that is induced by interpersonal conflict and personal loss; the biologic change may be the cause or the consequence of the psychologic processes. In contrast, in the phenomenologic approach, illness is defined by its symptoms, which are independent from the psychodynamic content. For the phenomenologist, a metabolic dysfunction underlies depression, while life circumstances determine marital, occupational, or psychological problems. In the physiologic view, biologic and psychologic processes are intimately and often causally related.

In depressed persons, biologic illnesses, if any, must be treated first because the correction of their metabolic alterations, such as PEA or serotonin deficit, is necessary for recovery and for psychotherapeutic learning. Psychologic interventions require the patient's ability to pay attention and to concentrate. Also, treating illness first is the one and only empathic intervention that behooves a health professional. This illustrates the priority of biologic processes. But the correction of metabolic dysfunctions often is not sufficient for full recovery, illustrating the supremacy of psychologic processes. The concept of biologic priority and psychologic supremacy is a central tenet of process theory (93,96). According to process theory, collective family and social processes have priority over individual psychology in evolution, history, and personal development. Hence, the clinician should attend to family and occupational conflicts and defeats before addressing cognitive and characterologic dysfunctions, if any. This is required by both therapeutic effectiveness and empathy. This bio-socio-psychologic method (76) contrasts with the pharmacologic approach currently dominating clinical practice and with the bio-psycho-social approach of system theories. In the process view, neurohormone replacement must be combined with conflict resolution and cocreative behavior (99).

Earlier concepts of homeostasis regarded health as equilibrium and depression as the result of neuroamine deficit. Actually, dysfunction and illness can also result from an excess, rather than a failure, of homeostasis. For instance, depression may be the consequence of an excessive inhibitory reaction to conflict and defeat (91). Likewise, the symptoms of mania appear to be the result of a magnification in homeostatic, periodic, chaotic, and creative processes (90). Within a process perspective, the evaluation of neuroamine changes in depression should include longitudinal observations of their turnover, rather than single measurements of their level at a particular time.

FUTURE RESEARCH AND PRESENT THERAPEUTIC USE

In conclusion, *PEA is the only neuroamine that produces stimulant effects and relieves depression*. The rapid and sustained relief of depression in over 60% of the patients studied indicates PEA may be an effective treatment of depression. Sixty percent is the same rate of effectiveness obtained with any antidepressant from imipramine to the latest marketed agent in clinical studies—psychiatric practice indicates a lower rate of success with any antidepressant. These positive results obtained with PEA should be considered with great caution in view of the size of the samples and the lack of controlled studies. At this time, only two pilot studies are available. If a double-blind, placebo-controlled study of PEA treatment supports these encouraging initial findings, then the effectiveness of PEA would have theoretical and practical implications.

The invitation to contribute to a series on alternative medicine at Massachusetts General Hospital and to this volume both was flattering and bewildering—PEA research developed within the context of medical science; what has made it alternative? Major research institutes have adhered for decades to the catecholamine theory of depression, and recent advances in pharmaceutical research have shifted the focus to serotonin. PEA treatment has been the object of only few clinical studies. PEA is the Cinderella of the neurohormones that regulate mood. It is an orphan without the parental support of a pharmaceutical manufacturer or a national research institute, beset by sibling rivalries and lack of funding. Having researched the field since the PEA hypothesis of affect was first proposed, the author is afraid to be overenthusiastic, as conviction is the worst enemy of truth according to Nietzsche. "*In the quest for truth ... the sentiment always has the initiative, it engenders the* a priori *idea or intuition; reason then develops the idea and deduces its logical consequences. But if the sentiment must be clarified by the light of reason, reason in turn must be guided by experiment*," explained Claude Bernard.

As a scientist, the author is aware that the available data are very preliminary. Yet the current evidence also supports, nay it demands, the development of large controlled, double-blind studies to establish when PEA is useful as a treatment for depression. The PAA test should be explored; no data exist correlating PEA effectiveness and PAA excretion. The PAA test does not diagnose depression, but it does distinguish some subtypes. In his modern classic, *Genesis and development of a scientific fact*, Fleck illustrates, using the history of the Wassermann reaction, how scientific progress results from incremental steps introduced by scientists who are determined to succeed in developing a useful test, rather than from the purported proof or purported refutation, which is often the symptom of scientific competition.

As a psychiatrist, the author's clinical experience indicates that *PEA is a simple, nontoxic, and often effective treatment of depression* that can be used continuously or as needed for long periods without fear of harmful consequences, such as weight gain, sexual inhibition, and other common side effects of antidepressant drugs. However, no data exist regarding its use in cardiovascular patients. PEA can be readily obtained for clinical use. *PEA should be used as the first treatment of depression* in otherwise healthy individuals.

ACKNOWLEDGMENTS

The unpublished data reported here were obtained in collaboration with Drs. Bennet Braun, Alyssa Levy, and Javaid Javaid and with the technical assistance of Nancy Hein. These studies were largely supported by the Society for the Advancement of Clinical Philosophy.

REFERENCES

1. Fischer E, Ludmer RI, Sabelli HC. The antagonism of phenylethylamine to catecholamines on mouse motor activity. *Acta Fisiol Latino Am* 1967;17:15–21.
2. Fischer E. The phenylethylamine hypothesis of thymic homeostasis. *Biol Psychiatry* 1975;10:667–673.
3. Sabelli HC, Giardina WJ, Mosnaim AD, Sabelli NH. A comparison of the functional roles of norepinephrine, dopamine and phenylethylamine in the central nervous system. *Acta Physiol Pol* 1973; 24:33–40.
4. Sabelli HC, Giardina WJ. Amine modulation of affective behavior. In: Sabelli H, ed. *Chemical modulation of brain function*. New York: Raven Press, 1973:225–259.
5. Sabelli HC, Mosnaim AD. Phenylethylamine hypothesis of affective behavior. *Am J Psychiatry* 1974;131:695–699.
6. Sabelli HC, Javaid JI. Phenylethylamine modulation of affect: therapeutic and diagnostic implications. *J Neuropsychiatry Clin Neurosci* 1995;7:6–14.
7. Paterson IA, Juorio AV, Boulton AA. 2-Phenylethylamine: a modulator of catecholamine transmission in the mammalian central nervous system? *J Neurochem* 1990;55:1827–1837.
8. Nakajima T, Kakimoto Y, Sano I. Formation of β-phenylethylamine in mammalian tissue and its effects on motor activity in mouse. *J Pharmacol Exp Ther* 1964;143:319–325.
9. Inwang EE, Mosnaim AD, Sabelli HC. Isolation and characterization of phenylethylamine and phenylethanolamine from human brain. *J Neurochem* 1973;20:1469–1473.
10. Mosnaim AD, Inwang EE, Sugerman JH, et al. Ultraviolet spectrophotometric determination of 2-phenylethylamine in biological samples and its possible correlation with depression. *Biol Psychiatry* 1973;6:235–257.
11. Mosnaim AD, Inwang EE, Sugerman JH, Sabelli HC. Identification of 2-phenylethylamine in human urine by infrared and mass spectroscopy and its quantification in normal subjects and cardiovascular patients. *Clin Chim Acta* 1973;46:407–413.
12. Mosnaim AD, Sabelli HC. Quantitative determination of the brain levels of a β-phenylethylamine-like substance in control and drug-treated mice. *Pharmacologist* 1971;13:283.
13. Durden DA, Phillips SR, Boulton AA. Identification and distribution of β-phenylethylamine in rat. *Can J Biochem* 1973;51:995–1002.
14. Reynolds GP, Sandler M, Hardy J, Bradford H. The determination and distribution of 2-phenylethylamine in sheep brain. *J Neurochem* 1976;34:213–1125.
15. Juorio AV. Brain β-phenylethylamine: localization, pathways and interrelation with catecholamines. In: Sandler M, Dahlstrom A, Belmaker RH, eds. *Progress in catecholamine research, central aspects, neurology and neuroradiology*, Vol. 42B. New York: Liss, 1988.
16. Oates JA, Nirenberg PZ, Jepson JB, et al. Conversion of phenylalanine to phenylethylamine in patients with phenylketonuria. *Proc Soc Exp Biol Med* 1963;112:1078–1081.
17. Shannon HE, Cone EJ, Yousefnejad D. Physiologic effects and plasma kinetics of β-phenylethylamine and its N-methyl homolog in the dog. *J Pharmacol Exp Ther* 1982;223:190–196.
18. Fuller RW, Rousch BW. Substrate-selective and tissue selective inhibition of monoamine oxidase. *Arch Int Pharmacodyn Ther* 1972;198:270–276.
19. Yang HYT, Neff NH. α-Phenyethylamine, a specific substrate for type B monoamine oxidase of the brain. *J Pharmacol Exp Ther* 1973;187:365–371.
20. Madubuike UP, Mosnaim AD, Sabelli HC. Brain phenylacetic acid, a major metabolite of 2-phenylethylamine in rabbit brain. Proceedings of the International Congress of Physiological Sciences. New Delhi, October 20–26, 1974.
21. Durden DA, Boulton AA. Identification and distribution of phenylacetic acid in the brain of the rat. *J Neurochem* 1982;38:1532–1536.
22. Shih JC, Chen K, Ridd MJ. Monoamine oxidase: from genes to behavior. *Annu Rev Neurosci* 1999; 22:197–217.
23. Edwards DJ, Blau K. Analysis of phenylethylamine in biological tissues by gas-liquid chromatography with electron-capture detection. *Anal Biochem* 1972;45:387–402.
24. Saavedra JM, Axelrod J. Demonstration and distribution of phenylethanolamine in brain and other tissues. *Proc Natl Acad Sci U S A* 1973;70:769–772.

25. Sabelli HC, Vazquez AJ, Flavin DF. Behavioral and electrophysiological effects of phenylethanol-amine, a putative neurotransmitter. *Psychopharmacologia (Berlin)* 1975;42:117–125.
26. Barroso N, Rodriguez M. Action of β-phenylethylamine and related amines on nigrostriatal dopamine neurons. *Eur J Pharmacol* 1996;297:195–203.
27. Gusovsky F. Phenylethylaminic mechanisms in animal behavioral stimulation and human affective disorders. Ph.D. dissertation. Rush University, 1984.
28. Mesfioui A, Math F, Jmari K, et al. Effects of amphetamine and phenylethylamine on catecholamine release in the glomerular layer of the rat olfactory bulb. *Biol Signals Receptors* 1998;7:235–243.
29. Giardina WJ, Pedemonte WA, Sabelli HC. Iontophoretic study of the effects of norepinephrine and 2-phenylethylamine on single cortical neurons. *Life Sci* 1973;12:153–161.
30. Sabelli HC, Mosnaim AD, Vazquez AJ, et al. Biochemical plasticity of synaptic transmission: a critical review of Dale's principle. *Biol Psychiatry* 1976;11:481–524.
31. Hendwood RW, Boulton AA, Phillis JW. Ionophoretic studies of some trace amines in the mammalian CNS. *Brain Res* 1979;164:347–351.
32. Paetsch PR, Greenshaw AJ. 2-Phenylethylamine-induced changes in catecholamine receptor density: implications for antidepressant drug action. *Neurochem Res* 1993;18:1015–1022.
33. Sato S, Tamura A, Kitagawa S, Koshiro A. A kinetic analysis of the effects of β–phenylethylamine on the concentrations of dopamine and its metabolites in the rat striatum. *J Pharm Sci* 1997;86:487–496.
34. Bailey BA, Philips SR, Boulton AA. In vivo release of endogenous dopamine, 5-hydroxytryptamine and some of their metabolites from rat caudate nucleus by phenylethylamine. *Neurochem Res* 1987;12:173–178.
35. Rockhold RW. Glutamatergic involvement in psychomotor stimulant action. *Prog Drug Res* 1998;50:155–192.
36. Sabelli HC, Mosnaim AD, Vazquez AJ. Phenylethylamine: possible role in depression and antidepressive drug action. In: Drucker-Colin RR, Myers RD, eds. *Advances in behavioral biology: neurohumoral coding of brain function.* New York: Plenum, 1974:331–357.
37. Paterson IA, Juorio AV, Boulton AA. 2-Phenylethylamine: a modulator of catecholamine transmission in the mammalian central nervous system? *J Neurochem* 1990;55:1827–1837.
38. Jackson DM, Temple DM. Temple β-phenylalanine as a cardiotonic constituent of tissue extracts. *Comp Gen Pharmacol* 1970;1:155.
39. Sabelli HC, Fawcett J. Gut flora and urinary phenylacetic acid. *Science* 1984;226:996.
40. Oldendorf WH. Brain uptake of radiolabelled amino acids, amines and hexoses after arterial infusion. *Am J Physiol* 1971;221:1629–1639.
41. Borison RL, Mosnaim AD, Sabelli HC. Biosynthesis of brain 2-phenylethylamine: influence of decarboxylase inhibition and D-amphetamine. *Life Sci* 1974;15:1837–1848.
42. Linnoila M, Karoum F, Potkin S, et al. Amelioration of psychosis with carbidopa. A case report. *Br J Psychiatry* 1984;144:428–431.
43. Sabelli HC, Fawcett J. *Carbidopa treatment of schizoaffective disorders.* 1989 CME Syllabus and Proceedings Summary. American Psychiatric Association 142nd Annual Meeting, San Francisco, May 6–11, 1989:105–106.
44. Borison RL, Sabelli HC, Ho B. Influence of a peripheral monoamine oxidase inhibitor (MAOI) upon the central nervous system levels and pharmacological effects of 2-phenylethylamine (PEA). *Pharmacologist* 1975;17:258.
45. Fischer E, Heller B, Miro AH. β-phenylethylamine in human urine. *Arzneim-Forsch* 1968;18:1486.
46. Fischer E, Spatz H, Saavedra J. Urinary elimination of phenylethylamine. *Biol Psychiat* 1972;5:139–147.
47. Boulton A, Milward L. Separation, detection and quantitative analysis of urinary β-phenylethylamine. *J Chromatography* 1971;57:287–296.
48. Inwang EE, Sugerman JH, DeMartini WJ, et al. Ultraviolet spectrophotometric determination of β-phenylethylamine-like substances in biological samples and its possible correlation with depression. *Biol Psychiatry* 1973;6:235–257.
49. Sabelli HC, Fawcett J, Gusovsky F, et al. Urinary phenylacetate: a diagnostic test for depression? *Science* 1983;220:1187–1188.
50. Sabelli HC, Fawcett J, Gusovsky F, et al. Phenylacetic acid as an indicator in bipolar affective disorders. *J Clin Psychopharmacol* 1983;3:268–270.
51. Gusovsky F, Fawcett J, Javaid JI, et al. A high pressure liquid chromatography method for plasma phenylacetic acid: a putative marker for depressive disorders. *Anal Biochem* 1985;145:101–105.
52. Karoum F, Potkin S, Chuang LW, et al. Phenylacetic acid excretion in schizophrenia and depression: the origins of PAA in man. *Biol Psychiatry* 1984;19:165–178.

53. Sandler M, Ruthven CRJ, Goodwin BL, et al. Decreased cerebrospinal fluid concentration of free phenylacetic acid in depressive illness. *Clin Chim Acta* 1979;93:169–171.
54. Zhou G, Shoji H, Yamada S, Matsuishi T. Decreased β-phenylethylamine in CSF in Parkinson's disease. *J Neurol Neurosurg Psychiatry* 1997;63:754–758.
56. Gusovsky F, Fawcett J, Javaid JI, et al. A high pressure liquid chromatography method for plasma phenylacetic acid: a putative marker for depressive disorders. *Anal Biochem* 1985;145:101–105.
57. Sabelli HC, Fawcett J, Gusovsky F, et al. Clinical studies on the phenylethylamine hypothesis of affective disorder: urine and blood phenylacetic acid and phenylalanine dietary supplements. *J Clin Psychiatry* 1986;47:66–70.
58. Braun BG, Sabelli HC, Javaid JI, et al. *Reduced phenylacetic acid in major and atypical depression but not in dysthmic disorder*. 145th Annual Meeting of the American Psychiatric Association, Washington, D.C., 1992.
59. Karege F, Rudolph W. High-performance liquid chromatographic determination of phenylacetic acid in human plasma extracted with ethylacetate. *J Chromatogr* 1991;70:376–381.
60. Gonzalez-Sastre F, Mora J, Guillamat R, et al. Urinary phenylacetic acid excretion in depressive patients. *Acta Psychiatr Scand* 1988;78:208–210.
61. DeLisi LE, Murphy DL, Karoum F, et al. Phenylethylamine excretion in depression. *Psychiatr Res* 1984;13:193–201.
62. Levy A. *A clinical study of the urinary phenylacetic acid (PAA) test of depression in prison inmates.* Doctoral thesis, 1991, Brigham Young University.
63. Sabelli HC, Carlson-Sabelli L, Levy A, Patel M. Anger, fear, depression and crime: physiological and psychological studies using the process method. In: Robertson R, Combs A, eds. *Chaos theory in psychology and the life sciences*. Mahwah, NJ: Laurence Erlbaum Associates, Inc., 1995:65–88.
64. Sandler M, Ruthven CRJ, Goodwin BL, et al. Phenylethylamine overproduction in aggressive psychopaths. *Lancet* 1978;ii:1269–1270.
65. Boulton AA, Davis BA, Yu PH, et al. Trace acid levels in the plasma and MAO activity in the platelets of violent offenders. *Psychiatr Res* 1983;8:19–23.
66. Sabelli HC, Vazquez AJ, Mosnaim AD, Madrid-Pedemonte L. 2-Phenylethylamine as a possible mediator for 9-tetrahydrocannabinol-induced stimulation. *Nature* 1974;248:144–145.
67. Sabelli HC, Pedemonte WA, Whally C, et al. Further evidence for a role of 2-phenylethylamine in the mode of action of 9-tetrahydrocannabinol. *Life Sci* 1974;14:149–156.
68. Shih JC, Chen K, Ridd MJ. Role of MAO A and B in neurotransmitter metabolism and behavior. *Pol J Pharmacol* 1999;51:25–29.
69. Karoum F, Linnoila M, Potter WZ, et al. Fluctuating high urinary phenylethylamine excretion rates in some bipolar affective disorder patients. *Psychiatr Res* 1982;6:215–222.
70. Sabelli HC, Durai UNB, Fawcett J, Javaid JI. High phenylacetic acid differentiates schizoaffectives from schizophrenics. *J Neuropsychiatr Clin Neurosci* 1989;1:37–39.
71. Sabelli HC, Javaid JI, Fawcett J, Kravitz HM. Urinary phenylacetic acid in panic disorder with and without depression. *Acta Psychiatr Scand* 1990;82:14–16.
72. Wynn P, Sabelli HC, Kravitz HM. Phenylacetate as a predictor of alprazolam effectiveness in panic attacks. *Pharmacologist* 1984;26:3.
73. Borison RL, Mosnaim AD, Sabelli HC. Brain 2-phenylethylamine as a mediator for the central actions of amphetamine and methylphenidate. *Life Sci* 1975;17:1331–1344.
74. Roth JA, CN Gillis. Deamination of β-phenylethylamine by monoamine oxidase-inhibition by imipramine. *Biochem Pharmacol* 1974;23:2537–2545.
75. Sabelli HC, Borison RL. Non-catecholaminic adrenergic modulators. In: Costa E, Giacobini E, Paoletti R, eds. *Advances in biochemical pharmacology: first and second messengers*. New York: Raven, 1976:69–74.
76. Sabelli HC, Borison RL, Diamond BI, et al. Phenylethylamine and brain function. *Biochem Pharmacol* 1978;27:1707–1711.
77. Borison RL, Sabelli HC, Diamond B, et al. *Lithium prevention of amphetamine-induced manic excitement and of reserpine-induced depression in mice: possible role of 2-phenylethylamine (PEA)*. Proceedings of the Society of Neuroscience, Toronto, November, 1977.
78. Yariyura-Tobias JA, Heller B, Spatz H, Fischer E. Phenylalanine for endogenous depression. *J Orthomol Psychiatry* 1975;3:80–81.
79. Beckmann H, Athen D, Olteanu M, Zimmer R. DL-phenylalanine versus imipramine: a double-blind controlled study. *Arch Psychiat Nervenkr* 1979;227:49–58.
80. Kravitz HM, Sabelli HC, Fawcett J. Dietary supplements of phenylalanine and other amino acid pre-

cursors of brain neuroamines in the treatment of depressive disorders. *J Am Osteopathic Assoc* 1984; 8:119–123.

81. Sabelli HC, Fawcett J, Javaid JI, Bagri S. The methylphenidate test to differentiate between desipramine-responsive (type I) and nortriptyline-responsive (type II) depressions. *Am J Psychiatry* 1983;140:212–219.

82. Sabelli HC. Rapid treatment of depression with selegiline-phenylalanine combination. *J Clin Psychiatry* 1991;52:137.

83. Malik M, Camm AJ. *Heart rate variability.* Armonk, NY: Futura, 1995

84. Sabelli HC, Carlson-Sabelli L, Patel M, et al. Psychocardiological portraits: a clinical application of process theory. In: Abraham FD, Gilgen AR, eds. *Chaos theory in psychology.* Westport, CT: Greenwood Publishing, 1995:107–125.

85. Sabelli HC, Javaid JI, Fawcett J. Phenylethylamine replacement and depletion in the treatment of depression, schizoaffective disorder and tardive dyskinesia. *Fed Proc* 1989;3:A1186.

86. Sabelli HC, Fahrer R, Doria Medina R, Ortiz Frágola E. Phenylethylamine replacement rapidly relieves depression. *J Neuropsychiatry* 1994;6:203.

87. Sabelli H, Fink P, Fawcett J, Tom C. Sustained antidepressant effect of PEA replacement. *J Neuropsychiatry Clin Neurosci* 1996;8:168–171.

88. Sabelli H. Phenylethylamine replacement as a rapid and physiological treatment for depression. *Psycheline* 1998;2:32–39.

89. Fawcett J, Kravitz HM, Sabelli HC. Stimulant challenge tests. In: Hall RCW, Beresford TP, eds. *Handbook of diagnostic procedures.* New York: Spectrum Publications, 1984:223–251.

90. Sabelli HC, Carlson-Sabelli L, Javaid JI. The thermodynamics of bipolarity: a bifurcation model of bipolar illness and bipolar character and its psychotherapeutic applications. *Psychiatry Interpersonal Biol Proc* 1990;53:346–367.

91. Sabelli HC, Carlson-Sabelli L. Process theory as a framework for comprehensive psychodynamic formulations. *Genetic Social Gen Psychol Monogr* 1991;117:5–27.

92. Sabelli A. *Escritos.* Buenos Aires: Private Edition, 1952.

93. Sabelli HC, Carlson-Sabelli L. Biological priority and psychological supremacy, a new integrative paradigm derived from process theory. *Am J Psychiatry* 1989;146:1541–1551.

94. Klein DF. Pathophysiology of depressive syndromes [letter]. *Biol Psychiatry* 1974;8:119.

95. Goldstein I. Male sexual circuitry. *Sci Am* 2000;283:70–75.

96. Sabelli H., Carlson-Sabelli L, Patel M, Sugerman A. Dynamics and psychodynamics. Process foundations of psychology. *J Mind Behav* 1997;18:305–334.

97. Cleare AJ, Bond A. The effect of tryptophan depletion and enhancement on subjective and behavioural aggression in normal male subjects. *Psychopharmacology* 1995;118:72–81.

98. Sabelli HC. Anticholinergic antidepressants decrease marital hostility. *J Clin Psychiatry* 1990;3: 127–128.

99. Sabelli H, Carlson-Sabelli L, Patel M, et al. Applying the process theory of systems to depressive illness: coupling neurohormone replacement with conflict resolution and co-creative behavior. In: Allen JK, Wilby J, eds. 42nd Annual Meeting of the International Society for the Systems Sciences, Atlanta, Georgia, 1998.

Chapter 7

Inositol in the Treatment of Psychiatric Disorders

Robert H. Belmaker, Jonathan Benjamin, and Ziva Stahl

INTRODUCTION

Inositol is a sugar alcohol and a structural (although not stereo-) isomer of glucose (Fig. 7.1). It differs from glucose because all six carbon atoms are found within the ring of the molecule. Located primarily within cell membranes, inositol is ubiquitous in biologic organisms; the average adult human consumes about 1 g in the daily diet. It is regarded by some as a vitamin (1) and by European folk wisdom as a remedy for neurasthenia and mild depression.

Berridge et al. (2) suggested that lithium acts in bipolar disorder by inhibiting the enzyme inositol-1-monophosphatase and causing a relative inositol deficiency. A possible excess of inositol in mania suggested its possible deficit in

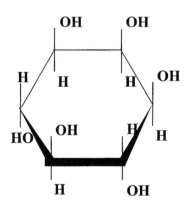

myo-inositol

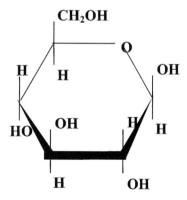

glucose

FIG 7.1. The structure of inositol and glucose.

111

depression. Barkai et al. (3) reported low levels of inositol in the cerebrospinal fluid of depressed patients. The authors therefore performed a pilot study of 6 g per day of inositol in patients with resistant depression; this was in addition to ongoing medication (4). The trial results were positive, and the only side effect reported was occasional mild flatulence. The authors then proceeded to a randomized, double-blind controlled trial of inositol, 12 g per day, versus a placebo in depression (5).

DEPRESSION STUDY

Patients who were referred to the study and who gave informed consent had all failed antidepressant treatment or had dropped out because of side effects. No medications other than inositol or the placebo were permitted during the trial, except for oxazepam, up to 15 mg daily, or an equivalent benzodiazepine if the patient had been taking it before the study began.

Twenty-seven patients completed the trial. All patients were given inositol or glucose in identical containers according to a prearranged random code. The drug was in powder form, and patients were instructed to take 2 teaspoons morning and evening in juice. A modified treatment emergent symptom scale was used to monitor side effects. Hematologic studies, blood chemistry, liver function, and kidney function were assessed at baseline and after 4 weeks of inositol treatment.

Scores on the Hamilton Depression Scale (HAM-D) declined from 32.9±5 at baseline to 28.7±7 at 2 weeks and to 28.9±10 at 4 weeks in the placebo group, and from 33.4±6 at baseline to 27.3±8 at 2 weeks and to 21.7±10 at 4 weeks in the inositol group. Analysis of variance of the final improvement scores (baseline minus week 4) for all subjects showed that inositol reduced the HAM-D significantly more than the placebo did ($F_{1,26}$=4.48, P=0.04). This difference was not yet apparent after 2 weeks of treatment.

PANIC STUDY

Because some antidepressant agents are also effective against panic disorder, the authors also decided on a trial of inositol treatment for panic disorder (6). Patients previously on medications withdrew from them at least 1 week before commencing a formal washout period; only two patients actually withdrew from medications this close to the study. Patients were prepared to go off conventional treatments in the hope of finding a new treatment without troubling side effects. The only medication allowed beside inositol and the placebo was oral lorazepam, 1 mg, as needed for anxiety.

The placebo was mannitol (N=10; N, number of subjects) or glucose (N=11). The treatments were supplied in an identical-appearing white powder form with similar taste and solubility. Patients took 6 g of medication twice a day dissolved in juice. All subjects began with a 1-week run-in period on open placebo (N=10) or no medication (N=11). Thereafter, each patient was randomly assigned to double-blind placebo or inositol for 4 weeks; he or she then crossed over to the alternate substance for another 4 weeks. Patients completed daily panic diaries in which they recorded the occurrence of panic attacks, the number of symptoms (from the American Psychiatric Association's *Diagnostic and statistical manual of mental disorders*, 3rd edition [DSM-III-R] list) in each attack, and the subjective severity of each attack. Investigators reviewed the diaries at each weekly assessment and completed the Marks-Matthews Phobia Scale, HAM-D, and the Hamilton Rating Scale for Anxiety (HAM-A). A panic score was calculated by taking the mean of severity of attacks (range, 0 to 10) and the number of symptoms per attack and multiplying this average by the number of attacks per week. The results at the end of the run-in week were used as baseline measures.

Twenty-five patients were enrolled; 21 patients completed the study. Nine men and 12 women participated, with a mean age of 35.8 years (standard deviation [SD], 7 years). Five patients had panic disorder, and 16 had panic disorder with agoraphobia. The mean duration of illness was 3.9 years (SD, 3 years). Every outcome measure improved more on inositol than on the placebo. For number of panic attacks, panic scores, and phobia scores, this difference was significant. The effect of inositol appeared to be clinically meaningful; the number of attacks per week fell from approximately 10 to approximately six on placebo and to approximately three and one-half on inositol. Ten of the 21 subjects were classified as true inositol responders, and three were placebo responders.

OBSESSIVE-COMPULSIVE DISORDER STUDY

The role of serotonin (5-hydroxytryptamine [5-HT]) in obsessive compulsive disorder (OCD) is supported by the specific effectiveness of serotonin reuptake inhibition in this illness and the ability of serotonin agonists to exacerbate the syndrome. Rahman and Neuman (7) reported that desensitization of 5-HT receptors is reversed by the addition of exogenous inositol. The authors therefore planned a trial of inositol in OCD. Since anti-OCD doses of selective serotonin reuptake inhibitors (SSRIs) are usually higher than antidepressant doses, the authors chose to give 18 g per day of inositol in OCD (8).

Fifteen patients entered the trial; 13 completed the study and were included in data analysis. The trial was of crossover design, with 6 weeks in each phase. Six patients started the trial on the placebo and seven patients on inositol. Patients were drug free for at least 1 week before beginning the trial. No washout occurred between the phases of the crossover. The dose of inositol (18 g per day) was given as 2 teaspoons in juice three times daily; the placebo was glucose. OCD was assessed using the Yale-Brown Obsessive-Compulsive Scale (Y-BOCS). Ratings were performed at baseline and at 3, 6, 9, and 12 weeks. The mean age of the subjects was 33.7 years (23 to 56 years), and eight women and five men participated. Mean duration of illness was 8.1±5 years (range, 1 to 17 years). Five patients had responded well in the past to SSRIs; five had had partial responses; three had had poor responses. None met the criteria for major depression. Only lorazepam, up to 2 mg daily, was allowed in addition to the study drug.

Mean improvement from baseline to 6 weeks in the Y-BOCS on inositol was 5.9±5.0 and on placebo 3.5±2.8 (P=0.04, paired t test). For the obsessions subscale, the mean improvement on inositol was 3.0±2.8 versus placebo, 2.0±1.6 (P=0.12, NS). For the compulsions subscale, the mean improvement on inositol was 3.0±2.8 and for the placebo 1.5±1.4 (P=0.03). Patients who had previously responded to SSRIs also responded to inositol; those who had been resistant in the past were resistant to inositol as well.

BULIMIA AND BINGE-EATING STUDY

Bulimia nervosa (BN) is a highly prevalent, but severe, eating disorder characterized by recurrent episodes of binge eating followed by purging. Binge eating disorder (BED) is a related disorder characterized by recurrent episodes of binge eating without the excessive weight and shape concern of BN. Several studies have reported that SSRIs yield therapeutic benefits in BN (9) and BED (10). Because the indications of inositol so far appeared to parallel those of SSRIs, the authors performed a study of inositol in BN and BED (11). The dose of 12 to 18 g per day of inositol was of a caloric value that is equivalent to 2 teaspoons of table sugar and thus was of negligible dietary impact for eating disorder patients. Patients with anorexia nervosa or patients with a body mass index less than 18 were excluded. The trial was of double-blind crossover design. Additional psychoactive medication was not permitted. After 1 week of single-blind run-in placebo, patients were randomized to inositol or placebo for 6 weeks. At the end of 6 weeks, the patients were crossed over to the alternative treatment for an additional 6 weeks. Evaluations were based on those used in the fluoxetine multicenter bulimia study (12). Patients were evaluated at baseline and every 2 weeks thereafter with the Eating Attitude Test (EAT) (13), the Visual Analogue Scale (14) of severity of binge eating (VAS-B), the clinician-administered Clinical Global Impression (CGI) for severity, the Eating Disorders Inventory (EDI) (15), the HAM-D, and the HAM-A. Twelve patients completed the trial.

Results showed significant effects of inositol treatment on CGI (main effect of treatment: $F_{1,11}$=6.8, P=0.02, with a post-hoc effect at week 6, P=0.046) (Fig. 7.2) and VAS (drug × time interaction $F_{2,22}$=4.2, P=0.03; main effect of treatment: $F_{1,11}$=5.5, P=0.04), a borderline significant effect on the EDI, and no effect on the EAT. Results in the subgroup of BN patients (N=9) were similar, with VAS-B main effect of treatment $F_{1,8}$=4.3, P=0.07 and treatment by week interaction $F_{2,16}$=3.7, P=0.04. Using the VAS-B and a criterion of at least 50% improvement from baseline, five patients improved to criterion on inositol and only one did so on the placebo (χ^2=3.6, P<0.06).

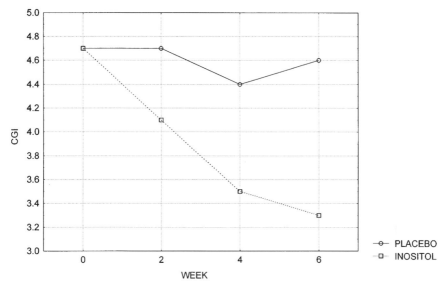

FIG. 7.2. The effect of inositol versus a placebo in bulimia on clinical global impression (CGI).

COMBINATION AND AUGMENTATION STUDIES OF INOSITOL WITH OTHER ANTIDEPRESSANT DRUGS

Antidepressant pharmacotherapy is ineffective in about one-third of depressed patients, and antidepressant medications take several weeks to ameliorate symptoms. Since several classes of antidepressant treatment exist, testing whether combinations of effective treatment might yield higher response rates or more rapid response than monotherapy has seemed logical. However, most studies show no advantage for a combination strategy in depression. This contrasts with the augmentation strategy in resistant depression (i.e., the second agent is added *after the failure of the first one* [16,17,18]). The failure of a second drug, which is effective by itself, to add benefit to a basic drug can possibly be taken as evidence that the two share a mechanism of action.

Inositol may act therapeutically in depression via the intracellular phosphatidyl inositol second messenger cycle, serving as a second messenger system for 5HT-2 receptors (see the following section). The SSRIs act via inhibition of serotonin reuptake within the synaptic cleft. The authors hypothesized that adding inositol to SSRIs might speed up the response to SSRIs or that it might significantly enhance the degree of patient response or the percentage of patients responding. Twenty-seven depressed patients completed a double-blind, controlled, 4-week trial of an SSRI plus a placebo or plus inositol (19). The HAM-D was used as an assessment tool at baseline and at 1, 2, 3, and 4 weeks. No significant difference was found between the two treatment groups. No serious side effects were exhibited by this combination compared to those with SSRI alone.

Similarly, current SSRI treatments for OCD provide only partial benefit. Given the positive previous study of inositol alone in OCD, ten *Diagnostic and statistical manual of mental disorders*, 4th edition (DSM-IV) OCD patients received 18 g of inositol for 6 weeks and a placebo for 6 weeks, in addition to ongoing SSRI treatment in a double-blind randomized crossover design. Weekly assessments included the YBOCS, the HAM-D, and the HAM-A. No significant difference was found between the two treatment phases (20).

The fact that lithium has proven to be of added value after 3 weeks of resistance to reuptake inhibition (16) suggests that changes in inositol metabolism via lithium inhibition of inositol monophosphatase could be involved in the amelioration of SSRI resistance. Thus the authors decided to study inositol therapy in a controlled design in an augmentation strategy in depressed patients failing a 3-week to 4-week trial of a SSRI, despite the absence of therapeutic benefit for inositol in the combination design (21). Patients could enter the study if they had had at least 3 weeks of treatment with an SSRI at clinically adequate doses (150 mg fluvoxamine, 20 mg fluoxetine, 20 mg paroxetine) and a score of at least 18 on the HAM-D (24-item scale), with, at most, mild improvement from the onset of SSRI treatment. They were randomly assigned to inositol, 12 g per day, or glucose. Forty-two patients entered the study. Twenty-three patients were treated with inositol augmentation of SSRI treatment; 19 patients were treated with SSRI and a placebo. Inositol had no effect for augmenting response to SSRIs. Thus, the study failed to find evidence that inositol might augment failed SSRI therapy in depression. Little improvement was seen in the first week, unlike what occurs with lithium augmentation where at least some patients show dramatic early improvement (17).

COMPARISON OF INOSITOL WITH A STANDARD SELECTIVE SEROTONIN REUPTAKE INHIBITOR

All previous controlled clinical studies compared inositol with a placebo. One consideration was that a direct comparison with an established drug would constitute a more severe test of efficacy. A double-blind, controlled, random-order, crossover study was undertaken to compare the effect of inositol with that of fluvoxamine in panic disorder (22). Twenty patients completed 1 month of inositol, to 18 g per day, and 1 month of fluvoxamine, to 150 mg per day. Improvements on the HAM-A scores, agoraphobia scores, and CGI scores were similar for both treatments (Fig. 7.3). In the first month, inositol reduced the number of panic attacks per week by 4.0±2, compared to a reduction of 2.4±2 on fluvoxamine (P=0.049). Analysis of 9 weeks of treatment showed no differences between the improvement on inositol and on fluvoxamine or between these effects in those who began with one or the other treatment on HAM-A and phobia scores. No main effects of the order of treatment or of the drug were observed on the change in frequency of panic attacks or in the CGI score, but significant interactions did occur between these factors on these two measures. Patients beginning on ino-

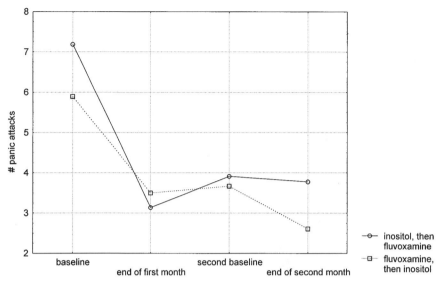

FIG. 7.3. Comparison of fluvoxamine versus inositol in panic disorder.

sitol had greater reductions in the number of panic attacks during inositol treatment than did those beginning on fluvoxamine during fluvoxamine treatment; during the second month, additional improvements were small and similar in both groups. Nausea and tiredness were more common on fluvoxamine than on inositol ($P=0.02$ and $P=0.01$, respectively); no side effect was more common on inositol than on fluvoxamine.

INDICATIONS FOR WHICH INOSITOL IS NOT EFFECTIVE

The spectrum of indications previously described bears a valid resemblance to that of antidepressant medications. The author's group has also examined the efficacy of inositol in schizophrenia, dementia, electroconvulsive treatment–induced memory impairment, attention deficit hyperactivity disorder (ADHD), and autism. Inositol showed no beneficial effects for these indications (23).

POSSIBLE MECHANISM OF ACTION

Inositol is a precursor for phosphatidyl-inositol (PI) biphosphate (Fig. 7.4). Cleavage of the phosphatidyl bond releases inositol triphosphate (IP_3) and diacylglycerol (DAG); the former stimulates release of calcium (Ca^{2+}), and the latter activates protein kinase C. These are second messengers. Cleavage of successive phosphates from IP_3 by inositol monophosphatase yields free inositol.

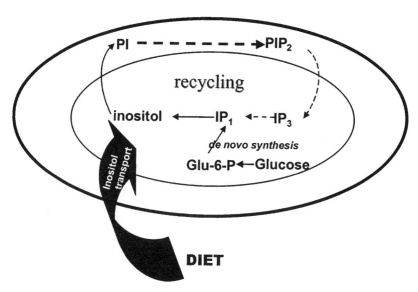

FIG. 7.4. Sources of inositol for cellular signaling. Abbreviations: Glu-6-P, glucose-6-phosphate; IP$_1$, inositol monophosphate; IP$_3$, inositol 1,4,5-triphosphate; PI, phosphatidyl inositol; PIP$_2$, phosphatidyl inositol diphosphate.

This sequence constitutes the PI cycle. Receptors for which the PI cycle is the second messenger system include cholinergic muscarinic, noradrenergic α1 (NA$_{\alpha 1}$) , 5-HT$_{2A}$ and 5-HT$_{2C}$, and dopaminergic D$_1$ receptors. The antidepressant effects of inositol in the Porsolt swim test animal model (see below) are blocked by a 5-HT antagonist and a 5-HT synthesis inhibitor but not by an NA toxin (24).

If SSRIs affect 5-HT$_{2A}$ and 5-HT$_{2C}$ receptors via effects on the 5-HT transporter, and this in turn induces chronic intracellular second messenger adaptations, then inositol might theoretically work more quickly by bypassing the synaptic change(s) that precede(s) the intracellular adaptation. In other words, the second messenger system is being directly affected without the need for changes in the function of the first messenger (the neurotransmitter). The authors have not found this to be the case. Acute administration of SSRIs often exacerbates anxiety in panic disorder (25), while chronic administration can block the anxiety induced by classic panicogens, such as lactate, carbon dioxide, and the 5-HT agonist mCPP (26). The authors gave a single 20-g dose of inositol 10 hours before challenging seven patients with panic disorder with 0.08 mg per kg of intravenous mCPP in a crossover placebo-controlled trial (26). mCPP had robust anxiogenic effects. No differences after acute pretreatment with inositol were observed compared to the placebo. A similar trial after chronic inositol has not been performed. Similarly, the authors saw no early effects of inositol in the positive studies of depression, panic, OCD, and bulimia. Conceivably, the later, intracellular changes following acute SSRI effects are the ones that are critical to their mechanism of action. The same unknown mechanism(s) might be required for inositol to take effect and might result in similar time courses of action.

ANIMAL MODELS

Inositol has been used in two animal models of depression. Reserpine-induced hypoactivity (27) is a pharmacologic model and is used to screen for new antidepressant drugs; typical antidepressants reverse the reserpine-induced hypoactivity. The Porsolt forced swim test (28) is a behavioral model; immobility and abandoning the struggle to remain afloat are depressive equivalents, and antidepressant agents reduce these effects. In the Porsolt test, Sprague-Dawley rats received 10% inositol or glucose-mannitol (control) in rat chow (29). The immobility time was reduced by inositol ($P<0.001$) (Fig. 7.5). In the reserpine-induced hypoactivity test, animals received intraperitoneal injections of 1.2 g per kg of inositol or the control (29). Immobility time after 0.25 mg per kg of reserpine was reduced by inositol compared to that in controls ($P <0.001$).

Inositol has been studied in an animal model of anxiety. The plus-maze (30) compares the frequency with which rodents enter the exposed and the closed arms of a maze and the amount of time they spend in these arms. Open arms are naturally aversive for rodents. Cohen et al. (31) gave rats daily intraperitoneal injections of inositol, 1.25 mg per kg, for 14 days. Rats treated with inositol spent significantly more time in the open arms than did control rats.

Inositol had no effect in the following two animal models of schizophrenia: amphetamine-induced hyperactivity and apomorphine-induced stereotypy (32). Thus, animal studies support the clinical studies in suggesting a spectrum similar to that of SSRIs. Inositol has not been studied in an animal model of OCD.

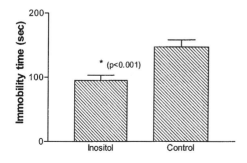

FIG. 7.5. The effect of inositol on immobility in the Porsolt test in the rat.

SIDE EFFECTS

Side effects in seven studies, all of which used a dose of 12 g per day, were reviewed by Belmaker et al. (33). Safety data in 107 patients, 61 of whom had had full laboratory assessments, revealed changes in blood chemistry in two patients, namely, mild increases in glucose. Other effects were flatus in two, nausea in one, and sleepiness and insomnia in two patients each. Studies performed since then (excluding those involving the coadministration of inositol with other agents) have included the bulimia study and the comparison with fluvoxamine in panic disorder (total N=33), both of which used a dose of 18 g per day, which was an increase of 150% over the dose in previous studies. Side effects on inositol in these studies were flatus in five patients, nausea in eight patients, dizziness in three patients, and sleepiness and headache in one patient each. All of these effects were mild. In the comparison with fluvoxamine (22), inositol was better tolerated (for nausea, the comparison showed $P=0.02$; for sleepiness, $P=0.01$).

EFFECTS ON NORMAL PERSONS

Only one small study of inositol (34) in normal volunteers has been done. Eleven volunteers were given a single dose of 12 g of inositol or a placebo in a randomized, crossover, double-blind design, with treatments separated by 1 week. Profiles of mood states showed a strong trend for inositol to reduce depression, hostility, tension, and fatigue compared with the placebo over 6 hours. This effect was significant in those normal individuals with high baseline depression or tension scores. These results are consistent with the traditional use of inositol as a folk remedy for anxiety and sadness.

SUMMARY

Present findings are consistent with the idea that inositol could be a natural substitute for an SSRI as follows: it is effective for depression, panic disorder, OCD, and bulimia; it is no faster in action than SSRIs; it has no additional benefit in combination or augmentation of SSRIs; it has equal efficacy in direct comparison with fluvoxamine; and it displays no beneficial effects in psychoses, ADHD, and autism. That nonresponders to SSRIs for OCD also failed to respond to inositol is disappointing, whereas those who had previously responded to SSRIs also responded to inositol in the same trial. Table 7.1 shows effect sizes (in SDs) of inositol and a placebo in studies of depression, panic disorder, OCD, and bulimia. The activity of inositol in animal models of depression allows further mechanistic study of its action. Synthetic derivatives of inositol could conceivably be more active than the parent compound and could constitute a novel direction of antidepressant research.

TABLE 7.1. *Effect sizes of placebo and inositol in five studies*

Study	Placebo	Inositol
Depression	0.52	1.53
Panic disorder	0.22	0.50
OCD	0.45	0.79
Bulimia	0.43	1.26
Panic disorder (comparison with fluvoxamine)	—	1.09
Mean	0.41	1.03

ES was calculated for each arm of each study as the difference in the main outcome measure from baseline to final assessment, divided by the pooled standard deviation for that measure in the relevant study. For additional efficacy estimations for the first three studies, see Levine J. Controlled trials of inositol in psychiatry. *Eur Neuropsychopharmacol* 1997; 7:147–155.

Abbreviations: ES, effect sizes; OCD, obsessive-compulsive disorder.

(From Cohen H, Kotter M, Kaplan Z, et al. Inositol administration has centrally-mediated behavioral effects with adaptation after chronic administration. *J Neural Transm* 1997;104:299–305, with permission.)

REFERENCES

1. Parfitt K, ed. *The complete drug reference*, 32nd ed. London: Pharmaceutical Press, 1999.
2. Berridge MD, Downes CP, Hanley MR. Neural and developmental action of lithium: a unifying hypothesis. *Cell* 1989;59:411–419.
3. Barkai A, Dunner DL, Gross HA, et al. Reduced myo-inositol levels in cerebrospinal fluid from patients with affective disorder. *Biol Psychiatry* 1978;13:65–72.
4. Levine J, Gonzalves M, Barbam I, et al. Inositol 6 gm daily may be effective in depression but not in schizophrenia. *Hum Psychopharmacol* 1993;8:49–53.
5. Levine J, Barak Y, Gonzalves M, et al. Double blind controlled trial of inositol treatment of depression. *Am J Psychiatry* 1995;152:792–794.
6. Benjamin J, Levine J, Fux M, et al. Double-blind, placebo-controlled, crossover study of inositol treatment for panic disorder. *Am J Psychiatry* 1995;152:1084–1086.
7. Rahman S, Neuman R. Myo-inositol reduces serotonin (5-HT2) receptor induced homologous and heterologous desensitization. *Brain Res* 1993;631:349–351.
8. Fux M, Levine J, Aviv A, Belmaker RH. Inositol treatment of obsessive-compulsive disorder. *Am J Psychiatry* 1996;153:1219–1221.
9. Kaye W, Gendall K, Strober M. Serotonin neuronal function and selective serotonin reuptake inhibitor treatment in anorexia and bulimia nervosa. *Biol Psychiatry* 1998;44:825–838.
10. Hudson JI, McElroy SL, Raymond NC, et al. Fluvoxamine in the treatment of binge-eating disorder: a multicenter placebo-controlled, double-blind trial. *Am J Psychiatry* 1998;155:1756–1762.
11. Gelber D, Levine J, Belmaker RH. Effect of inositol on bulimia nervosa and binge eating. *Int J Eating Disord* 2001;29:345–348.
12. Fluoxetine bulimia nervosa collaborative study group. Fluoxetine in the treatment of bulimia nervosa: a multi center, placebo controlled, double blind study. *Arch Gen Psychiatry* 1992;49:139–147.
13. Garner DM, Olmstead MP, Bohr Y, et al. The eating attitude test: psychometric features and clinical correlates. *Psychol Med* 1982;12:871–878.

14. McCormak HM, Horne DJ, Sheather S. Clinical applications of visual analogue scales: a critical review. *Psychol Med* 1998;18:1007–1009.

15. Garner DM, Olmstead MP, Plivy J. Development and validation of multidimensional eating disorder inventory for anorexia nervosa and bulimia. *Int J Eating Disord* 1983;2:15–34.

16. de Montigny C, Grunberg P, Mayer A, et al. Lithium induces a rapid relief of depression in tricyclic antidepressants drug non responders. *Br J Psychiatry* 1981;138:252.

17. de Montigny C, Cournoyer G, Morissette R, et al. Lithium carbonate addition in tricyclic antidepressant-resistant unipolar depression. *Arch Gen Psychiatry* 1983;40:1327–1334.

18. de Montigny C, Elie R, Caille G. Rapid response to the addition of lithium in iprindole-resistant unipolar depression: a pilot study. *Am J Psychiatry* 1985;142:220–223.

19. Levine J, Mishory A, Susnosky S, Martin M, Belmaker RH. Combination of inositol and serotonin reuptake inhibitors in the treatment of depression. *Biol Psychiatry* 1999;45:270–273.

20. Fux M, Benjamin J, Belmaker RH. Inositol versus placebo augmentation of serotonin reuptake inhibitors in the treatment of obsessive-compulsive disorder: a double blind crossover study. *Int J Neuropsychopharmocol* 1999;2:193–195.

21. Nemets B, Mishory A, Levine J, Belmaker RH. Inositol addition does not improve depression in SSRI treatment failures. *J Neural Trans* 1999;106:795–798.

22. Palatnick A, Frolov K, Fux M, Benjamin J. Double-blind controlled crossover trial of inositol versus fluvoxamine in panic disorder. *J Clin Psychopharmacol* 2001;21:335–339.

23. Levine J. Controlled trials of inositol in psychiatry. *Eur Neuropsychopharmacol* 1997;7:147–155.

24. Einat H, Clenet F, Shaldubina A, et al. The antidepressant activity of inositol in the forced swim test involves 5-HT2 receptors. *Behav Brain Res* 2001;118:77–83.

25. Ramos R, Gentil V, Gorenstein C. Clomipramine and initial worsening in panic disorder: beyond the jitteriness syndrome. *J Psychopharmacol* 1993;7:265–269.

26. Benjamin J, Nemetz B, Fux M, et al. Acute inositol does not attenuate m-CPP-induced anxiety, mydriasis and endocrine effects in panic disorder. *J Psychiatr Res* 1997;3:489–495.

27. Bourin M. Is it possible to predict the activity of a new antidepressant in animals with simple psychopharmacological tests? *Fund Clin Pharmacol* 1990;4:49–64.

28. Porsolt RD, Anton G, Blavet N, Jalfre M. Behavioral despair in rats, a new model sensitive to antidepressant treatments. *Eur J Pharmacol* 1978;47:379–391.

29. Einat H, Karbovski H, Korik J, et al. Inositol reduces depressive-like behaviors in two different animal models of depression. *Psychopharmacol* 1999;144:158–162.

30. Rodgers RJ. Animal models of anxiety: where next? *Behav Pharmacol* 1997;8:477–496.

31. Cohen H, Kotler M, Kaplan Z, et al. Inositol administration has centrally-mediated behavioral effects with adaptation after chronic administration. *J Neural Transm* 1997;104:299–305.

32. Einat H, Belmaker RH. The effects of inositol treatment in animal models of psychiatric disorders. *J Affect Disord* 2001;62:113–121.

33. Belmaker RH, Bersudsky Y, Benjamin J, et al. Manipulation of inositol-linked second messenger systems as a therapeutic strategy in psychiatry. In: Gessa GL, Fratta W, Pani L, Serra G (eds). *Depression and mania: from neurobiology to treatment.* New York: Raven Press, 1995:67–84.

34. Levine J, Pomerantz T, Belmaker RH. The effect of inositol on cognitive processes and mood states in normal volunteers. *Eur Neuropsychopharmacol* 1994;4:418–419.

PART II

Treatment of Anxiety and Sleep Disorders

8

Homeopathy, Kava, and Other Herbal Treatments for Anxiety

Kathryn M. Connor and Jonathan R.T. Davidson

INTRODUCTION

In 1993, Eisenberg et al. (1) observed that approximately one-third of the United States population was using complementary and alternative medicine (CAM), either through professional prescription or via over-the-counter and self-administration. Importantly, in this study, anxiety was one of the most frequent diagnoses in people who were seeing their regular medical doctor and who also admitted using CAM treatments. In a recent survey, Astin (2) also found that anxiety-related problems were common reasons for subjects using CAM. Jacobs and Crothers (3) observed that anxiety neurosis and stress reactions were high in the list of diagnostic categories among subjects seeking treatment in their homoeopathic practices. Davidson et al. (4) assessed the psychiatric diagnoses of 83 subjects presenting for complementary medical treatment in the United Kingdom and the United States and found that anxiety disorders were present in 25% of their sample, with generalized anxiety being the most common. Given the further growth of popular interest and consumption of complementary treatments since 1993, one may make the assertion that the use of CAM for anxiety disorders represents an important public health issue. Recently, Knaudt et al. (5) found that, among psychiatric outpatients with depression or anxiety, 54% had used some form of CAM regularly in the previous year, with the use of herbal treatments (38%) being most common. Their general attitude regarding the benefits for CAM was favorable. Further information is clearly needed as to the foundation and efficacy of CAM, as well as to its overall contribution to the welfare of those who suffer from anxiety disorders. Two particularly well established methods of treatment are those deriving from the homoeopathic system of medicine, as well as the use of phytochemicals (botanical preparations).

HOMOEOPATHIC TREATMENT FOR ANXIETY

As a system of therapeutics, homeopathy has stood up to the test of time, and after almost being persecuted out of existence, it is now making a modest resurgence, particularly outside of North America (6). Nonetheless, the field remains poorly understood and quickly dismissed. Perhaps the most obvious reason for its apparent absurdity is the fact that many homeopathic medicines contain no material substance beyond water, yet they are claimed to be therapeutically effective. Paradoxically, the proponents of homeopathy would even go so far as to say that the more dilute the remedy, the more potent it becomes. Leaving aside this admittedly major objection, a number of interesting parallels are found between homeopathy and psychiatry (7).

The Principle of Similars

A central belief of homeopathy is that like is cured by like. This means that the most effective treatment for a particular clinical state is the treatment that induces these same symptoms when given at higher doses in healthy individuals (6). Parallels to this phenomenon exist in psychiatry, particularly with respect to dynamic psychotherapies and cognitive and behavioral treatments. For instance, in anxiety, psychotherapy usually strives to induce graduated levels of the symptoms for which the person is seeking help, in the belief that exposure to these symptoms will ultimately lead to their reduction or elimination. Inducing breathlessness or palpitations, which occurs in panic control treatment for panic disorder, is a good example. An example of this principle at work with biologic treatments in psychiatry is the use of sleep deprivation to treat depression, in which sleep loss is one of the cardinal symptoms (8).

The Principle of Self-Healing

Homeopathy teaches that symptoms represent the body's attempt to restore health or balance in the face of a pathologic challenge. This is referred to as the *self-healing principle* and is thought to reflect the working of an underlying vital force in the organism. An interesting recent neurobiologic parallel has been advanced by Post and Weiss (9), who opined that some symptoms of major depression could be the body's attempt to self-treat and induce restitution in response to the disease process. In other words, symptoms might be seen as "good guys" rather than "bad guys." Perhaps, they say, the symptoms are compensatory or adaptive. They offer some examples with respect to changes in the hypothalamo-pituitary-thyroid axis, from this perspective.

The Rollback Phenomenon

Constantine Hering, a leading homeopath in the 19th century and the founder of Hahnemann Medical College in Philadelphia, noted that symptoms tend to remit in the reverse order of their appearance, a term referred to as rollback. Detre and Jarecki (10) have observed the same phenomenon in psychiatry with respect to affective disorders.

Recognition of Patterns

Lastly, homeopathic practice is based on the total clinical picture, or recognition of patterns. These patterns constitute symptoms, signs, temperamental characteristics, behaviors, emotions, attitudes, taste, and physical preferences. For the most part, psychiatry still remains a pattern-based practice that certainly pays acknowledgment to the importance of features beyond symptoms. For example, in a scale predictive of the response to electroconvulsive therapy (11), inclusion of the pyknic body type is seen as a positive predictor and hysterical personality features as a negative predictor. Equally, tendencies to show rejection sensitivity as a premorbid personality trait have been linked to the positive effects of monoamine oxidase inhibitors in depression (12). While the extent to which today's psychiatry has retained the value of pattern recognition in this sense is unclear, it has certainly done so in the past; and the different effects of noradrenergic and serotonergic drugs suggest that psychiatry is reawakening its awareness to such things.

With the previous considerations as background, perhaps a convincing case can be made to examine whether homeopathic treatments have anything to offer in psychiatry. Unfortunately, not a single controlled double-blind trial has been conducted to date, and the authors' group set about acquiring some preliminary experience with this form of treatment in an open-label, clinical use framework.

In 12 patients with anxiety or depression, homeopathic treatment was either added to conventional therapy or offered as monotherapy. Treatment ranged from 7 to 18 weeks according to the patient, and response was measured by means of a Clinical Global scale (CGI), the SCL-90 self-rating, or the Brief Social Phobia Scale (BSPS). Patients were treated in accordance with typical homeopathic clinical practice, meaning that a careful and detailed individual assessment was initially completed, upon which the remedy of choice was selected. Six of 12 patients responded well on the CGI; this was also the case using the secondary outcome measures, such as Symptom Checklist (SCL-90) or BSPS. The results of this study were reported previously (13) and suggested that, under some circumstances, subjects could benefit from such treatment. In a number of cases, the remedy selected changed over time, according to the salience of particular symptoms. Whether the patient had specifically requested such treatment or whether the practitioner recommended it to patients made little difference to the outcome.

Overall, while the results were somewhat encouraging, this investigator felt that a response of 50% in an open-label trial fell short of what is typically seen in many open-label studies. Whether this was a reflection of the elements of chronicity or treatment resistance in the sample is not clear, but one could certainly say that many of the subjects responded well to subsequent treatment with conventional therapy. This, of course, leads to the next suggestion, which is the importance of conducting a clinical trial in which homeopathy is compared to conventional antidepressant drug therapy and a placebo. To the authors' knowledge, no such trials are under consideration for anxiety disorder.

HERBAL TREATMENT FOR ANXIETY

Kava

A considerable increase in the use of phytochemicals for treating psychiatric conditions has occurred. In the case of anxiety disorders, the best known and most popular of these plant-derived medicines is Kava kava, or *Piper methysticum*. The medicine is derived from the root of this plant, which is native to the Pacific Islands. In Polynesian tribes, kava was traditionally prepared by virgins, who chewed kava roots, placed the mash in a fermenting pot, and prepared a hot tealike drink for the tribe members.

Approximately 200 years ago, investigators noted the relaxing effect of kava liquid obtained from the roots of the *P. methysticum* plant. The presumed active anxiolytic ingredients were subsequently isolated by Hansel (14); they include the following so-called kava-lactones: kavain, methysticin, yangonin, dihydro-kavain, dihydro-methysticin, and desmethoxy-yangonin.

An extensive animal literature suggests that the possible sites and mechanism of action for kava relate to its effect as a glutamate suppressant, its effects on the sodium and calcium voltage–dependent channels, or possibly its γ-aminobutyric acid–like (GABAergic) effects (15–17). Kava also possibly enhances the effects of 5-hydroxytryptamine (5-HT)1A agonists (18). Based on animal studies, one would expect that kava is anxiolytic, that tolerance and withdrawal would be unlikely, and that the drug may work through the inhibition of sodium or calcium channels via an antiglutamate effect or GABAergic effects. Possible serotonergic effects are also under consideration.

Kava has been studied in double-blind clinical trials in Europe, which have suggested that clinical benefits are evident as early as 4 weeks (19,20) and that the effect is sustained over several months of therapy (21). A 25-week multicenter, randomized, placebo-controlled, double-blind trial with a special extract of kava assessed 101 outpatients suffering from different types of *Diagnostic and statistic manual for mental disorders*, 3rd edition, (DSM-III-R) anxiety disorders, including agoraphobia, specific phobia, generalized anxiety disorder, and adjustment disorder with anxiety. In various anxiety scales, a significant superiority of kava appeared from week 8 onward (22), compared to the placebo. More recently, a 4-week placebo-controlled study of kava by Singh et al. (23) showed substantially greater effects for kava than for a placebo on symptoms of daily stress in symptomatic volunteers without an axis I disorder.

Relative to the benzodiazepine oxazepam, kava seems to be equally effective (24) but without many of the problems associated with benzodiazepines, such as sedation and decrement in performance. Herberg (25) found that kava did not potentiate performance-impairing alcohol effects but that it did enhance concentration in those receiving kava and alcohol, compared to those who received the placebo and alcohol.

Side effects from kava are uncommon; they may include gastrointestinal upset, allergic skin reactions, headaches, and dizziness (21,26). However, toxic reactions with very high doses (up to 300–400 g per week) have been reported; these include ataxia, skin rash, hair loss, redness of the eyes, problems with visual accommodation, respiratory problems, loss of appetite, and acute hepatitis (21,27,28). In many of these cases, the doses were at least 100 times higher than those typically consumed.

Prolonged use of kava may cause kava dermopathy (29), a transient yellowing of the skin. A survey of Aboriginal kava users (30) found that kava users were more likely to complain of poor health and a puffy face and to have a typical scaly rash and slightly increased patellar reflexes. Other characteristics of heavy kava users included subnormal weight, abnormal liver function test results, hematuria, poorly acidified urine, and abnormal blood indices. Shortness of breath in kava users was associated with tall P waves on a resting electrocardiogram, suggesting possible pulmonary hypertension. Some reports of adverse interactions between kava and benzodiazepines do exist (31).

The above toxic effects are generally reversible if the use of kava is discontinued. Nonetheless, the duration of kava use is not recommended to exceed 3 months (32). No studies address the question of safety in pregnancy, and for this reason, kava is not recommended for use in pregnant women.

The studies reviewed suggest that kava may be more effective than a placebo for mild anxiety states, but it does not appear to be helpful for panic disorder or for more severe anxiety states. Major problems with the published studies of kava in anxiety include a failure to define the diagnostic group systematically or to stipulate which diagnostic criteria were used. In any case, kava was well tolerated in these trials, and patient dropout was minimal. While kava seems to be safe in combination with other compounds, the full profile of possible herb-drug and herb–herb interactions for kava needs to be better understood.

Although kava appears to be effective at doses ranging from 60 to 300 mg kava lactones per day (32), the effect of different doses of kava is unknown, as are the minimum or maximum doses for use in anxiety or for safety with long-term use (e.g., greater than 25 weeks). *The recommended maximum dose is unnecessarily low.* More placebo-controlled controlled studies and studies comparing kava to the conventional anxiolytics are needed to better clarify kava's safety and efficacy. Comprehensive accounts of kava can be found elsewhere (33).

Other Medications

While other herbal products have traditional uses in treating anxiety disorders, currently a lack of empirical data about these exists; the authors see the field as one in which considerable activity may be expected in the years ahead. A limited literature can be found and is summarized here. Among other studies, an interesting report has been made of the fact that, in traffic-related stress, valerian is more effective than a placebo in a double-blind, placebo-controlled, single-dose trial (34). The benefits reported included increased performance and reduced tremor and tension. Traditionally, valerian has been used for sleep disturbances, which are commonly reported in those with anxiety disorders. Thus, further study of possible antianxiety effects for valerian is encouraged (valerian is reviewed in detail in Chapter 9).

In a study by Bourin et al. (35), the combination herbal product Euphytose, which contains valerian, passion flower, crataegus, ballota, cola, and Paullina, was more effective than the placebo in adjustment disorder with anxious mood.

One further possible application of an herbal product for anxiety is suggested by Taylor and Kobak (36), who found a promising effect of St. John's wort in an open-label trial of obsessive-compulsive disorder. Given that St. John's wort has demonstrated serotonergic activity, this stands to reason and warrants further investigation.

Other herbal remedies, such as passion flower, hops, and lemon balm, are widely used in central Europe for anxiety, but empirical data to support these practices are lacking.

CONCLUSIONS

Public and professional interest in complementary and alternative treatments for anxiety is growing; it is focused particularly in the areas of homeopathy and herbal medicine. Much more information is needed as to the efficacy, safety, tolerance, and relative merits of such treatments compared to that of the standard drugs available and the proven effectiveness of psychotherapy. Also, establishing guidelines as to when an individual is justified in self-treating and when seeking professional help are more appropriate are important. For physicians to become more familiar and skillful in the use of herbal medicines, training, which is sorely lacking at present, needs to be made available.

REFERENCES

1. Eisenberg DM, Kessler RC, Foster C, et al. Unconventional medicine in the United States. *New Engl J Med* 1993;328:246–252.
2. Astin JA. Why patients use alternative medicine: results of a national study. *JAMA* 1998;279: 1548–1553.
3. Jacobs J, Crothers D. Who sees homeopaths? *Br J Homeopathy* 1991;80:57–58.
4. Davidson JR, Rampes H, Eisen M, et al. Psychiatric disorders in primary care patients receiving complementary medical treatments. *Compr Psychiatry* 1998;39:16–20.
5. Knaudt PR, Connor KM, Weisler RH, et al. Alternative therapy use by psychiatric outpatients. *J Nerv Ment Dis* 1999;187:692–695.
6. Ullman D. *Discovering homeopathy: medicine for the 21st century*. Berkeley, CA: North Atlantic Books, 1991:16–18.
7. Davidson JRT. Psychiatry and homoeopathy: basis for a dialogue. *Br Homoeopathic J* 1994;83:78–83.
8. Wu JC, Bunney WE Jr. The biological basis of an antidepressant response to sleep deprivation and relapse: review and hypothesis. *Am J Psychiatry* 1990;147:14–21.
9. Post RM, Weiss SRB. Endogenous biochemical abnormalities in affective illness: therapeutic versus pathogenic. *Biol Psychiatry* 1992;32:469–484.
10. Detre TP, Jarecki HG. *Modern psychiatric treatment*. Philadelphia: Lippincott, 1971:53–54.
11. Roth M, Gurney C, Mountjoy CQ. The Newcastle rating scales. *Acta Psychiatr Scand* 1993;310:42–54.
12. Quitkin FM, Harrison WM, Liebowitz MR, et al. Delineating the boundaries of atypical depression. *J Clin Psychiatry* 1984;45:19–21.

13. Davidson JRT, Morrison RM, Shore J, et al. Homeopathic treatment of depression and anxiety. *Alt Ther Health Med* 1997;3:46–49.
14. Hänsel R. Therapie mit phytopharmaka. *Deutsche Apoth Z* 1964;104:459.
15. Glietz J, Fricse J, Beile A, et al. Anticonvulsant action of (+1-) kavain estimated from its properties on stimulated symptoms and Na⁺ channel receptor sites. *Eur J Pharmacol* 1996;315:89–97.
16. Glietz J, Fiele A, Peters T. (+1-)-kavain inhibits veratridine-activated voltage-dependent Na⁺-channels in synaptoptosomes prepared from rat cerebral cortex. *Neuropharmacology* 1995;34:1133–1138.
17. Jussofie A, Schmiz A, Hiemke C. Kavapyrone enriched extract from Piper methysticum as modulator of the GABA binding site in different regions of the rat brain. *Psychopharmacology* 1994;16:469–474.
18. Walden J, von Wagener J, Winter U, et al. Effects of kavain and dihydromethysticum on field potential changes in the hippocampus. *Prog Neuropsycholopharmacol Biol Psychiatry* 1997;21:697–706.
19. Lehmann E, Kinzler E, Friedemann J. Efficacy of a special kava extract (Piper methysticum) in patients with states of anxiety, tension and excitedness of non-mental origin. *Phytomedicine* 1996;2:113–119.
20. Warneke G. Psychosomatische dysfunction en im weiblichen klimakterium. Klimische wirksamkeit und vertraplichkeit van kava-extrakt WS-1490. *Fortsch Med* 1991;109:119–122.
21. Volz HP, Kieser M. Kava-kava extract WS-1490 versus placebo in anxiety disorders. A randomized placebo-controlled 25-week outpatient trial. *Pharmacopsychiatry* 1997;30:1–5.
22. Kinzler E, Kromer J, Lehmann E. Effect of a special kava extract in patients with anxiety, tension, and excitation states of non-psychotic genesis. Double blind study with placebos over 4 weeks. *Arzneimittel Forsch* 1991;41:584–588.
23. Singh NN, Ellis CR, Singh YN. *A double-blind, placebo-controlled study of the effects of kava (Kavatrol) on daily stress and anxiety in adults.* Presented at the 3rd annual Alternative Therapies Symposium. San Diego, April 1998.
24. Lindenberg D, Pitule-Schodel H. [D,L-kavain in comparison with oxazepam in anxiety disorders. A double-blind study of clinical effectiveness]. *Fortschr Med* 1990;108:49–50, 53–54.
25. Herberg KN. Effects of kava-special extract (WS 1490) combined with ethyl alcohol on safety-relevant performance parameters. *Blutalkohol* 1993;30:96–105.
26. Hansel R, Keller K, Rimpler H, Schneider G, eds. *Hagers handbuch der pharmazeutischen praxis,* 6th ed. New York: Springer Verlag, 1994:201–221, 268–292.
27. Strahl S, Ehret V, Dahm HH, Maier KP. Necrotizing hepatitis after taking herbal remedies. *Dtsch Med Wochenschr* 1998;123:1410–1414.
28. Miller LG. Herbal medicinals: selected clinical considerations focusing on known or potential drug-herb interactions. *Arch Intern Med* 1998;158:2200–2211.
29. Norton SA, Ruze P. Kava dermopathy. *J Am Acad Dermatol* 1994;31:89–97.
30. Mathews JD, Riley MD, Fejo L, et al. Effects of the heavy usage of kava on physical health: summary of a pilot survey in an aboriginal community. *Med J Aust* 1988;148:548–555.
31. Almeida JC, Grimsley EW. Coma from the health food store: interaction between kava and alprazolam [letter]. *Ann Intern Med* 1996;125:940–941.
32. Schulz V, Hansel R, Tyler VE. *Rational phytotherapy: a physicians' guide to herbal medicine,* 4th ed. Berlin: Springer, 2001.
33. Connor KM, Vaughan DS. *Kava: nature's stress relief.* New York: Avon Books, 1999.
34. Moser L. Arzneimittel bei stress am steur? *Deutsche Apoth Z* 1981;121:2651–2654.
35. Bourin M, Bougerol T, Guitton B, Broutin E. A combination of plant extracts in the treatment of outpatients with adjustment disorder with anxious mood: controlled study versus placebo. *Fund Clin Pharmacol* 1997;11:127–132.
36. Taylor L, Kobak KA. *An open-label trial of St. John's wort in obsessive-compulsive disorder.* Poster presentation at the National Institutes of Health (NIH) New Clinical Drug Evaluation Unit (NCDEU) meeting. Boca Raton, Florida, June 1999.

9

Valerian: Its Value as a Sedative Hypnotic

Roberto A. Dominguez

INTRODUCTION

Interest in the medicinal use of botanical products is rising. In the United States, approximately 1,800 herbal remedies are now available, and recent estimates project an annual increase of 25% in sales. In Europe, the pharmacopeia of herbal medicine is more advanced and better organized (1). For example, decades ago in Germany, the Federal Health Agency formed Commission E. This group's mandate was to combine the efforts of scientists and practitioners to assess the efficacy of and to propagate the safe use of these products. More than 300 monographs, describing constituents and preparations, modes of administration, dosage, indications, and the adverse effects of botanicals have been published. In Germany, the natural product market exceeds 3.0 billion dollars annually. Other European countries where botanical remedies are popular include the United Kingdom, Italy, The Netherlands, Belgium, and Spain (2).

A large number of plants have putative sedative properties. A short list would include almonds, oats, poppy seed, hops, chamomile, skullcap, Indian hemp, Melissa, passion flower, and valerian. Of these, the sedative and calmative properties of valerian are one of the best studied (3). The name valerian is thought to be derived from the Latin *valere*, which means "to be in good health." It is a perennial plant, 3 to 5 feet tall, whose many species grow in temperate and temperate-to-warm climates throughout the world. Valerian's flowers, which typically bloom during the summer months, are mostly white or pale pink. Approximately 200 species have been identified (4). One of the most common is the *edulis*, or Mexican valerian. Others include valerian *wallichi* (Indian valerian) and *faurei* (Japanese valerian) (5). Valerian is also commonly referred to in the German literature as "Baldrian" (3).

BACKGROUND

The most common species of valerian used for its medicinal purposes is *Valeriana officinalis*, or common valerian. The *officinalis* variety is cultivated mostly in western Europe. Its unique odor comes from volatile oils, which most regard as unpleasant or even repugnant. For this reason some patients immediately decline its use. However, some regular users find it aromatic. Nevertheless, the odor from a closed bottle of valerian can easily permeate the volume of a small drawer. Users also describe its distinctive and unpleasant taste and aftertaste.

More than 100 over-the-counter preparations of valerian are available throughout the world. Commercial preparations are often combined with other botanicals. Valerian is blended with passion flower, Melissa, hypericum, or kava because these natural products are also reported to have sedative, calmative, or other psychotropic effects. It is most commonly promoted as a sedative-hypnotic (6), but some use it for the relief of anxiety (7). Historically, it was typically ingested as a tea, but today valerian is readily available as tablets and capsules at the health food store, pharmacy, large discount stores, and even at the corner supermarket.

CHEMICAL PROFILE

The fragments of the valerian plant that yield its putative medicinal properties are its rhizome and roots. Their chemical constituents can vary widely depending on the species or the mixture of species blended within a preparation. In addition, the extraction methods employed and the geographical region where the plants were cultivated influence its chemistry even when they are of the same species. Valerians' chemical constituents can be divided into the following four major groups: (a) monoterpenes and sesquiterpenes, which include bornyl acetate, valerenic acid and its derivatives, isovaleric acid, valeranone, and valerenal; (b) iridoids, which include valtrate and isovaltrate; (c) alkaloids, which include baldrinal; and (d) a number of amino acids (3,8–12). Those amino acids found in the highest concentrations are arginine and glutamine. Others include alanine and γ-aminobutyric acid (GABA) (9). Derivatives of almost all of these principal chemical groups or the combination of them have been thought responsible for the sedative-hypnotic effects of valerian. Iridoid esters, such as valtrate and isovaltrate, have received some attention. Others believe that the many sesquiterpenes, principally valerene derivatives, such as valerenic and acetoxyvalerenic acids, account for its action. These are abundant in the *officinalis* variety (13). The valepotriates, which are found in minimal concentrations in the *officinalis* variety, do not appear to be related to valerian's therapeutic action (14). Many chemists also suspect that multiple constituents of valerian with medicinal properties still have not been identified.

The European monograph on valerian from Commission E that was published in 1985 lists indications for valerian that include restlessness and nervous disturbance of sleep (9). The monograph also characterizes valerian as calming and sleep-inducing. It describes how to prepare an infusion, tinctures, and extracts from valerian root and their recommended doses. The monograph reports no known contraindications, side effects, or interactions. It also lists possible modes of administration, including external application as a bath additive (13).

In an effort to study and authenticate their therapeutic use, the National Institutes of Health and other scientists worldwide have attempted to characterize the central nervous system receptor activity of herbal products, including valerian (15,16). For example, of particular interest to the mental health professional is ginkgo, whose traditional use is for asthma and circulatory disorders but which also appears to be beneficial in the treatment of dementia (17). Ginkgo has significant activity at the GABA (A and B), 2-(aminomethyl)phenylacetic acid, and cholecystokinin (CCK) receptors. Valerian also demonstrates some affinity for GABA (A and B), AMPA, *N*-methyl-D-aspartate, and CCK receptors. How this receptor activity relates to its medicinal benefits remains under investigation.

Recent valerian receptor–binding studies have focused on GABA. This receptor activity could help explain its sedative properties and other pharmacologic effects (18). Studies have reported interactions with both GABA-A and GABA-B receptors (19). However, valerian extracts can have high concentrations of GABA, which may obscure these receptor-binding effects (9,20,21). In addition, *in vitro* studies do not always explain *in vivo* effects, since many of valerian's constituents fail to cross the blood-brain barrier (20). Valerian's amino acid content may also explain its sedative effects. Some studies suggest that its high concentrations of glutamine (9,20,21), as well as of adenosine (22), could be related to its hypnotic properties. Studies of valerian's effects on benzodiazepine receptor binding have yielded conflicting results (22,23).

ANIMAL STUDIES

Animal studies have shown that various constituents of valerian root seem capable of producing CNS-depressant effects. Specific valerian extracts can increase phenobarbital and other barbiturate-induced sleep time (24,25). In some of these studies, sedative effects have been dose dependent and comparable to those produced by phenothiazines and benzodiazepines. Valerian's sedative properties have been attributed to its sesquiterpenes, including valeranone and valerinal (25,26). Other studies in mice have suggested that certain specific metabolites of the valepotriates possess most of its sedative action (27). Valerian has also been described as slightly less potent than diazepam in rats (28). Based on their results, these authors suggest that valerian could be effective in the treatment of benzodiazepine withdrawal. However, physicians are strongly cautioned against using valerian for symptoms of benzodiazepine withdrawal because no confirmatory clinical studies have been reported. To demonstrate these sedative effects, many animal studies use maximum doses or routes of administration that are not possible in humans.

Multiple reviews in some scientific, but mostly in lay, publications exalt valerian's efficacy and safety (29). Some statements are misleading since they often fail to separate opinion from relevant scientific findings. For example, the author has read commentaries such as "...scientific studies have confirmed its ability to improve sleep quality and relieve insomnia..." and "...as effective in reducing sleep latency as...barbiturates and benzodiazepines...." Some of these reviews provide no references to support these statements. In some cases, the references provided are of similar review articles that are either opinions or unreferenced. In other cases the opinions are based on animal studies, which may have limited relevance to humans. Finally, some statements about valerian's efficacy and safety are based on human studies in which the methods and resultant conclusions may be flawed. Other favorable, but unsubstantiated, statements about valerian occasionally found in lay reviews include "...there is no hangover effect..." and "...after nighttime dosing there is an alerting effect in the morning."

POLYSOMNOGRAPHIC EFFECTS

If valerian is a predictable hypnotic, its electroencephalographic (EEG) effects may resemble those of the well known sedatives. Results from the few published studies are mixed. A very well designed and recently published polysomnographic study compared the objective and subjective effects of Valdispret forte, a product containing 405 mg of valerian, in poor sleepers who were elderly (30). The herbal preparation was given on a thrice-daily regimen for 7 days. After an adaptation night, polysomnographic recordings were obtained for two nonconsecutive nights in eight subjects. Valerian showed a consistent increase in slow-wave sleep, a decrease in stage-1 sleep, and no effect in REM sleep. However, no improvement in subjectively rated sleep latency or quality was observed. The small sample size may not have allowed the detection of favorable subjective sleep effects.

Another polysomnographic study assessed the efficacy of Euvegal forte, a preparation that contains both valerian and Melissa balm, in a small number of patients from a medical practice (31). In this one-night crossover design versus triazolam and a placebo, the valerian preparation proved overall to be inferior to triazolam (0.125 mg), but it was superior to the placebo in improving the sleep efficiency of poor sleepers. An increase in slow-wave sleep in poor sleepers was also seen. However, this study also failed to demonstrate an improvement in sleep latency from the valerian/balm combination. A third sleep EEG study compared the effects of 60 and 120 mg of a valerian preparation (Harmonicum much) to a placebo in 11 subjects (32). Only one night of recording was obtained. In contrast to the two studies already reviewed (30,31), the 120 mg dose significantly decreased stage 4, as well as REM, sleep.

A recently published abstract of a polysomnographic trial tested the valerian product Sedonium (33). It included 16 patients with a diagnosis of primary insomnia. The study had a double-blind crossover design over a 2-week period. In concert with other studies, the authors report a significant increase in slow-wave sleep, as well as a decrease in slow-wave sleep latency. Subjectively, a modest improvement in sleep onset was also noted.

An often cited subjective (using rating scales to assess sleep effects, N=10; N, number of subjects) and objective (using sleep EEG, N=8) sleep study was conducted in nonsymptomatic volunteers using Leathwood's (see "Clinical Trials") valerian extract (34). The subjective trial had three arms as follows: valerian 450 mg, 900 mg, and a placebo. Each treatment was administered before bedtime for only one night. Significant reduction in sleep latency and wake-time after sleep onset was reported for each valerian dose in comparison to the placebo. No effect on the number of nighttime awakenings was observed. The results also suggest a dose-response relationship, but this comparison did not reach statistical significance. The polysomnographic study also reported subjective improvement in both sleep latency and wake-time. However, no significant effects in sleep architecture were apparent. A numerical advantage in some EEG parameters favoring the valerian arms occurred for items such as wake-time after onset, total sleep time, and latency to stage 2. From these subjective and sleep EEG results, the authors conclude that "...valerian ...exerts a mild hypnotic action."

CLINICAL TRIALS

Open-Label Trials

Although relatively few controlled trials in patients with insomnia have been published, two large promotional open-label trials are available from the German literature (35,36). These trials were almost identical in their design. They tested a product that contains valerian root extract, Baldrian Dispert, and focused on its hypnotic efficacy during 10 consecutive days of administration. Patients were recruited from the general and pediatric practices of more than 1,000 German physicians. The symptomatic inclusion criteria were vague, using general terms such as *problems going to sleep*, *problems sleeping through the night*, and *sleep disturbances*.

The first of these naturalistic trials included 11,168 patients (35). The hypnotic efficacy of this valerian product was clearly apparent for most patients within the first 2 nights of administration. Physicians rated subjective improvement in broad symptomatic categories (as good or very good) for more than 70% of their patients. The second trial included 1,689 patients from both general and pediatric practices (36). Data were collected from children as young as 1 year of age. The efficacy results were similar; more than 70% of patients were judged to have a good or very good response. A rapid therapeutic effect was also noted because improvement was apparent after the first or second night of treatment.

Open-label trials are difficult to interpret because of multiple factors, most important being the lack of controls. These trials present other concerns. For example, the reader does not learn what incentives were offered to physicians or patients for their participation. Informed consent is not mentioned for either trial, even for the one that included the pediatric patients. Yet, although the efficacy results must be viewed with some skepticism, most clinicians at least value the safety data. These results provide the greatest surprise. In the smaller trial of 1,689 patients, only eight reported a side effect, and apparently none discontinued treatment because of intolerance (36). The safety results from the larger study (35) are even more incredible as, of the 11,168 patients treated over a 10-day period, a single adverse reaction was reported. Thus, these two promotional trials, which included almost 13,000 patients, are of very limited clinical value.

A recent abstract included 518 patients also treated in an open-label design (37). The preparation studied was Sedacur forte, which combines valerian with other botanicals. Patients were selected from general practices because of complaints of nervous restlessness or difficulties in going to sleep. Physicians rated more than 90% of patients to have achieved good and very good results after 4 weeks. Side effects were not discussed.

Controlled Trials

Several controlled studies have also been published. A subjective trial of valerian's hypnotic effect was conducted under the assumption that the valepotriates and sesquiterpenes contribute to its sedative effects (38). Two treatment groups were used. Each of the 27 subjects was given each of the preparations for only one night. One preparation was Valerina natt (which contains 400 mg of valerian and other botanicals). Perhaps to mask valerian's odor and aftertaste, the alternate preparation contained the other herbal ingredients of Valerina natt but only 4 mg of valerian. Subjects (74% women) were recruited from a medical clinic. They reported chronic symptoms and only 4 to 6 hours of total sleep each night. Fifty percent were taking other sedatives. Twenty-one of the 27 subjects (78%) rated Valerina natt as superior to the control preparation ($P<0.001$). These results from a relatively well designed study strongly suggest valerians' sedative effects. No adverse effects were reported.

In various reviews discussing valerian's hypnotic effects, the two most commonly cited clinical trials were published by Leathwood et al. in the 1980s (39,40). This investigator was employed at the research department of the Nestle Products Company in Switzerland. Both were placebo-controlled studies, and they suggest the safety and efficacy of the particular aqueous extract of valerian under study (33). However, each trial has design flaws that limit its interpretation and generalizability. Nevertheless, these studies provide the most convincing evidence of valerian's efficacy as a hypnotic.

The weaker of the two studies compared the hypnotic efficacy of an aqueous extract of valerian in three treatment groups as follows: (a) valerian, 450 mg; (b) valerian, 900 mg; and (c) a placebo (39). Eight volunteers who complained that they usually had problems getting to sleep participated in the trial. Participants, who were members of the research staff or their families, took each treatment 1 hour before bedtime. Each preparation was given for four nonconsecutive nights, over a period of 18 nights, in a random-order design. Weekend nights were excluded for unknown reasons, and no mention was made as to how the authors protected the blind in light of valerian's strong odor and aftertaste. During the study nights, the participants used untested wrist-worn activity meters in an attempt to confirm sleep onset objectively (41).

Three of the eight activity meters broke down at some time during the trial, resulting in missing data.

For this study, the most convincing efficacy comparison was the apparent reduction in sleep latency. Both valerian groups (450 and 900 mg) reported a significant (one-tailed paired t test) improvement in sleep latency compared to placebo. Yet, during the trial, the placebo group's mean sleep latency was only 15.8 minutes, suggesting a clinically asymptomatic group of participants. No dose-response relationship was apparent, since the mean improvement in sleep latency with the 900-mg dose was numerically lower than that with the 450-mg dose. Subjective ratings of improved sleep quality, depth, and latency significantly favored the 450-mg dose over the placebo, but no statistical significance was seen between placebo and the 900-mg dose. Valerian had no significant effect on total sleep time. The report also provides essentially no discussion as to side effects, except that the authors equated the subjective hangover effect reported by some of the subjects in the 900-mg group as similar to that of benzodiazepines and barbiturates.

A larger and more convincing subjective study to test the efficacy of valerian as a hypnotic was published by the same group in 1982 (40). In their introduction, the authors state that, until their report, valerian's clinical efficacy was almost entirely anecdotal. They mention their own small and apparently unpublished animal studies, as well as their partially published EEG studies, which suggest valerian's sedative effects (42). A total of 166 asymptomatic volunteers participated in the trial. They had three treatment groups as follows: (a) Leathwood's aqueous extract of valerian (400 mg); (b) another commercial preparation of valerian marketed in Switzerland (Hova), which contains 60 mg of valerian; and (c) a placebo (brown sugar). Subjects served as their own controls as each product was taken in random order for three nonconsecutive nights. The authors discuss no specific inclusion or exclusion criteria for entering the trial except that the volunteers agreed to take part. The manuscript is not clear on whether the strong and distinct odor of valerian may have jeopardized the blind, although aqueous extracts of valerian typically lack the marked odor, taste, and an aftertaste found in other preparations. The authors provide a rather generic description of their statistical analysis. For example, how missing data were handled is uncertain.

The results presented are from 128 (77% of the initial sample) participants who returned their posttreatment questionnaires. Forty-eight percent described themselves as poor or irregular sleepers, but this categorical definition was not defined. Sleep latency for the valerian group was significantly shorter than usual ($P<0.05$) in comparison to the placebo. Although numerically superior, Hova failed to separate from placebo. Sleep quality was also significantly better for valerian, especially for the group who considered themselves habitually poor or irregular sleepers. Fifty-four percent of those poor sleepers after valerian reported that their sleep quality was better than usual in contrast to 28% of those on the placebo. In comparison to the placebo, sleep quality with valerian was best for women and younger subjects who were poor sleepers.

In this study valerian failed to have a significant effect in reducing the number of nighttime awakenings. In addition, valerian use was not associated with residual sedative daytime effects. Reported adverse effects are not further discussed except for the mention of one subject who withdrew from the trial because of nausea (the authors report that they do not know which medication was to blame). From their results, the authors conclude that an aqueous extract of valerian root improved the sleep quality of poor or irregular sleepers without producing a detectable hangover effect the next morning.

Another controlled valerian study treated 78 older patients (mean age, 70.0 years) using a parallel balanced design (43). Patients with disturbances of subjective well-being and behavioral disorders of nervous origin were randomly assigned to receive Valdispert (also known as Baldrian Dispert) or a matching placebo for 2 weeks. The tablets were identical in external appearance, but no mention of differences in odor or taste is made. Apparently, some patients were discontinued from concomitant psychotropics to enter this trial. No specific inclusion or exclusion criteria were formulated, except for the judgment of the participating physicians that the test product could be helpful. In this study, women outnumbered men by a ratio of 3 to 1.

Various rating instruments were used to assess change in subjective well-being and behavioral disturbances. However, the most convincing results from this trial are in the subjective reduction of sleep problems. All patients who entered the trial complained of insufficient sleep. A robust, statistically significant ($P<0.001$) improvement for Valdispert over the placebo for both sleep latency and nighttime awakenings was reported over the 2-week period. Very few side effects were reported, none of which appeared to be related to valerian.

Results in a Psychiatric Population

Insomnia is a frequent complaint from patients who suffer from mood or anxiety disorders (44). Some ethnic groups commonly use botanicals to treat a variety of physical and emotional symptoms. At the author's University-affiliated public hospital, 80% of the patients are Hispanic. Some report the regular use of natural products. Within this setting, one group encouraged a small number of patients to try valerian for their chronic insomnia. To the author's knowledge, this is the first published case series that has assessed the usefulness of valerian in an adult psychiatric population with insomnia (45). Without altering the patient's established psychotropic regimen, the clinicians wanted to learn how helpful a popular preparation of valerian root in the United States could be in this setting. They also wished to have an estimate of the best dose, sustained effect, and overall safety of valerian to advise others of its value. Participants were urged to use the valerian preparation available at the local General Nutrition Centers, a popular national chain of health food stores. Their brand name is Nature's Way. These bottles are labeled as containing capsules of valerian root, the strength of which is 470 mg per capsule.

The case series included 23 participants. Three failed to return for any of the brief weekly assessments. The remaining 20 completed the 2-week trial. Eighty percent (16 out of 20) were women, and their mean age was 55.9 years (range, 43–72 years). All were born in Latin America, and 60% were of Cuban origin. They reported a mean of 5.7 years of mental health treatment. All were unemployed. Most (11 out of 20) had a working diagnosis of *Diagnostic and statistical manual of mental disorders*, 4th edition, (DSM-IV) major depression, four of generalized anxiety disorder, two of schizoaffective disorder, two of primary insomnia, and one of dysthymic disorder. At baseline, 65% were being prescribed medications with potential sedative effects. Four were taking benzodiazepines regularly. Participants were asked to continue all concomitant medications, including those with a sedative effect, during the 2-week follow-up period.

No specific severity threshold for insomnia was required for participants to be asked to try valerian. However, most reported moderate to marked insomnia. For example, 55% reported that their insomnia interfered extremely with their household or social activities. Most also reported some difficulty in initiating sleep. Fifty-five percent endured a sleep delay between 61 and 120 minutes, with an additional 35% reporting a delay between 31 and 60 minutes. Subjective mean total sleep time for the group was 4.75 hours, and 30% reported never feeling rested and refreshed in the morning.

Participants were asked to begin taking valerian at a dose of one capsule at bedtime. They were also asked to increase their dose gradually to three capsules at night and to remain on this dose during the second week. An ordinal scale between 1 and 5 was used to measure improvement after each week. Results after 1 week were encouraging. At week 1, 80% reported that valerian was at least moderately helpful. The subjective week 2 results were surprisingly favorable. The overall week 2 global improvement was statistically superior to that of week 1 ($P=0.005$). Eighty percent again reported that valerian was at least moderately helpful, but 30% thought it was extremely helpful. Most (80%) also reported that they were at least somewhat likely to purchase valerian in the future.

Valerian demonstrated a sustained positive effect on global sleep ratings during the 2-week follow-up period. Most participants who reported the product as at least moderately helpful after week 1 endorsed similar or higher ratings at week 2. Side effects were assessed by general inquiry after each week. Surprisingly, no adverse effects were attributed to valerian, including residual daytime effects. Few mentioned valerian's odor as a deterrent. However, one of the original 23 participants who failed to return for her follow-up visits later told us that the odor was so strong that she decided not to take the capsules.

This case series suggests that valerian may be helpful as an herbal supplement for some Hispanic patients with chronic insomnia. These results may not be generalized to other populations. Initially, all (23 out of 23) patients asked to try valerian believed that using a natural product for their insomnia was extremely attractive. Thus, a strong selection bias was present, which undoubtedly contributed to the unexpected favorable results. Interestingly, concomitant benzodiazepine use was not a predictor of poor response to valerian. All patients on concomitant benzodiazepines rated valerian as either moderately to extremely or extremely helpful at week 2.

These results also suggest a dose-response relationship, as significantly more patients reported a favorable effect with the higher dose. Other trials have used higher doses of valerian, but since commercial preparations vary, making specific dosing recommendations based on these results is impossible (30,35,36). In this case series, valerian seemed to retain its favorable effect for most patients for at least 14 consecutive nights. Patients with an acute or a recent history of psychotic symptoms were excluded from the sample. Two patients with schizoaffective disorder whose psychotic symptoms were in remission were asked to try valerian. Both reported the botanical as moderately helpful. The short-term use of valerian did not exacerbate their psychotic symptoms. Another advantage of valerian is its cost. A 30-day supply of valerian, at the maximum recommended nighttime dose, costs approximately $6.50.

OTHER POSSIBLE PSYCHOTROPIC AND MEDICINAL EFFECTS

Some clinical studies suggest valerian's antidepressant efficacy (46,47). These 6-week, double-blind trials compared a specific herbal preparation (Sedariston Product) to tricyclic antidepressants. One trial found valerian superior to desipramine (46). The other trial used amitriptyline as the reference antidepressant and found both equally effective (47). Unfortunately, these studies were poorly designed. In addition, Sedariston combines valerian with Rose of Sharon (another name for St. John's wort). Thus, interpreting valerian's antidepressant effect is impossible. One animal study, using a common paradigm that predicts antidepressant action, also suggests valerian's antidepressant activity (48). However, even though massive doses of valerian were used, its effect was much weaker than that of imipramine.

Other clinical studies have reported valerian's antianxiety and calmative effects. Some of these, although controlled, are extremely weak (7,43). One of these trials suggested valerian's stress-reducing effects using a simplistic challenge paradigm in a small number of asymptomatic volunteers (7). Another 2-week study reported on valerian's antianxiety effect in a larger group of patients (49). It compared valerian, in combination with hypericum (St. John's wort), to small doses of diazepam. The botanical mixture reduced anxiety symptoms and was judged by the authors as superior when considering the risks-versus-benefits ratio.

A recently published 4-week, double-blind clinical trial reports on the efficacy of the valerian preparation Euphytose (50). This preparation contains five other botanicals with putative psychotropic effects. By using the change in the Hamilton Anxiety Scale over time, it demonstrated the superiority of the herbal combination to the placebo in patients with adjustment disorder with anxiety. However, only a cursory discussion of the methods is provided. Of the 182 patients entered, incredibly no premature discontinuations or apparently missing data were observed. In addition, the self-evaluation questionnaires used were not relevant to the presenting symptoms.

Some of the author's Hispanic patients use valerian for its tranquilizing effects. In addition, several families report a decisive calmative effect from valerian in the untoward behavioral symptoms of their adult relatives with autism or mental retardation. The group has not systematically studied these putative effects. Many other therapeutic effects for valerian have been suggested. Among these are reports of valerian's possible weak anticonvulsant effects (18,24). In addition, reports of smooth muscle relaxation also exist, making some valerian preparations perhaps helpful for gastrointestinal colic and cramps (51,52).

ADVERSE EFFECTS

One published small case series questioned valerian's safety (53). The author linked valerian to severe liver damage. A follow-up letter to the editor questioned valerian's association with any of the reported cases (54). Another report described the acute effects from valerian poisoning in 23 patients (55). Although a variety of valerian preparations were ingested, no hepatotoxic effects were observed. Finally, another case report found the clinical course after a valerian overdose to be benign (56).

A recently published case report describes a 58-year-old patient who suffered from delirium following the abrupt discontinuation of valerian (57). The authors also suggest that valerian use may have worsened the patient's preexisting heart disease. In their commentary the authors warn that "...valerian root may be associated with serious withdrawal symptoms following abrupt discontinuation." However, they also add that "Since this patient was taking multiple medications and had undergone a surgical procedure, we cannot casually link valerian root to his symptoms." The authors accept the history of valerian use from the family (which the patient apparently concealed), yet rely on the patient's self-report in which he denied the use of alcohol or other drugs. Apparently, no urine toxicologic studies were performed, and the authors overlook the possibility that this classic sedative withdrawal reaction may have been mediated by alcohol, abusable drugs, or both. More importantly, the authors fail to recognize that the patient was clearly misusing valerian. According to the report, the patient had been ingesting for it for many years at a daily dose that most herbalists would consider 10 to 20 times the maximum recommended dose. The report is unclear, but it appears that the authors inexplicably discharged the patient on a maintenance dose of a benzodiazepine.

Side effects, such as headaches, increased anxiety, palpitations, and dyspepsia, have been associated with valerian in some trials (3). Although contrary to the results of published studies (39), the caution that a dose-dependent effect in alertness may exist is also reasonable (58). The untoward effects of valerian when ingested during pregnancy, in nursing mothers, or in children are also not known. Otherwise, no clear adverse event profile has emerged.

Valerian does not appear to potentiate the sedative and psychomotor effects of alcohol significantly (59,60). In addition, in comparison with benzodiazepines, single doses do not produce residual daytime or specific cognitive effects (61). However, *in vitro* studies have suggested that it may have a cytotoxic and muta-genic effect (3). These toxic effects may be solely associated with the valepotri-ates derivatives, which are probably absent or present only in insignificant amounts in aqueous commercial preparations. Finally, in contrast to the weak anticonvulsant effects previously mentioned, others have described an epilepto-genic effect in mice (25).

RECOMMENDATIONS

Some general recommendations about valerian should be shared with patients prior to suggesting its use. Its unique and strong odor, as well as its aftertaste, should be mentioned. Perhaps even more advisable is for the health care provider to purchase a bottle of valerian and note its smell. Some manufacturers recom-mend refrigerating the bottle after it is opened. For those who plan to use valer-ian occasionally and for whom a supply may last several months, refrigeration is recommended. While in the refrigerator, as long as the container is closed, its odor does not seem to permeate other foods.

The optimal dose of valerian that may be helpful as a hypnotic is equivocal. Available preparations vary widely. At present, if three tablets or capsules at bed-time do not seem at least partially helpful, the author recommends that the patient discontinue use of the product. Others encourage the use of higher doses, but this recommendation is not based on controlled studies (35,36). No system-atic studies address the question of loss of efficacy after an initial response. In the case series presented (45), valerian maintained its favorable hypnotic effect for 2 consecutive weeks of nightly use. At present, the authors are conducting a larger 4-week, parallel comparative study with valerian. Preliminary results reveal that, for those patients who initially benefit from its use, valerian main-tains its favorable effect on sleep during 4 weeks of nightly use. Finally, the rec-ommendation during the first trial was for patients to take valerian 30 to 60 min-utes prior to retiring. This advice seems to work well.

Of the many botanical products with putative sedative effects, valerian is one of the best studied. The extract of valerian's root contains a wide variety of chemicals, many of which have been linked to its hypnotic properties. Various preparations of valerian and valerian in combination with other botanicals are commercially available in the United States. Some animal, as well as EEG stud-ies, suggest that it has a mild sedative effect. However, few, if any, large scien-tifically sound and convincing clinical trials have been published. A frequently cited 1982 large, short-term, controlled trial (40) reports a significant effect in reducing sleep latency without residual daytime effects. The author's 2-week case series in psychiatric outpatients reveals that patients with chronic insomnia may benefit from its use, even when using other sedatives (45). Clinicians should consider valerian as an alternative to prescription hypnotics, particularly for those who believe that natural products are an attractive option (62).

REFERENCES

1. Cott J. NCDEU Update: natural product formulations available in Europe for psychotropic indications. *Psychopharmacol Bull* 1995;31:745–751.
2. Muller JL, Clauson KA. Pharmaceutical considerations of common herbal medicine. *Am J Managed Care* 1997;3:1753–1770.
3. Hobbs C. Valerian. *HerbalGram* 1989;21:19–34.
4. Combest WL. Valerian. *Pharmacist* 1997;Dec:62–68.
5. Oshima Y, Matsuoka S, Ohizumi Y. Antidepressant principles of valeriana fauriei roots. *Chem Pharm Bull (Tokyo)* 1995;43:169–170.
6. Insomnia. In: Murray MT, Pizzorno JE, eds. *Encyclopedia of natural medicine.* Rocklin, CA: Prima Publishing, 1991:393–394.
7. Kohnen R, Oswald D. The effects of valerian, propranolol, and their combination on activation, performance, and mood of healthy volunteers under social stress conditions. *Pharmacopsychiatry* 1988; 21:447–448.
8. Houghton PJ. The biological activity of valerian and related plants. *J Ethnopharmacol* 1988;22: 121–142.
9. Santos M, Ferreira F, Cunha AP, et al. An aqueous extract of valerian influences the transport of GABA in synaptosomes. *Planta Med* 1994;60:278–279.
10. Stoll A, Seebeck E, Stauffacher D. New investigations on valerian. *Schweiz Apotheker Z* 1957;95: 115–120.
11. Bos R, Hendricks H, Bruins AP, et al. Isolation and identification of valerenane sesquiterpenoids from valeriana officinalis. *Phytochemistry* 1986;25:133–135.
12. Thies PW. Active component of valerian. Valerodidatum, an iridoid ester glycoside from valeriana species. *Tetrahedron Lett* 1968;28:2471–2474.
13. Valerianae radix. In: Bisset NG, Wichtl M, eds. *Herbal drugs and phytopharmaceuticals: a handbook for practice on a scientific basis.* Boca Raton, FL: CRC Press, 1994:513–516.
14. Krieglstein J, Grusia D. Valepotraite, valerenic acid, valeranone, and volatile oil are ineffective after all. *Deutsche Apotheker Z* 1988;128:2041–2046.
15. Proposals for European monographs on the medicinal use of Valerianae radix. European Scientific Cooperative for Phytotherapy (ESCOP). Presented at the ESCOP symposium. Brussels, 1990, Vol 1.
16. Cott J. Efforts in natural products research. In: Koslow SH, Murthy RS, Coehlo GV, eds. *Decade of the brain: India/USA research in mental health and the neurosciences.* Rockville, MD: U.S. Department of Health and Human Services, 1995:173–183.
17. Le Bars PL, Katz MM, Berman N, et al. A placebo-controlled, double-blind, randomized trial of an extract of Ginkgo biloba for dementia. *JAMA* 1997;278:1327–1332.
18. Hiller KO, Zetler G. Neuropharmacological studies on ethanol extracts of valeriana officinalis: behavioral and anticonvulsant properties. *Phytotherapy Research* 1996;10:145–151.
19. Mennini T, Bernasconi P, Bombardelli, Morazzoni P. In-vitro study on the interaction of extracts and pure compounds from valeriana officinalis roots with GABA, benzodiazepine, and barbiturate receptors in rat brain. *Fitoterapia* 1993;64:291–300.
20. Schulz H, Stoltz C, Muller J. The effect of valerian extract on sleep polygraphy in poor sleepers: a pilot study. *Pharmacopsychiatry* 1994;27:147–151.
21. Battaglioli G, Martin D. Glutamine stimulates aminobutyric acid synthesis in synaptosomes but other putative astrocyte-to-neuron shuttle substrates do not. *Neurosci Lett* 1996;209:129.
22. Balduini W, Cattabeni F. Displacement of (3H)-N6-cyclohexyladenosine binding to rat cortical membranes by an extract of valeriana officinalis. *Med Sci Res* 1989;17:639–640.
23. Holzl J, Godau P. Receptor binding studies with valeriana officinalis on the benzodiazepine receptor. *Planta Med* 1989;55:642.
24. Leuschner J, Muller J, Rudman M. Characterization of the central nervous depressant activity of a commercially available valerian root extract. *Arzneimittelforschung* 1993;43:638–641.
25. Hendriks H, Bos R, Woerdenbag HJ, Koster AS. Central nervous system depressant activity of valerenic acid in the mouse. *Planta Med* 1985;51:28–31.
26. Hendriks H, Bos R, Allersma DP, et al. Pharmacological screening of valeranal and some other components of the essential oil of Valeriana officinalis. *Planta Med* 1981;42:62–68.

27. Veith J, Schneider G, Lemmer B, Willems M. Einfluss einiger Abbauprodukte von Velepotriaten auf die Motilitat licht-dunkel synchronisieter Mause. *Planta Med* 1986;53:179–183.
28. Andreatini R, Leite J. Effect of valepotriates on the behavior of rats in the elevated plus maze during diazepam withdrawal. *Eur J Pharmacol* 1994;260:233–235.
29. Ravitzky M. Focus on herbs: valerian, nature's antianxiety agent. *Alt Comp Ther* 1994;1:48–49.
30. Schulz H, Stolz C, Muller J. The effect of valerian extract on sleep polygraphy in poor sleepers: a pilot study. *Pharmacopsychiatry* 1994;27:147–151.
31. Dressing H, Riemann D, Low H, et al. Insomnia: are valerian/balm combinations of equal value to benzodiazepine? *Therapiewoche* 1992;42:726–736.
32. Gessner KD, Klasser M. The effect of harmonicum much on human sleep-a polygraphic EEG-investigation. *EEG EMG Z Elektroenzephalogr Elektromyogr Verwandte Geb* 1984;15:45–51.
33. Balderer G, Borbely AA. Effect of valerian on human sleep. *Psychopharmacology* 1985;87:406–409.
34. Quispe Bravo S, Diefenbach K, Donath F, et al. The influence of valerian on objective and subjective sleep in insomniacs. *Eur J Clin Pharmacol* 1997;52:A70.
35. Schmidt-Voigt J. Treatment of nervous sleep disturbances and inner restlessness with a purely herbal sedative: results of a study in general practice. *Therapiewoche* 1986;36:663–667.
36. Seifert T. Therapeutic effects of valerian in nervous disorders: a field study. *Therapeutikon* 1988;2: 94–98.
37. Friede M, Liske E, Wustenberg P, Woelk H. Results of a multicentric non-interventional trial with a phytosedative in elderly patients. *Eur J Clin Pharmacol* 1997;52:A84.
38. Lindahl O, Lindwall L. Double-blind study of a valerian preparation. *Pharmacol Biochem Behav* 1989;32:1065—1066.
39. Leathwood PD, Chauffard F. Aqueous extract of valerian reduces latency to fall asleep in man. *Planta Med* 1985;2:144–148.
40. Leathwood PD, Chauffard F, Heck E, Munoz-Box R. Aqueous extract of valerian root (Valerina officinalis L.) improves sleep quality in man. *Pharmacol Biochem Behav* 1982;17:65–71.
41. Borbely AA, Neuhaus HU, Mattman P, Waser PG. Long term recording of motor activity: its use in research and clinical situations. *Schweiz Med Wochenschr* 1981;111:730–735.
42. Leathwood PD, Chauffard F. Quantifying the effects of mild sedatives. *J Psychiatr Res* 1983;17: 115–122.
43. Kamm-Kohl AV, Jansen W, Brockmann P. Modern valerian therapy of nervous disorders in elderly patients. *Medwelt* 1984;35:1450–1454.
44. Mellinger GD, Balter MB, Uhlenhuth EH. Insomnia and its treatment: prevalence and correlates. *Arch Gen Psychiatry* 1985;42:225–232.
45. Dominguez RA, Bravo-Valverde RL, Kaplowitz BR, Cott JM. Valerian as a hypnotic for Hispanic patients. *Cult Divers Ethnic Minority Psychology* 2000;6:84–92.
46. Steger W. Depressions: a randomized double blind study to compare the efficaciousness of a combination of plant derived extracts with a synthetic antidepressant. *Ther Erfahrungen* 1985;61:914–918.
47. Kniebel R, Burchard JM. Therapy of depression in the clinic: a multicenter double blind comparison of herbal extracts from valerian roots and roses of sharon with the standard antidepressant amitriptyline. *Ther Erfahrungen* 1988;64:689–696.
48. Sakamoto T, Mitani Y, Nakajima K. Psychotropic effects of Japanese valerian root extract. *Chem Pharm Bull (Tokyo)* 1992;40:758–761.
49. Panijel M. Therapy of symptoms of anxiety. *Therapiewoche* 1985;41:4659–4668.
50. Bourin M, Bougerol T, Guitton B, Broutin E. A combination of plant extracts in the treatment of outpatients with adjustment disorder with anxious mood: controlled study versus placebo. *Fund Clin Pharmacol* 1997;11:127–132.
51. Morazzoni P, Bombardelli E. Valeriana officinalis: traditional use and recent evaluation of activity. *Fitoterapia* 1995;66:99–112.
52. Wagner H, Juric K. About the spasmolytic activity of valerians. *Planta Med* 1979;37:84–86.
53. MacGregor FB, Abernethy VE, Dahabra S, et al. Hepatotoxicity of herbal medicines. *BMJ* 1989; 299:1156–1157.
54. Farrel RJ, Lamb J. Herbal remedies. *BMJ* 1990;300:47–48.
55. Chan TY, Tang CH, Critchley JA. Poisoning due to an over-the-counter hypnotic, Sleep-Qik. *Postgrad Med J* 1995;71:227–228.
56. Willey LB, Mady SP, Cobaugh DJ, Wax PM. Valerian overdose: a case report. *Vet Hum Toxicol* 1995; 37:364–365.
57. Garges HP, Varia I, Doraiswamy PM. Cardiac complications and delirium associated with valerian root withdrawal. *JAMA* 1998;280:1566–1567.

58. Valerian. In: Jellin JM, ed. *Natural medicines comprehensive database*. Stockton, CA: Therapeutic Research Faculty, 1999:926–928.
59. von Eickstedt KW. Modification of the alcohol effect by valepotriate. *Arzneimittelforschung* 1969;19: 995–997.
60. Mayer B, Springer E. Psychoexperimental studies on the effect of a valepotriate combination as well as the combined effects of valtratum and alcohol. *Arzneimittelforschung* 1974;24:2066–2070.
61. Gerhard U, Linnenbrink N, Georghiadou CH, Hobi V. Effects of two plant-based sleep remedies on vigilance. *Schweiz Rundschau Med* 1996;85:473–481.
62. Astin JA. Why patients use alternative medicine. *JAMA* 1998;279:1548–1553.

10

Melatonin for Treatment of Sleep and Mood Disorders

Irina V. Zhdanova and Leah Friedman

INTRODUCTION

Melatonin (*N*-acetyl-5-methoxytryptamine) is a phylogenetically primitive molecule that is found in such diverse species as unicellular organisms, plants, and vertebrates. In vertebrate animals, the main source of melatonin is the pineal gland (epiphysis cerebri). This small structure, located approximately in the center of the human brain, has fascinated anatomists and philosophers for over two millennia. The first description is believed to have occurred around 300 B.C. by Herophilous, an Alexandrine Greek physician. It received its name, pineal organ, from Galen (A.D. 130–200), the Greek anatomist, to whom its shape resembled a pine cone. Galen thought that this unpaired structure near the base of the third ventricle served as a valve for regulating the flow of thought. Expanding on Galen's ideas, the French philosopher Rene Descartes (1596–1650) assigned psychic activity to the pineal gland, considering it "the seat of imagination and common sense" (1). In light of modern knowledge about the pineal gland, that Descartes linked its function with the optic nerves and eyes is remarkable (Fig. 10.1). Since all early conceptions of the physiologic role of the pineal organ had little scientific data to support them, it was primarily considered a vestigial appendix of the brain throughout the eighteenth to nineteenth centuries.

At the beginning of the twentieth century, studies by McCord and Allen showed that mammalian pineal tissue contained a substance that caused the skin of tadpoles to blanch (2). In the 1950s, Aaron Lerner, a professor of dermatology at Yale University, became interested in this effect, hoping that such a substance could help in treating vitiligo, a human skin pigmentation disorder. Pursuing this goal, Lerner et al. identified an active compound of the pineal gland that was responsible for a blanching effect in amphibians and coined the name melatonin (3). Although melatonin proved to be without effect in human skin pigment distribution, Lerner was the first to observe and to report a sedative effect of the pineal hormone in humans.

Since then, studies conducted in dozens of laboratories all over the world have revealed much about melatonin, although many questions regarding its role in human and animal physiology remain either unanswered or unaddressed. Yet, the

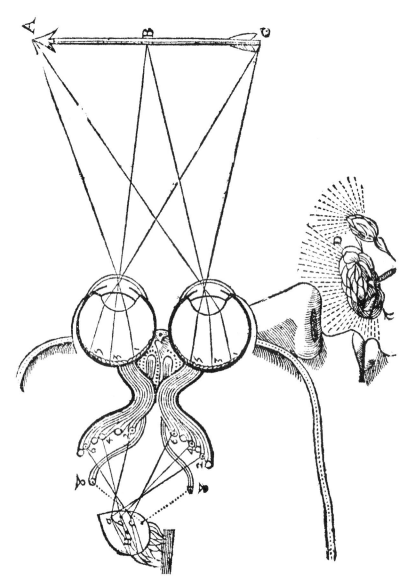

FIG. 10.1. Drawing by Rene Descartes in *De Homine*, 1662. The pineal gland is marked *H*.

widely publicized claims about melatonin's multiple positive effects and the fact that this hormone has received the label "food supplement" have encouraged millions of people to consume melatonin on a daily basis without medical control in quantities that increase circulating hormone levels 10-fold to 50-fold over those that normally occur in human blood.

The goal of this chapter is to present both basic and clinical information about melatonin to help promote understanding of its role in supporting the physiologic harmony of the organism and the importance of the appropriate use of melatonin therapy.

MELATONIN: A KEY HORMONE OF THE CIRCADIAN PHOTONEUROENDOCRINE AXIS

The major structures of the human circadian system, including the eyes, the suprachiasmatic nuclei (SCN) of the hypothalamus, and the pineal gland, all develop from the roof of the diencephalon. They are involved in the perception or translation of photic information and thereby facilitate an organism's adaptive adjustment to the rhythmic changes in environmental illumination due to the earth's daily rotation under the sun. A near–24-hour (circadian) rhythm of melatonin secretion from the human pineal gland depends on a periodic signal from SCN, the master biologic clock. The neurons of this small brain structure are normally active during the day and slow down at night, and they are capable of sustaining a circadian pattern of activity even in the absence of rhythmic environmental input. The activation of SCN neurons has an inhibitory effect on the pineal gland, defining a nocturnal pattern of melatonin secretion. If, for example, SCN neurons are activated at night by environmental light perceived by the retina, melatonin production declines. Melatonin, in turn, can attenuate the activity of SCN. This melatonin action is likely to support a normal decline in the activity of the SCN at night, further promoting melatonin secretion and contributing to an overall increase in the amplitude of circadian body rhythms.

Melatonin can also produce a shift in the circadian phase of SCN activity, either advancing or delaying it. The direction of the phase-shift depends on the time of melatonin treatment; for instance, administration of melatonin in the late afternoon can advance the circadian clock, while early-morning treatment can cause a phase delay (4).

A temporal and functional interplay between melatonin and the SCN and their response to environmental light promote a temporal alignment of multiple circadian body rhythms with each other (internal synchronization) and with the periodic changes in the environment (external synchronization).

MELATONIN PRODUCTION AND METABOLISM

The 24-hour pattern of melatonin production in humans (Fig. 10.2) is characterized by a nocturnal increase. It is typically initiated about 2 hours before the

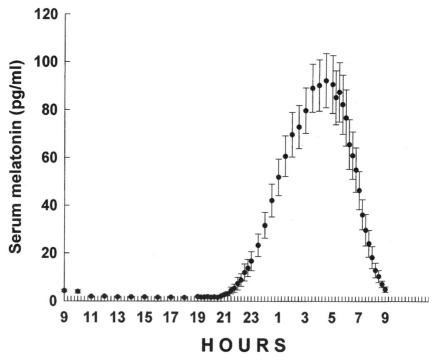

FIG. 10.2. Daily profile of endogenous serum melatonin levels in young adults (mean ± standard error of the mean [SEM], N=23).

individual's habitual bedtime, unless it is blocked by environmental light; and it then declines in the morning. This rhythmic pattern of melatonin secretion persists in people maintained in constant darkness. Exposure to darkness during the daytime does not induce melatonin production; however, the abrupt imposition of bright light at night can suppress it.

The circulating amino acid L-tryptophan is the precursor of melatonin (Fig. 10.3). Within cells in the pineal gland, it is converted to serotonin (5-hydroxytryptamine) by a two-step process that is catalyzed by the enzymes tryptophan hydroxylase and 5-hydroxytryptophan decarboxylase. This process involves serotonin's *N*-acetylation, catalyzed by *N*-acetyltransferase, and then its methylation by hydroxyindole-O-methyltransferase to produce melatonin. The hormone is released directly into the bloodstream and the cerebrospinal fluid as it is synthesized, and, as it is lipid soluble, it has ready access to every cell of the body. Approximately 50% to 70% of circulating melatonin is reportedly bound to plasma albumin; the physiologic significance of this binding is as yet unknown. Inactivation of melatonin occurs in the liver where it is converted to 6-hydroxymelatonin by the P-450–dependent microsomal mixed-function oxidase enzyme system. Most of the 6-hydroxymelatonin is excreted in the urine

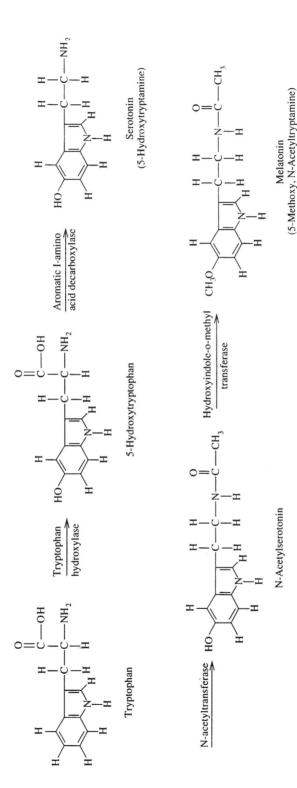

FIG. 10.3. Biosynthesis of melatonin from tryptophan.

and feces as a sulfate conjugate (6-sulfatoxymelatonin) and the rest, a much smaller amount, as a glucuronide. Some melatonin may be converted to *N*-acetyl-5-methoxykynurenamine in the central nervous system. Approximately 2% to 3% of the melatonin produced is excreted unchanged in the urine.

CIRCULATING MELATONIN LEVELS IN HEALTH AND DISEASE

The human fetus and newborn infant do not produce melatonin; they instead rely on the hormone supplied via the placental blood and, postnatally, via the mother's milk. After infants are 9 to 12 weeks old, rhythmic melatonin production increases rapidly; the highest nocturnal melatonin levels are attained in children under 5 years of age. Thereafter, melatonin levels decrease, with perhaps the most dramatic changes occurring during adolescence (5). Although exceptionally healthy elderly persons sometimes maintain high melatonin production (6), the majority of aged individuals have low circulating melatonin levels (7–9). Typical nocturnal peak serum concentrations of melatonin in young humans are around 100 pg per mL, while daytime levels are as low as 1 to 3 pg per mL. Although the circulating melatonin pattern for a given individual tends to remain surprisingly constant from day to day, marked interindividual variations in nocturnal melatonin levels are observed in all age groups (Fig. 10.4).

Some, although not all, studies have found that middle-aged and elderly insomniacs have lower melatonin production than good sleepers of the same age (10). Similarly, a controversial body of data exists on the melatonin levels in psychiatric patients. Early studies proposed that low nocturnal melatonin levels could be a trait-dependent marker for major depressive disorder (11); conversely, others reported that melatonin was elevated during manic states (12). Such trends have been considered a possible reflection of contrast changes in noradrenergic activity in depression and mania, since melatonin production in the

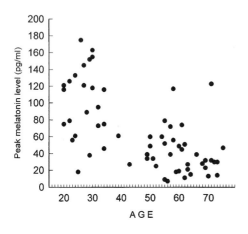

FIG. 10.4. Individual peak endogenous melatonin levels in people of different ages.

pineal gland depends on its sympathetic innervation. Further studies, however, either failed to document significant differences between depressed patients and control subjects or found even higher melatonin levels associated with depression (13,14). Decreased nocturnal melatonin levels were also reported in both drug-free schizophrenics and those treated with antipsychotic drugs (15,16). The inconsistent reports regarding melatonin production in patients with psychiatric disorders might be explained by pronounced interindividual and age-related variability in melatonin levels, a heterogeneity of affective disorders, the effects of environmental illumination during test procedures, or the relatively small number of patients studied. These factors require rigorously controlled studies to determine whether alterations in endogenous melatonin levels might indeed be characteristic of psychiatric disorders.

MELATONIN TREATMENT

Even if extreme changes in circulating melatonin levels are not part of the pathogenesis of age-related insomnia or psychiatric diseases, a number of clinical symptoms characteristic of these disorders, such as sleep alterations, circadian rhythm disturbances, and anxiety, might benefit from timely melatonin treatment.

Effects of Melatonin on Sleep

Melatonin and Sleep in Healthy Individuals

Indirect signs of a close relationship between melatonin and sleep in humans do exist. The hours of increased melatonin secretion are concurrent with the habitual hours of sleep, and the onset of melatonin secretion correlates with the onset of evening sleepiness (17–19). Studies of circadian phase shifts in humans also show that change in the timing of the onset of melatonin secretion correlates with change in the timing of evening sleepiness, a phenomenon widely observed in shift workers and in transmeridian jet-travelers. An increase in endogenous circulating melatonin levels resulting from infusion of its precursor tryptophan (20) or a suppression in melatonin metabolism (21) is reported to increase sleepiness and to promote sleep. In contrast, suppression of melatonin production by treatment with beta-blockers disturbs the sleep process (22).

Melatonin treatment is typically found to produce either subjective or objective sleep-promoting effects in healthy research subjects when administered during the day or to improve overnight sleep in insomniacs (23). Depending on the methods of sleep assessment used and the baseline sleep patterns characteristic of the various populations tested, the effects of melatonin treatment have been described as increased reaction time, diminished subjective alertness, increased fatigue or sleepiness, increased sleep propensity, a reduction in latency to sleep onset, a decrease in the number of nocturnal awakenings, or an increase in sleep efficiency. These effects are observed in response to doses that induce physiological (around 100 pg per mL) and pharmacologic (over 200 pg per mL) circulating levels of the hormone. Remarkably, the effects of both physiologic and pharmacologic doses of melatonin are not accompanied by any dramatic changes in electrophysiologic sleep architecture, a common complication encountered with many existing hypnotics and anxiolytics. Collectively, the available data on the effects of melatonin on sleep suggest that a nocturnal surge in melatonin production may be an important factor in normal human sleep regulation and that melatonin deficiency might contribute to an altered sleep pattern.

Melatonin Treatment in the Geriatric Population

Persistent insomnia in the elderly is strongly associated with a depressed mood, while improvement in sleep can positively affect daytime vigilance and performance (24). However, conventional hypnotic drugs, often used in the elderly to promote sleep, can cause daytime sedation and impair motor coordination and memory function. For example, amnestic and performance-disruptive effects are reported to parallel the hypnotic effects of the benzodiazepines (25,26). Although the reasons for the substantial increase in mood and sleep disorders found in elderly humans are not entirely clear and they may involve a number of factors, low amplitude of the circadian signal (27), including a decline in melatonin production, may well contribute to altered nighttime sleep quality and low daytime mood and performance. Melatonin treatment, used in both physiologic and pharmacologic doses, can improve sleep in aged insomniacs (28,29). One should note, however, that the sleep-promoting effects of melatonin demonstrate substantially higher variability in older individuals compared to young healthy adults, presumably due to age-related changes in the sensitivity of melatonin receptors or to alterations in melatonin metabolism. This finding bears on the important issue of whether melatonin doses should be individualized for therapeutic purposes.

Melatonin Treatment in Children with Neurologic Disorders and Mental Retardation

Studies in children with severe insomnia, which is associated with multiple neurologic disorders, showed that the administration of melatonin could substantially improve their sleep patterns and increase sleep duration (30). Similarly, the author's study of children with Angelman syndrome (AS), a rare genetic disorder characterized by severe mental retardation, hyperactivity, and disturbed sleep, found that timely administration of low melatonin doses both promoted nighttime sleep and advanced the circadian rhythm of melatonin production (31). Furthermore, some children with AS showed a reduction in hyperactivity, as well as enhanced attention. Whether these are consequences of improved nighttime sleep or they represent additional results of melatonin treatment that could be beneficial to other populations suffering from attention deficits needs further investigation.

Melatonin Treatment in Psychiatric Disorders

Sleep and mood are intimately linked physiologic processes, and sleep deprivation in healthy adults results in increased anxiety or depression (32). The majority of mood disorders are associated with significant sleep alterations, which often manifest as the first behavioral symptoms of the disease (33). The increase in subjective sleep disturbance may also be the first signal of relapse in remitted depressed patients. Difficulty falling asleep, frequent nighttime awakenings, or nightmares are present in such diverse mental illnesses as depression, schizophrenia, and anxiety disorders. Moreover, individuals with chronic insomnia have significantly higher risks for incident depression (34). Successful treatment of psychiatric symptoms is typically associated with sleep improvement (35), while effective management of insomnia in depressed patients can markedly improve their mood (36). Thus, insomnia might be part of a pathophysiologic complex that predisposes one to psychiatric disease, or it might be an important factor in precipitating or sustaining alterations in mood and cognitive functions.

A few studies have attempted to use melatonin to treat patients suffering from psychiatric disorders. Such treatment was found to improve sleep in patients with major depression, although it did not significantly affect their mood (37,38). Both sleep and mood were improved by melatonin treatment in patients suffering from winter depression or from mania (39,40). Sleep in schizophrenia patients who were experiencing chronic insomnia was also enhanced by melatonin administration (15). Conversely, no changes after melatonin treatment in sleep or mood were documented in patients with rapid-cycling bipolar disorder (41). All these studies involved relatively small numbers of patients, especially considering the heterogeneity of these disorders. Clearly, more studies are needed to evaluate the efficacy of melatonin treatment for insomnia in psychiatric patients and to compare it to conventional therapy with hypnotic medications.

Effects of Melatonin on Circadian Body Rhythms

Both sleep and mood are under the control of the biologic clock, located in the SCN (42). Alterations in biologic rhythms and lack of their synchronization with each other or with the environment might result in sleep and mood disorders or might exacerbate existing pathologic conditions. The role of melatonin in synchronizing circadian body rhythms or increasing the amplitude of circadian oscillation suggests that the pineal hormone might have beneficial effects in psychiatric and sleep disorders that are associated with a disruption in body rhythms.

Circadian Alterations in Psychiatric Disorders

Some, although not all, studies assessing chronobiologic measures in psychiatric patients found increased variability, lower amplitude, or internal desynchronization of circadian body rhythms (43–46). However, whether these changes observed in psychiatric patients reflect alterations in their sleep-wake cycle or social schedule, result from faulty feedback mechanisms in their hypothalamo-pituitary-adrenal and somatotropic axes, or indicate changes in their intrinsic circadian clock system is not clear.

Some studies in seasonal affective disorder (SAD) patients suggest that this condition is associated with, and perhaps results from, a circadian phase delay (47,48). Melatonin treatment in the afternoon can improve both mood and sleep in patients with SAD (49). Whether the effect on mood in this population results from an observed modest phase shift in patients' circadian body rhythms or from improved nighttime sleep needs further clarification.

Circadian Alterations in Sleep Disorders

In humans, the major sleep episode is normally synchronized with the dark phase of the environmental light-dark cycle and with melatonin production by the pineal gland. If this alignment is altered, sleep quality and quantity declines and, with it, the normal daytime mood and performance. As a result, circadian sleep disorders are invariably associated with educational, occupational, financial, social, and marital problems, which may in turn lead to psychiatric problems.

Multiple determinants of a misalignment of circadian rhythms could exist. Some are related to abrupt advances or delays in the sleep period relative to the environmental light-dark cycle, such as those due to transmeridian flight or shift work. Others reflect an intrinsic impairment of circadian and homeostatic regulation of sleep. The latter include a non–24-hour sleep-wake syndrome that is rare in normally sighted persons but common in the blind and the delayed or advanced sleep-phase syndromes (DSPS and ASPS) that are associated with much later (DSPS) or much earlier (ASPS) sleep onset and morning awakening than what is expected according to social cues or individuals' circadian temperature patterns (50). The most dramatic alteration of circadian regulation of sleep manifests as an irregular sleep-wake pattern, characterized by several daytime sleep periods and lack of a consolidated nighttime sleep episode. This circadian disorder is most commonly observed in patients with developmental or degenerative neurologic conditions.

Non–24-hour Sleep-Wake Syndrome

Because light is the primary zeitgeber (time giver) of the endogenous circadian pacemaker, the fact that, in most blind persons, the pacemaker is not synchronized with the 24-hour day is not surprising. Therefore, despite maintaining regular schedules of sleep, work, and social contact, many blind people have free-running circadian rhythms with a period that typically is slightly longer than 24 hours. As a result, they tend to suffer cyclic bouts of insomnia as their circadian pacemakers move in and out of phase with the environmental cues that determine their habitual bedtime (51,52). The way to treat such disorders is to offer the individual a strong zeitgeber other than environmental light. Contradictory reports have been received regarding the ability of timely melatonin administration to phase shift and entrain the free-running rhythms in blind individuals. Some studies found improved sleep quality but not a circadian phase shift after melatonin treatment, while others documented both the entrainment of previously free-running circadian rhythms and an increase in sleep efficiency in blind subjects receiving melatonin (53–56).

Delayed or Advanced Sleep-Phase Syndromes

Several studies described different degrees of success in treating DSPS patients with melatonin to achieve phase advance (57). The recent studies, whose designs were more refined and which involved a greater number of subjects than the earlier ones, showed significant sleep-wake cycle phase advances (58,59). Interestingly, studies in adolescents, an age group that frequently develops DSPS, suggest that a substantial decline in melatonin production at this age might be one of the predisposing factors for the onset of this sleep disorder (60). Indeed, a rapidly developing deficit in both the circadian and homeostatic effects of melatonin on sleep initiation could cause a delay of their nighttime sleep period. Although no clinical trials of the effects of melatonin on ASPS have been conducted so far, the hypothesis that melatonin treatment in the morning could phase delay the onset of evening sleepiness in patients with this disorder is plausible.

Irregular Sleep-Wake Pattern

Melatonin treatment might be beneficial in individuals with neurologic disorders that are associated with the irregular sleep-wake pattern. The preliminary data suggest that severely altered sleep patterns in patients with Alzheimer disease can be improved by timely melatonin treatment (61). Similarly, nighttime melatonin treatment in children with AS, a developmental neurologic disorder, has been found to modify their irregular sleep-wake patterns by significantly increasing their nighttime sleep period and reducing sleep fragmentation (31). In addition, the authors found a substantial delay in melatonin secretion onset in some of the children with AS. Such phase delay may result from irregularities in the sleep-wake or environmental light-dark cycles, or it could be a sign of a weakened circadian clock function as part of the general developmental disorder. Whatever the reason, daily melatonin treatment succeeded in readjusting patients' sleep-wake and melatonin rhythms and synchronized them with the children's bedtimes (Fig. 10.5).

Jet Lag

Difficulty falling asleep at night and staying alert during the day are the major symptoms of a circadian desynchrony following a rapid transition between time zones. Jet-lag syndrome can also include mood alterations. The ability of mela-

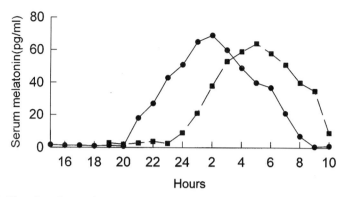

FIG. 10.5. Circadian phase advance in the pattern of melatonin secretion in the Angelman syndrome child after 4 weeks of daily melatonin treatment. Square: before treatment; circle: after treatment.

tonin to produce a circadian phase shift suggests that it can help facilitate a resetting of the circadian clock to match the new environmental time after a transmeridian flight. Some studies have documented an improvement in subjective measures of sleep and performance when subjects received melatonin treatment after a real transmeridian flight or its simulation under laboratory conditions (62–65). Others, however, did not find melatonin treatment efficacious in eliminating jet-lag symptoms compared to a placebo (66,67). Such discrepancies might result from the low sensitivity of subjective measures of sleep and alertness used in these studies, from differences in the doses and preparations of melatonin used, or from the masking effects of environmental light (which typically was not well controlled in the field studies). Furthermore, the positive effects observed could be, to a large extent, explained by an acute sleep-promoting effect of the hormone, which would prevent an accumulation of sleep debt and would thus improve daytime performance.

Shift Work

A chronic state of circadian desynchrony developed in response to shift work often leads to chronic sleep disruption during daylight off-shift hours and to diminished alertness and performance during nighttime work hours. Depression, which is also more common in this population, may be a consequence of truncated sleep or disruption of circadian rhythms. Most nightshift workers, even if they maintain a permanent night work schedule, fail to achieve complete physiologic adaptation of their endogenous circadian rhythms (68). Administration of exogenous melatonin has been reported to improve shift workers' tolerance of the night shift (69). This may result from the entraining effects of melatonin and the synchronization of sleep hours with a period of normal melatonin production. Alternatively, in addition to a phase-shifting effect, melatonin may help shift workers to override the alerting signal of their intrinsic circadian system and to improve their sleep during their subjective day when their endogenous melatonin is low.

MECHANISMS OF MELATONIN ACTION

Understanding of the mechanisms of action of melatonin at the cellular level has advanced substantially over the past few years. Studies conducted in many laboratories demonstrate that melatonin has specific binding sites in various central and peripheral tissues of different animal species (70). The recent cloning of a family of G-protein–coupled melatonin receptors (71) has opened new possibilities for understanding melatonin's action in various target cells. These receptors inhibit cyclic adenosine monophosphate accumulation via a pertussis-toxin–sensitive G-protein in most of the tissues tested, but, in some tissues, they can also affect other signal transduction pathways, such as those involving cyclic guanosine monophosphate, diacylglycerol, or γ-aminobutyric acid (72). Melatonin's high lipid solubility also suggests that this hormone may well have some direct actions inside cells in addition to its actions on cellular membrane receptors.

The exact mechanisms underlying melatonin's effects on sleep, circadian body rhythms, and mood remain to be elucidated. The two major ways in which melatonin might improve the sleep process include the following: it could act acutely to affect the mechanisms involved in sleep homeostasis, thereby making one sleepy; or it could modulate the mechanisms that impart circadian rhythmicity to the temporal pattern of sleep propensity (73,74). The contribution of each of these actions to the hormone's net effect would be expected to depend on the time of its administration and the individual's sensitivity to melatonin.

Studies conducted *in vitro* suggest that a chronobiologic effect of melatonin (i.e., the induction of circadian phase shift) is likely to be explained by its direct effect on SCN neurons (75,76). Such a phase shift in the circadian oscillation of SCN activity may alter the physiologic and behavioral rhythmicity of the entire organism. The suppression of SCN activity by melatonin may also contribute to the acute sleep-promoting effect of the pineal hormone by relieving the mechanisms controlling sleep from the activating pressure of the circadian pacemaker during the day and by promoting a normal nocturnal decline in its neuronal activity. However, that melatonin can directly act on brain structures involved in the regulation of sleep initiation and maintenance is also plausible.

Other lines of evidence suggest that the effect of melatonin on sleep might be related to the hormone's ability to induce hypothermia (77–79). Indeed, the nocturnal decline in body temperature is concurrent with the increase in melatonin release from the pineal gland. Both of these rhythmic patterns are remarkably stable, and they maintain their characteristic phase relationships after light-induced circadian shifts. At present, the mechanisms through which melatonin can decrease core body temperature are not clear. The hypothermic effect of melatonin might result from an overall reduction in alertness, or it may entirely depend on the peripheral action of the hormone since it has been shown to enhance heat loss, perhaps via peripheral vasodilation (80).

The anxiolytic effects of melatonin (discussed below) may also play an important part in its sleep-promoting effects. As was reported earlier, an increase in circulating melatonin levels within the physiological range is not an imperative signal for sleep but rather a gentle promoter of general relaxation and sedation, elements of sleepiness that, in favorable conditions, might significantly facilitate sleep onset and that are typical of a period that is conventionally called "quiet wakefulness" (19). Interestingly, when a person is adequately motivated, he or she can readily overcome these feelings and can remain both alert and productive for some time, regardless of blood melatonin level.

MELATONIN THERAPY: DOSES, TIMING, AND SIDE EFFECTS

Both the acute and the entraining effects of melatonin might provide a useful tool for improving sleep and mood in those people who suffer from psychiatric disease, circadian sleep disorders, or insomnia of other origin. An obvious benefit of using melatonin is that, with such a treatment, organisms are exposed to a familiar substance that is normally involved in their physiologic processes. The major risks of such a treatment may stem from the same reason. Misused exogenous melatonin could simultaneously alter all the known and unknown functions in which the pineal hormone is normally involved. Whether melatonin is used to treat sleep, mood, or circadian rhythm disorder, administering it at the right circadian time in doses that would induce physiologic levels of the hormone and under conditions of low environmental illumination is important.

Therapeutic Doses of Melatonin

Available data show that physiologic doses of melatonin, which raise plasma melatonin to levels within its normal nocturnal range (60 to 200 pg per mL), can significantly promote daytime sleep onset in healthy individuals, improve overnight sleep in people suffering from age-related insomnia, shift the circadian phase of body rhythms, or attenuate the subjective effects of drug withdrawal (81). Pharmacologic doses of melatonin typically do not increase the effects of melatonin above those achieved by physiologic doses, and they might even be less effective (82).

The amount of melatonin that will enter a patient's bloodstream within a certain time following oral ingestion depends on several factors, including the amount of melatonin in the preparation and the diluent employed. Preparations that use oil as a vehicle, for example, produce much higher concentrations of melatonin in the blood due to rapid absorption, but for considerably shorter periods of time, than those preparations containing lactose, microcellulose, or simi-

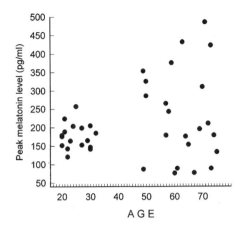

FIG. 10.6. Peak serum melatonin levels in people of different ages after the ingestion of a 0.3-mg dose of melatonin at daytime.

lar diluents. Within a 0.1-mg to 0.3-mg range of oral doses, the latter type of solid formulations typically induce physiologic serum melatonin levels.

Another factor that might affect blood melatonin levels is the patient's age. Mean melatonin levels following the administration of the same dose (0.3 mg) of the hormone may be substantially higher among older individuals compared to young people (83). The range of interindividual variation may also be significantly higher among older subjects. Thus, even a low, 0.3-mg melatonin dose may induce supraphysiologic circulating levels of the hormone in some people over 50 years of age (Fig. 10.6).

Considering differences in the pharmacokinetics of the so-called fast-release and slow-release melatonin preparations, each of which has its benefits and drawbacks, is also important. The available pharmacologic doses of fast-release melatonin (e.g., 3 mg) (Fig. 10.7) and low-dose, slow (controlled) release

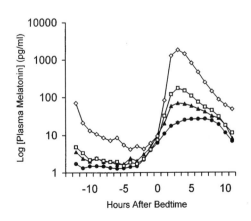

FIG. 10.7. Increase in 24-hour melatonin levels after the administration of different melatonin doses or a placebo 30 minutes before bedtime. Placebo, ●; 0.1 mg, ▲; 0.3 mg, □; 3 mg, ◇.

preparations (e.g., 0.5 mg) tend to increase hormone levels over a 24-hour period, thus altering the circadian pattern of circulating melatonin (84). This complication does not occur with the physiologic doses of a fast-release preparation (i.e., 0.3 mg or less). However, depending on the individual's characteristic rate of melatonin metabolism, a fast-release preparation may not be able to sustain a high enough level of the hormone in the second half of the night. If this is the case and the symptoms of the sleep disorder include early morning awakening, an additional half-dose of melatonin (e.g., 0.1 mg) upon awakening may be recommended.

Melatonin is currently sold in the United States labeled as a dietary supplement because, supporters argue, of its presence in some food products. Indeed, melatonin's presence in living organisms, including plants, appears to be almost ubiquitous. However, the amounts of melatonin in food are so negligibly low that, to consume enough food to match the lowest physiologic oral dose used in human studies (e.g., 0.1 mg), one would need to ingest hundreds of bananas or tomatoes or hundreds of pounds of rice during one meal. Furthermore, melatonin, with a half-life less than an hour, is rapidly metabolized in the body, making its accumulation over days or weeks from the consumption of melatonin-containing food impossible. The body never gets meaningful amounts of melatonin from food; normally, it produces its own. Hence, dietary control of circulating melatonin levels is unrealistic, and calling the pineal hormone a food supplement is misleading.

If melatonin is administered for its sleep-promoting or circadian effects, this should be recognized as hormone replacement therapy and should be handled accordingly (i.e., without causing circulating melatonin levels in excess of those normally found in humans). The benefit of treating a disorder using a normal physiologic agent in concentrations that are normal in humans is that the physiologic harmony of the organism is less likely to be disrupted and side effects are less likely to occur. Sensitive methods are now available for measuring melatonin levels in blood, saliva, and urine, thus making possible the detection of melatonin deficiencies and the adjustment of the therapeutic dose of melatonin so as to not to raise its levels beyond the normal range during treatment.

Timing of Melatonin Treatment

The circadian pattern of melatonin production, with high nighttime and low daytime levels, and the ability of the pineal hormone to affect the phase and amplitude of circadian body rhythms dictate that special attention should be paid to the timing of melatonin treatment.

The effect of melatonin on sleep is typically manifest within 30 to 60 minutes after oral administration (85). If melatonin is used to improve nighttime sleep, it should be taken about 30 minutes before bedtime. This allows orally administered melatonin to increase the hormone level substantially in general circulation before the desired time of sleep onset. Although the acute effect of melatonin on sleep does not seem to depend on the time of administration, coordinating treatment with the time of melatonin's normal increase in secretion would minimize the possibility of an undesired circadian phase-shift.

By contrast, the timing of the hormone's administration is crucial for the exploitation of its phase-shifting effect. Melatonin tends to produce a phase advance when it is administered in the late afternoon, while early morning melatonin treatment tends to cause a phase delay (4). The mid-afternoon administration of melatonin does not pose a chronobiologic effect. If melatonin is being used therapeutically to induce phase advance, it should be administered 4 to 5 hours before the onset of the individual's nocturnal melatonin secretion. In a healthy person, this would correspond to about 5 to 6 hours before the habitual bedtime. However, in a patient with DSPS whose sleep propensity rhythm might be delayed relative to other circadian body rhythms, including that of melatonin, the timing of melatonin treatment should be determined using serum or salivary melatonin measurements (83).

If melatonin is administered to counteract the effect of an eastward transmeridian flight that results in a 3- to 6-hour time difference, administering a physiologic dose (0.1 to 0.3 mg) at the local bedtime following the flight might be useful. Such treatment will restore the deficit in melatonin that the traveler will experience on his or her subjective afternoon, and it might also promote a desired phase advance in the endogenous rhythmic pattern of melatonin secretion. Following a westward flight, ingesting melatonin in the evening, when the endogenous level of the hormone during a subjective night is already increased and the person feels very sleepy, might not be advised. However, taking a half dose (e.g., 0.1 mg) immediately following the midnight or early morning awakening typical of westward flights might be helpful. This could help to facilitate the resumption of sleep acutely, as well as its maintenance for the next several hours, and to support a phase-delay of the circadian pacemaker by exploiting the phase-delaying effect of the hormone when it is administered during the subjective morning. Using melatonin for jet-lag syndrome when more than seven time zones have been crossed is more challenging, since the time when melatonin treatment might produce a phase shift is likely to overlap with the daytime period at the destination site. Consequently, the sleep-promoting effect of melatonin would be undesirable, and the environmental light would be likely to attenuate the effect of melatonin administration significantly.

In undertaking the treatment of shift workers with melatonin, documenting the individual's initial endogenous melatonin pattern and its responsiveness to an actual work schedule is important. The variability between people in the capacity to adapt to shift work is pronounced, and this capacity is influenced by many factors, including the subject's age, sex, and the magnitude and direction of the shift work schedule, as well as the intensity and timing of the individual's light exposure. Thus, the specific treatment of a circadian phase disorder in a particular shift worker requires substantial knowledge of the person's physiologic responses and the environmental factors to which he or she is exposed.

Possible Side Effects of Melatonin Therapy

The publicity surrounding the pineal hormone and its over-the-counter availability in the United States has encouraged millions of people to consume melatonin on a daily basis in quantities that elevate their circulating hormone levels many-fold over those that occur normally. The notion that uncontrolled use of melatonin, especially in pharmacologic doses, is utterly safe rests on little research and on the common public experience of a lack of short-term toxic effects of the pineal hormone. Long-term clinical and experimental studies are needed to address this important question.

Even the present, limited knowledge of melatonin's effects raises concerns about its excessive use. Abnormally high melatonin levels at night and in the day following the consumption of a pharmacologic dose of the hormone may disrupt the delicate mechanism of the circadian system and may dissociate mutually dependent circadian body rhythms, as a recent study describes (86). Thus, if administered in high doses or at inappropriate times, melatonin might induce a circadian rhythm disorder, rather than cure one.

Pharmacologic doses of melatonin also significantly lower body temperature (87) in a dose-dependent manner, reflecting acute changes in either energy metabolism or temperature regulation. Both of these fundamental functions are critical for adaptation and health, and their disruption could be especially damaging in children and the elderly.

Certain reproductive disorders in humans are reportedly associated with an increase in melatonin production, including some cases of male primary hypogonadism or female amenorrhea (88,89). Patients with pineal tumors, which increase melatonin secretion, might display delayed puberty, while non-parenchymal tumors, which may destroy pinealocytes and may thus diminish melatonin production, are sometimes associated with precocious puberty. Thus, uncontrolled use of high melatonin doses could conceivably provoke unwanted modifications in human reproductive function.

As with any other treatment, children might be more sensitive not only to the primary effects of melatonin but also to possible untoward side effects of the hormone. Children typically have the highest circulating melatonin levels of any age group. This fact might be extremely important for their normal development and may contribute to their efficient sleep. However, until much more is known about the effects of melatonin on the growing human organism, melatonin treatment in children should be used only extremely conservatively (i.e., in physiologic doses administered at night, in cases of documented and obvious melatonin deficiency, or in special cases where the benefits of melatonin treatment clearly outweigh any possible ill effects) (30,31,55).

To say that one of the areas where the least is known about the clinical effects of melatonin is in its possible interaction with other medications would perhaps be fair. A complication may arise from the use of a common metabolic pathway by both melatonin and other drugs. Melatonin inactivation occurs in the liver where it is converted to 6-hydroxymelatonin by the P-450–dependent microsomal mixed-function oxidase enzyme system. Thus, any medication that might either slow down (e.g, methoxypsoralen) or facilitate (e.g., valproic acid) this pathway could significantly influence circulating melatonin levels. Similarly, the melatonin load may influence the rate of metabolism and, therefore, the circulating concentrations of other drugs taken concomitantly. On the other hand, psychotropic drugs affecting norepinephrine or serotonin levels might alter the pattern of melatonin production, which depends on increased noradrenergic innervation of the pineal gland at nighttime with serotonin serving as a direct precursor for melatonin synthesis. Furthermore, in addition to its direct actions, melatonin is likely to modulate the effects of other endogenous or exogenous substances. In a number of *in vitro* studies, melatonin treatment that was inactive when administered alone was shown to potentiate the effects of other agents, such as vasointestinal peptide or norepinephrine (90,91). Such potential modulating effects of melatonin call for thoughtful use of the pineal hormone, careful consideration of the appropriate doses, and judicious timing of other treatments relative to the time of melatonin administration.

Finally, avoiding bright light exposure during melatonin treatment (i.e., keeping the environmental illumination at less than 50 lux, or dim light) is important. Under natural conditions, high circulating melatonin levels and bright light do not coexist because melatonin production in the pineal gland is acutely suppressed by environmental light, limiting it to the dark phase of a 24-hour light-dark cycle (92). Even regular room light at night can rapidly suppress melatonin production in the pineal gland. In contrast, melatonin administration induces high circulating levels of the hormone that cannot be opposed by light, thus permitting these two stimuli to coincide in time. Such combination of bright light and high circulating melatonin levels is likely to cancel or to attenuate significantly the effect of melatonin treatment. More importantly, this could produce an adverse effect on the visual system, since melatonin has been reported to increase photoreceptor susceptibility to light-induced damage in animals (93,94), and it might have a similar effect in humans (95).

NEW DIRECTIONS FOR STUDY

Numerous questions regarding the physiologic functions of melatonin and its potential therapeutic applications remain to be addressed. These questions include the role of melatonin in human development; the long-term effects of melatonin treatment on sleep and mood in the elderly suffering from age-related insomnia or degenerative disorders; and possible benefits of melatonin therapy in children with mental retardation, attention deficit, and hyperactivity. Further studies are needed to elucidate the mechanisms of the acute sleep-promoting and phase-shifting effects of melatonin in humans.

Another potentially important area of research is the possible therapeutic value of melatonin in anxiety disorders, such as those associated with acute withdrawal from drugs of abuse. That repeated exposure to addictive substances results in profound changes in multiple physiologic processes in humans is well established, while their withdrawal is known to cause anxiety, insomnia, depression, and circadian rhythm disorders. The intensification of such symptoms can lead to the perpetuation of the addictive behavior, yet drugs that reduce the intensity of those symptoms (e.g., benzodiazepines) are often characterized by abuse liability. The recent observation that the daytime administration of low-dose (0.3 mg) melatonin can significantly attenuate anxiety, irritability, and other subjective symptoms of nicotine withdrawal (Fig. 10.8) in habitual smokers during acute 10-hour abstinence (81) suggests that melatonin might be useful for the treatment of mood disorders associated with drug withdrawal. Consistent with this observation, preliminary data show that the nighttime low-dose oral melatonin treatment has an anxiolytic-like effect in rats withdrawn from chronic cocaine administration, while

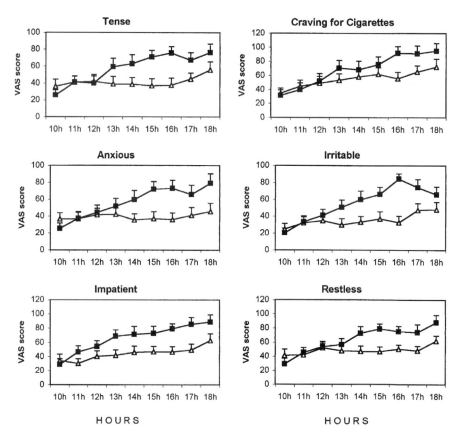

FIG. 10.8. Changes in mood and craving for cigarettes in habitual smokers during acute nicotine abstinence. Melatonin (Δ) or placebo (■) was administered at 11:30 hours. Abbreviation: VAS, visual analog scale. (From Zhdanova IV, Piotrovskaya VR. Melatonin reduces symptoms of acute nicotine withdrawal in humans. *Pharm Biochem Behav* 2000;67:131–135, with permission.)

it does not alter the behavior of control animals. Importantly, unrestricted free-choice, oral-melatonin self-administration revealed a lack of melatonin preference in rats, and its withdrawal did not result in significant changes in the animals' behavior, suggesting that the hormone is devoid of dependence liability.

SUMMARY

As the major hormone of the circadian system, melatonin helps the organism to structure physiologic and behavioral processes adaptively in a periodically changing environment. Furthermore, several lines of evidence suggest that melatonin has a physiologic role in human sleep initiation and maintenance, perhaps serving as a humoral link between circadian and homeostatic sleep mechanisms. Thus, the combined sleep-promoting and chronobiologic effects of melatonin treatment could be of substantial assistance to those suffering from insomnia of different origins, including age-related sleep disturbances or circadian rhythm sleep disorders characterized by an advanced or delayed sleep phase. Importantly, melatonin might be a treatment of choice for blind individuals with free-running circadian rhythms and for patients with severe developmental or degenerative brain disorders associated with irregular sleep-wake patterns, such as children with Angelman syndrome or the elderly with Alzheimer disease.

At present, the idea that changes in melatonin patterns are part of the pathogenesis of the major psychiatric disorders appears unlikely, although more studies are needed to determine whether alterations in melatonin levels during development or aging might represent a risk factor for mental disease. Nevertheless, the observed effects of melatonin treatment on sleep and mood might be of substantial benefit to patients suffering from a variety of psychiatric disorders that are typically associated with insomnia and anxiety, including major depression, seasonal affective disorder, schizophrenia, or drug withdrawal syndrome.

The combined action of melatonin on vigilance and mood, as well as the coupling of multiple circadian body rhythms, might fully justify the use of melatonin as a therapeutic agent. However, dealing with something so multipurpose suggests that using great care is advisable, especially if long-term treatment is considered. The fact that melatonin is a normal human hormone means that it is produced and used by the organism under specific circumstances and in specific concentrations. Similarly, the optimal use of melatonin treatment requires that the patient receive the correct dose of the hormone at the proper time of day. Effective melatonin therapy should consider the characteristic individual melatonin-related parameters, including the endogenous levels, the rate of metabolism, and the phase of its circadian rhythm.

REFERENCES

1. Descartes R. *Treatise of man*. Cambridge, MA: Harvard University Press, 1972:36.
2. McCord CP, Allen FP. Evidences associating pineal gland function with alterations in pigmentation. *J Exp Zool* 1917;23:207–224.

3. Lerner AB, Case JD, Heinzelman RV. Structure of melatonin. *J Am Chem Soc* 1959;81:6084–6087.
4. Lewy AJ, Ahmed S, Jackson JML, Sack L. Melatonin shifts human circadian rhythms according to a phase-response curve. *Chronobiol Int* 1992;9:380–392.
5. Waldhauser F, Weiszenhacher G, Frisch H, et al. Fall in nocturnal serum melatonin during prepuberty and pubescence. *Lancet* 1984;1:362–365.
6. Zeitzer JM, Daniels JE, Duffy JF, et al. Do plasma melatonin concentrations decline with age? *Am J Med* 1999;107:432–436.
7. Iguchi H, Kato KI, Ibayashi H. Age-dependent reduction in serum melatonin concentrations in healthy human subjects. *J Clin Endocrinol Metab* 1982;55:27–29.
8. Sack L, Lewy AJ, Erb DL, et al. Human melatonin production decreases with age. *J Pineal Res* 1986; 3:379–388.
9. Sharma M, Palacios-Bois J, Schwartz G, et al. Circadian rhythms of melatonin and cortisol in aging. *Biol Psychiatry* 1989;25:305–319.
10. Haimov I, Laudon M, Zisapel N, et al. Sleep disorders and melatonin rhythms in elderly people. *BMJ* 1994;309:167.
11. Beck-Friis J, Kjellman BF, Aperia B, et al. Serum melatonin in relation to clinical variables in patients with major depressive disorder and a hypothesis of a low melatonin syndrome. *Acta Psychiatr Scand* 1985;71:319–330.
12. Kennedy SH, Tighe S, McVey G, Brown GM. Melatonin and cortisol switches during mania, depression, and euthymia in a drug-free bipolar patient. *J Nerv Ment Dis* 1989;177:300–303.
13. Rubin RT, Heist EK, McGeoy SS, et al. Neuroendocrine aspects of primary endogenous depression. XI. Serum melatonin measures in patients and matched control subjects. *Arch Gen Psychiatry* 1992; 49:558–567.
14. Shafii M, MacMillan DR, Key MP, et al. Nocturnal serum melatonin profile in major depression in children and adolescents. *Arch Gen Psychiatry* 1996;53:1009–1013.
15. Shamir E, Laudon M, Barak Y, et al. Melatonin improves sleep quality of patients with chronic schizophrenia. *J Clin Psychiatry* 2000;61:373–377.
16. Monteleone P, Natale M, La Rocca A, Maj M. Decreased nocturnal secretion of melatonin in drug-free schizophrenics: no change after subchronic treatment with antipsychotics. *Neuropsychobiology* 1997;36:159–163.
17. Tzischinsky O, Shlitner A, Lavie P. The association between the nocturnal sleep gate and nocturnal onset of urinary 6-sulfatoxymelatonin. *J Biol Rhythms* 1993;8:199–209.
18. Akerstedt T, Froberg JA, Friberg Y, Wetterberg L. Melatonin excretion, body temperature and subjective arousal during 64 hours of sleep deprivation. *Psychoneuroendocrinology* 1979;4:219–225.
19. Zhdanova IV, Wurtman RJ, Morabito C, et al. Effects of low oral doses of melatonin, given 2-4 hours before habitual bedtime, on sleep in normal young humans. *Sleep* 1996;19:423–431.
20. Hajak G, Huether G, Blanke J, et al. The influence of intravenous L-tryptophan on plasma melatonin and sleep in men. *Pharmacopsychiatry* 1991;24:17–20.
21. Souetre E, Salvati E, Belugou JL, et al. 5-Methoxypsoralen increases evening sleepiness in humans: possible involvement of the melatonin secretion. *Eur J Clin Pharmacol* 1989;36:91–92.
22. Brismar K, Hylander B, Eliasson K, et al. Melatonin secretion related to side-effects of beta-blockers from the central nervous system. *Acta Med Scand* 1988;223:525–530.
23. Zhdanova IV, Lynch HJ, Wurtman RJ. Melatonin: a sleep promoting hormone. *Sleep* 1997;20: 899–907.
24. Henderson JG Jr, Pollard CA. Prevalence of various depressive symptoms in a sample of the general population. *Psychol Rep* 1992;71:208–210.
25. Roehrs T, Merlotti L, Zorick F, Roth T. Sedative, memory, and performance effects of hypnotics. *Psychopharmacology (Berl)* 1994;116:130–134.
26. Coenen AM, van Luijtelaar EL. Effects of benzodiazepines, sleep and sleep deprivation on vigilance and memory. *Acta Neurol Belg* 1997;97:123–129.
27. Van Coevorden A, Mockel J, Laurent E, et al. Neuroendocrine rhythms and sleep in aging men. *Am J Physiol* 1991;260:E651–E661.
28. Haimov I, Lavie P, Laudon M, et al. Melatonin replacement therapy of elderly insomniacs. *Sleep* 1995;18:598–603.
29. Zhdanova IV, Wurtman RJ, Regan MM, et al. Melatonin treatment for age-related insomnia. *J Clin Endoc Metab* 2001;86:4727–4730.
30. Jan JE, Espezel H, Appleton RE. The treatment of sleep disorders with melatonin. *Dev Med Child Neurol* 1994;36:97–107.

31. Zhdanova IV, Wurtman RJ, Wagstaff J. Effects of low dose of melatonin on sleep in children with Angelman syndrome. *J Pediatr Endocrinol Metab* 1999;12:57–67.
32. Pilcher JJ, Walters AS. How sleep deprivation affects psychological variables related to college students' cognitive performance. *J Am Coll Health* 1997;46:121–126.
33. Gillin JC. Are sleep disturbances risk factors for anxiety, depressive and addictive disorders? *Acta Psychiatr Scand Suppl* 1998;393:39–43.
34. Breslau N, Roth T, Rosenthal L, Andreski P. Sleep disturbance and psychiatric disorders: a longitudinal epidemiological study of young adults. *Biol Psychiatry* 1996;39:411–418.
35. Lee JH, Reynolds CF III, Hoch CC, et al. Electroencephalographic sleep in recently remitted, elderly depressed patients in double-blind placebo-maintenance therapy. *Neuropsychopharmacology* 1993;8: 143–150.
36. Kupfer DJ. Pathophysiology and management of insomnia during depression. *Ann Clin Psychiatry* 1999;11:267–276.
37. Dolberg OT, Hirschmann S, Grunhaus L. Melatonin for the treatment of sleep disturbances in major depressive disorder. *Am J Psychiatry* 1998;155:1119–1121.
38. Dalton EJ, Rotondi D, Levitan RD, et al. Use of slow-release melatonin in treatment-resistant depression. *J Psychiatry Neurosci* 2000;25:48–52.
39. Robertson JM, Tanguay PE. Case study: the use of melatonin in a boy with refractory bipolar disorder. *J Am Acad Child Adolesc Psychiatry* 1997;36:822–825.
40. Bersani G, Garavini A. Melatonin add-on in manic patients with treatment resistant insomnia. *Prog Neuropsychopharmacol Biol Psychiatry* 2000;24:185–191.
41. Leibenluft E, Feldman-Naim S, Turner EH, et al. Effects of exogenous melatonin administration and withdrawal in five patients with rapid-cycling bipolar disorder. *J Clin Psychiatry* 1997;58:383–388.
42. Boivin DB, Czeisler CA, Dijk DJ, et al. Complex interaction of the sleep-wake cycle and circadian phase modulates mood in healthy subjects. *Arch Gen Psychiatry* 1997;54:145–152.
43. Rao ML, Strebel B, Halaris A, et al. Circadian rhythm of vital signs, norepinephrine, epinephrine, thyroid hormones, and cortisol in schizophrenia. *Psychiatry Res* 1995;57:21–39.
44. Abelson JL, Curtis GC. Hypothalamic-pituitary-adrenal axis activity in panic disorder. 24-hour secretion of corticotropin and cortisol. *Arch Gen Psychiatry* 1996;53:323–331.
45. Posener JA, DeBattista C, Williams GH, et al. 24-Hour monitoring of cortisol and corticotropin secretion in psychotic and nonpsychotic major depression. *Arch Gen Psychiatry* 2000;57:755–760.
46. Wehr TA, Goodwin FK. Biological rhythms in manic-depressive illness. In: Wehr TA, Goodwin FK, eds. *Circadian rhythms in psychiatry*. Pacific Grove, CA: The Boxwood Press, 1983:129–184.
47. Lewy AJ, Bauer VK, Cutler NL, et al. Morning vs evening light treatment of patients with winter depression. *Arch Gen Psychiatry* 1998;55:890–896.
48. Thalen BE, Kjellman BF, Morkrid L, Wetterberg L. Melatonin in light treatment of patients with seasonal and nonseasonal depression. *Acta Psychiatr Scand* 1995; 92:274–284.
49. Lewy AJ, Bauer VK, Cutler NL, Sack RL. Melatonin treatment of winter depression: a pilot study. *Psychiatry Res* 1998;77:57–61.
50. Coleman RM, Roffwarg HP, Kennedy SJ, et al. Sleep-wake disorders based on a polysomnographic diagnosis. A national cooperative study. *JAMA* 1982;247:997–1003.
51. Miles LEM, Wilson MA. High incidence of cyclic sleep/wake disorders in the blind. *Sleep Res* 1977; 6:192.
52. Nakagawa H, Sack RL, Lewy AJ. Sleep propensity free-runs with the temperature, melatonin and cortisol rhythms in a totally blind person. *Sleep* 1992;15:330–336.
53. Folkard S, Arendt J, Aldhous M, Kennett H. Melatonin stabilizes sleep onset time in a blind man without entrainment of cortisol or temperature rhythms. *Neurosci Lett* 1990;113:193–198.
54. Arendt J, Aldhous M, Wright J. Synchronisation of a disturbed sleep-wake cycle in a blind man by melatonin treatment. *Lancet* 1988;2:772–773.
55. Palm L, Blennow G, Wetterberg L. Long-term melatonin treatment in blind children and young adults with circadian sleep-wake disturbances. *Dev Med Child Neurol* 1997;39:319–325.
56. Sack RL, Brandes RW, Kendall AR, Lewy AJ. Entrainment of free-running circadian rhythms by melatonin in blind people. *N Engl J Med* 2000;343:1070–1077.
57. Kayumov L, Zhdanova IV, Shapiro CM. Melatonin, sleep, and circadian rhythm disorders. *Semin Clin Neuropsychiatry* 2000;5:44–55.
58. Nagtegaal JE, Kerkhof GA, Smits MG, et al. Delayed sleep phase syndrome: a placebo-controlled cross-over study on the effects of melatonin administered five hours before the individual dim light melatonin onset. *J Sleep Res* 1998;7:135–143.

59. Kayumov L, Buttoo K, Shapiro CM. Delayed sleep phase syndrome: a randomized crossover placebo-controlled study of effect of exogenous melatonin administered at a partially fixed time. *Sleep* 1999;22:160–161.
60. Carskadon MA, Vieira C, Acebo C. Association between puberty and delayed phase preference. *Sleep* 1993;16:258–262.
61. Brusco LI, Fainstein I, Marquez M, Cardinali DP. Effect of melatonin in selected populations of sleep-disturbed patients. *Biol Signals Recept* 1999;8:126–131.
62. Arendt J, Aldhous M, Marks V. Alleviation of jet lag by melatonin: preliminary results of controlled double blind trial. *BMJ* 1986;3:1170.
63. Nickelsen T, Demisch K, Demisch K, et al. Influence of subchronic intake of melatonin at various times of the day on fatigue and hormonal levels: a placebo-controlled, double-blind trial. *J Pineal Res* 1989;6:325–334.
64. Petrie K, Coraglen JV, Thompson L, et al. Effect of melatonin on jet lag after long haul flights. *BMJ* 1989;298:705–707.
65. Petrie K, Dawson AG, Thompson L, et al. A double-blind trial of melatonin as treatment for jet lag in international cabin crew. *Biol Psychiatry* 1993;33:526–530.
66. Spitzer RL, Terman M, Williams JB, et al. Jet lag: clinical features, validation of a new syndrome-specific scale, and lack of response to melatonin in a randomized, double-blind trial. *Am J Psychiatry* 1999;156:1392–1396.
67. Edwards BJ, Atkinson G, Waterhouse J, et al. Use of melatonin in recovery from jet-lag following an eastward flight across 10 time-zones. *Ergonomics* 2000;43:1501–1513.
68. Sack RL, Blood ML, Lewy AJ. Melatonin rhythm in night shift workers. *Sleep* 1992;15:434–441.
69. Folkard S, Arendt J, Clark M. Can melatonin improve shift workers' tolerance of the night shifts? Some preliminary findings. *Chronobiol Int* 1993;10:315–320.
70. Sugden D. Melatonin: binding site characteristics and biochemical and cellular responses. *Neurochem Int* 1994;24:147–157.
71. Reppert SM. Melatonin receptors: molecular biology of a new family of G protein-coupled receptors. *J Biol Rhythms* 1997;12:528–531.
72. Vanecek J. Cellular mechanisms of melatonin action. *Physiol Rev* 1998;78:687–721.
73. Sack RL, Hughes RJ, Edgar DM, Lewy AJ. Sleep-promoting effects of melatonin: at what dose, in whom, under what conditions, and by what mechanisms? *Sleep* 1997;20:908–915.
74. Zhdanova IV, Wurtman RJ. Efficacy of melatonin as a sleep-promoting agent. *J Biol Rhythms* 1997; 12:644–650.
75. Shibata S, Cassone VM, Moore RY. Effects of melatonin on neuronal activity in the rat suprachiasmatic nucleus in vitro. *Neurosci Lett* 1989;13:140–144.
76. Gillette MU, McArthur AJ. Circadian actions of melatonin at the suprachiasmatic nucleus. *Behav Brain Res* 1996;73:135–139.
77. Saarela S, Reiter RJ. Function of melatonin in thermoregulatory processes. *Life Sci* 1994;54:295–311.
78. Reid K, Van den Heuvel C, Dawson D. Day-time melatonin administration: effects on core temperature and sleep onset latency. *J Sleep Res* 1996;5:150–154.
79. Hughes RJ, Badia P. Sleep-promoting and hypothermic effects of daytime melatonin administration in humans. *Sleep* 1997;20:124–131.
80. Krauchi K, Cajochen C, Wirz-Justice A. A relationship between heat loss and sleepiness: effects of postural change and melatonin administration. *J Appl Physiol* 1997;83:134–139.
81. Zhdanova IV, Piotrovskaya VR. Melatonin reduces symptoms of acute nicotine withdrawal in humans. *Pharm Biochem Behav* 2000;67:131–135.
82. Dollins AB, Zhdanova IV, Wurtman RJ, et al. Effect of inducing nocturnal serum melatonin concentrations in daytime on sleep, mood, body temperature, and performance. *Proc Natl Acad Sci U S A* 1994;91:1824–1822.
83. Zhdanova IV, Wurtman RJ, Balcioglu A, et al. Endogenous melatonin levels and the fate of exogenous melatonin: age effects. *J Gerontol Biol Sci* 1998;53A:B293–B298.
84. Hughes RJ, Sack RL, Lewy AJ. The role of melatonin and circadian phase in age-related sleep-maintenance insomnia: assessment in a clinical trial of melatonin replacement. *Sleep* 1998;21:52–68.
85. Zhdanova IV, Wurtman RJ, Lynch HL, et al. Sleep inducing effects of low melatonin doses ingested in the evening. *Clinical Pharmacol Ther* 1995;57:552–558.
86. Middleton B, Arendt J, Stone BM. Complex effects of melatonin on human circadian rhythms in constant dim light. *J Biol Rhythms* 1997;12:467–477.

87. Cagnacci A, Soldani R, Romagnolo C, Yen SS. Melatonin-induced decrease of body temperature in women: a threshold event. *Neuroendocrinology* 1994;60:549–552.
88. Walker AB, English J, Arendt J, MacFarlane IA. Hypogonadotrophic hypogonadism and primary amenorrhoea associated with increased melatonin secretion from a cystic pineal lesion. *Clin Endocrinol (Oxf)* 1996;45:353–356.
89. Luboshitzky R, Shen-Orr Z, Ishai A, Lavie P. Melatonin hypersecretion in male patients with adult-onset idiopathic hypogonadotropic hypogonadism. *Exp Clin Endocrinol Diabetes* 2000;108:142–145.
90. Krause DN, Barrios VE, Duckles SP. Melatonin receptors mediate potentiation of contractile responses to adrenergic nerve stimulation in rat caudal artery. *Eur J Pharmacol* 1995;276:207–213.
91. Lopez-Gonzalez MA, Calvo JR, Osuna C, et al. Melatonin potentiates cyclic AMP production stimulated by vasoactive intestinal peptide in human lymphocytes. *Neurosci Lett* 1992;136:150–152.
92. Lewy AJ, Wehr T, Goodwin FK, et al. Light suppresses melatonin secretion in humans. *Science* 1980; 210:1267–1269.
93. Wiechmann AF, Yang XL, Wu SM, Hollyfield JG. Melatonin enhances horizontal cell sensitivity in salamander retina. *Brain Res* 1988;453:377–380.
94. Wiechmann AF, O'Steen WK. Melatonin increases photoreceptor susceptibility to light-induced damage. *Invest Ophthalmol Vis Sci* 1992;33:1894–1902.
95. Arushanian EB, Ovanesov KB. Melatonin lowers the threshold of light sensitivity of the human retina. *Eksp Klin Farmakol* 1999;62:58–60.

PART III

Treatment of Other Disorders

11

The Uses of Black Cohosh in Menopause and Chaste Tree Fruit in Premenstrual Syndrome

Steven Dentali

INTRODUCTION

Black cohosh, primarily a New World remedy that has been exported to and studied in Germany, is now the subject of a National Institutes of Health (NIH) investigative work for treating menopausal conditions. Chaste tree's use in the treatment of premenstrual syndrome (PMS) has been imported to North America from Europe, where it is now receiving similar attention. This chapter presents the nomenclature and history, actions and indications, constituents, pharmacology, dosage and toxicity, and some clinical reports for the medicinal uses of black cohosh root and rhizome and chaste tree fruit.

BLACK COHOSH

The nomenclature of black cohosh begins with North American Indians. The term *cohosh* is thought to be an Algonquian word meaning rough, with reference to the texture of the roots. A New World plant used by Native Americans, it was most abundant in the Ohio River Valley, but it could also be found from Maine to Wisconsin, south along the Allegheny Mountains to Georgia, and west to Missouri.

Various common names have been used to refer to black cohosh, including black snakeroot, bugbane, rattleroot, squawroot, and macrotys. It is a member of the *Ranunculaceae,* or buttercup, family, which includes other medicinal plants such as aconite, goldenseal, and pulsatilla. Its best known scientific name is *Cimicifuga racemosa*. However, it recently may have been assigned back to *Actaea racemosa*. The generic name *Cimicifuga* derives from the Latin cimex (a kind of bug) and fugare (to put to flight), which is perhaps indicative of the use of some strongly smelling close relatives to repel insects. The species name *racemosa* refers to the flowering stalk, termed a raceme. The designation of rattleroot is indicative of the rattling sound made by the dry seeds in their pods. This plant prefers the shade of rich open hardwood forests, but it will tolerate some sunny spots.

The part of the black cohosh plant used in medicinal preparations is the root and rhizome (which is technically an underground stem). It was officially part of the United States Pharmacopeia (USP) from the first edition in 1820 to 1936 and in the National Formulary from 1936 to 1950. The Eclectic physicians used a preparation of black cohosh called macrotys. It was considered one of the best known, specific medicines for heavy, tensive, aching pains as it had a direct influence on the female reproductive organs.

Phytochemically, black cohosh has not yet been well studied. Its identified constituents include triterpene glycosides, principally the xylosides actein and cimicifugoside. The aglycones that remain after the cleavage of the xylose sugar from each of these glycosides are acetylacteol and cimigenol, respectively. The glycoside 27-deoxyactein and its aglycone (27-deoxyacetylacteol), which are remarkable due to their cyclopropane ring feature, have also been reported, as have the following: the isoflavone formononetin; aromatic acids, including isoferulic and salicylic acids; and tannins, resin, fatty acids, starches, and sugars. Recently, phytochemical work on the triterpene glycosides of black cohosh reported the discovery of eight new cimiracemosides and eight previously known compounds (1). The presence of the phytoestrogen formononetin, which binds to estrogen receptors, reportedly has not been confirmed in commercial black cohosh preparations (2).

Black cohosh is indicated for women displaying symptoms of PMS, menopause, dysmenorrhea, and uterine spasm. Two aspects of its action are observed. Black cohosh has a direct antineuralgic effect (some also ascribe vasomotor relaxation) with antidepressant actions. Traditionally, it has been used as an antispasmodic and antirheumatic with special applicability to the musculoskeletal symptoms of menopause, as well as hot flushes. Its characterization as a menopausal remedy, which is recent, is a significant diminution of traditional indications. It has also been used for painful or delayed menstruation, ovarian cramping, muscular and neurologic pain, and inducing labor at the end of pregnancy. Such a broad range of indications is consistent with the general action of medicinal plants that offer systemic impacts from a variety of active compounds.

Black cohosh's medicinal actions are sometimes considered endocrine in nature. It promotes bleeding as an emmenagogue, although it is also used as an antirheumatic. It is listed in the German Commission E monograph as having an estrogen-like action, with suppression of lutenizing hormone and binding to estrogen receptors. Although recent work on rats and mice (3) and in humans (4) does not support an estrogenic binding and activating mechanism, clinically black cohosh has had an estrogen-like effect, as it is believed to relieve hot flashes and vaginal dryness. If further research confirms the nonbinding and nonactivation of estrogen receptors, then a nonhormonal mechanism of action, possibly neurotransmitter-mediated, may be involved. In fact, recent *in vitro* work has demonstrated black cohosh's complete lack of binding to, or activity on, estrogen and progesterone receptors or on an estrogen-inducible gene (presenelin-2) in S30 breast cancer cells (5).

Earlier pharmacologic work on black cohosh has shown a selective reduction of the serum concentration of lutenizing hormone (LH) and the ability to bind to the estrogen receptors of rat uteri. As the researchers said, "It is assumed that triterpene glycosides such as cimicifugoside have an effect on the hypothalamus-pituitary system, leading to secondary effects on the reproductive and central/peripheral nervous systems." They reported endocrine activity using ovariectomized rats and observed a reduction in pituitary LH serum concentration without changes in the follicle-stimulating hormone (FSH) or prolactin release. This activity was lost after glycoside hydrolysis of the tested extract. At least three active compounds, including formononetin, were determined to be involved. Formononetin itself was active in an *in vitro* estrogen receptor binding assay, but it did not reduce LH serum levels *in vivo* (6,7).

The German Commission E monograph and the British Herbal Pharma-copoeia specify a dose of 40 to 200 mg of dried rhizome and root or of alcohol extracts made with 40% to 60% ethanol corresponding to this amount. Although black cohosh has a history of safe use, no long-term controlled human studies longer than 6 months have been conducted. No serious side effects have been observed in clinical studies, although some instances of minor gastrointestinal disturbances have been reported. When overdoses were ingested, the following adverse effects were seen: frontal headache, dizziness, nausea, and vomiting.

Published clinical studies of black cohosh include seven reports or trials from 1960 through 1991. In the first of these, which is essentially a combined case history from 4 years of experience with 517 female patients, a hormone-like action with a slightly euphoric effect was described (8). This influence was con-sidered beneficial, and it was particularly evident in "autonomic-psychic change-of-life phenomena." No adverse side effects were noted.

In two open studies (N=36 and N=50; N, number of subjects), 40 drops of tincture (alcohol extract) was administered twice daily for 3 months for menopausal complaints in the gynecologic practices of Daiber and Vorberg (9,10). Their subjects included cases where hormone therapy was contraindi-cated (30 of 50 patients) or refused (31 of 36 patients). Clear improvements in complaints were reported as early as 4 weeks. A decrease in the Kupperman Menopausal Index, a positive Clinical Global Impression (CGI), and improve-ment in psychologic symptoms, such as a decrease in weariness, despondency, and ill humor and an increase in motivation-mood state, were recorded.

Stolze reported on a study carried out by 131 general practitioners with 629 patients treated for menopausal complaints (11). Of these 629 patients, 367 were not previously treated; 204 had been treated with hormones, 35 with psy-chopharmaceutical agents, and 11 with hormone and psychopharmaceutical combinations; and 12 lacked specific data. The tincture, 40 drops twice a day, was administered for 6 to 8 weeks. Clear improvement in 80% of the patients was reportedly seen in as early as 4 weeks. The tincture was considered well tol-erated in 93% of the cases, with 7% reporting transitory stomach complaints.

Warnecke reported an open, controlled, comparative study on 60 patients over the course of 12 weeks (12). One group received 40 drops of black cohosh tinc-ture twice a day; another group received 0.625 mg of conjugated estrogens daily, and a third took 2 mg of diazepam daily. Somatic measurements were made, and positive estrogen-like stimulation of the vaginal mucosa was seen in the black cohosh and conjugated estrogen groups, with a clear increase in cytologic indices in as early as 4 weeks. Significant reductions in hot flashes, night sweats, nervousness, headaches, and heart palpitations were seen with all forms of therapy. The authors stated that black cohosh appeared to be a low-risk effective therapy with no toxic side effects and that it should be the first choice for mild-to-moderate menopausal ailments.

Stoll conducted a randomized, double-blind trial with 80 women split into three groups over 12 weeks (13). The first group received two 8-mg tablets of a commercial black cohosh extract (Remifemin) daily. As in the previous study, the second group received conjugated estrogens (0.625 mg daily), while the third was administered a placebo. The black cohosh group produced a significant increase in the degree of vaginal epithelium proliferation over the placebo. Cytologic changes similar to that expected for estrogen treatment were seen, while significant decreases in the Menopausal Index and Hamilton anxiety (HAM-A) score (<15), indicating an antidepressant action, were also reported for the black cohosh group. No clear improvement was noted in the control group. The estrogen dose was too low to show a clear benefit.

A randomized study involving 60 patients under 40 years of age with ovarian functional deficits after hysterectomy with at least one ovary remaining were treated over a 6-month period in a university gynecologic clinic (14). This study involved four groups as follows: (a) two tablets two times daily (Remifemin); (b) estriol, 1 mg daily; (c) conjugated estrogens, 1.25 mg daily; and (d) an estrogen-progestin combination. Therapy was evaluated at 4, 8, 12, and 24 weeks with a modified Kupperman-Index, including trophic disorders of the genitals, and serum FSH and LH levels. At the end of the study, the Kupperman-Index was lower in all groups. No decrease in LH and FSH levels were noted, and no significant differences were observed between the groups.

Another group studied the same commercial product in 110 menopausal women who took either two tablets twice a day or a placebo. The researchers reported a significant reduction in LH levels after 8 weeks (15). They followed up this finding with animal studies and showed that black cohosh had the ability to reduce LH secretion in ovariectomized rats and to compete *in vitro* with 17-β-estradiol binding. They identified at least three different endocrinologically active principles. One suppressed LH without demonstrating estrogen receptor binding; a second was active in both test systems; and a third group actively bound to estrogen receptors without suppressing LH with chronic treatment, but it was shown to inhibit LH upon acute injection.

A recent randomized, placebo-controlled, double-blind trial of black cohosh for treating hot flashes among breast cancer survivors found it to be no more efficacious than the placebo in treating hot flashes and other menopausal symptoms (16). Placebo effects are quite strong for the treatment of menopausal symptoms, although they tend to wear off in time. The 60-day duration of this study may have been insufficient for distinguishing the effects, if any, of black cohosh compared to those from the placebo over time. FSH and LH levels were measured in a subset of patients. Black cohosh did not appear to affect these serum hormone levels. This, combined with the lack of *in vitro* activity (5) for black cohosh, supports the conclusion that it is safe for treating women with estrogen-sensitive cancer.

Definitive chemical, pharmacologic, and clinical work has not been done with black cohosh. However, what is known about the chemistry and the bioactivity of this long-standing remedy tends to support the wider traditional anti-neuralgic and antidepressant uses and the more recent menopausal applications. To obtain a better understanding of the medicinal effects of this plant, more work is needed. One step in this regard would be to identify active compounds, to standardize extracts according to that consideration, and to conduct additional clinical trials. This work is now being carried out at the University of Illinois at Chicago (UIC)/NIH Center for Botanical Dietary Supplement Research in Women's Health. A randomized, double-blinded, placebo-controlled phase II trial is planned to examine the use of black cohosh for the reduction of menopausal symptoms in healthy menopausal women. The study duration will be 1 year.

Black cohosh is currently regulated as a dietary supplement. One of the main thrusts of the Dietary Supplement Health and Education Act of 1994 that established this position was to provide the American public with information so that they could make informed choices as to their self-care. This appears to be working because many women already treat themselves with black cohosh preparations for symptoms associated with menopause, and the remedy seems to be growing in popularity. Black cohosh is also found in formulations intended to have an antispasmodic effect on skeletal muscles, especially the lower back.

Clinicians who choose to inform their patients of black cohosh can offer a relatively low-cost nonprescription alternative to conventional treatments. This can be a reasonable option for patients seeking such an alternative and as a first choice before transitioning to prescription hormonal treatments if they become necessary or preferred by the patient. The standard dose of black cohosh based on a clinical trial of a commercial product is one tablet twice daily, corresponding to 40 mg of the crude drug. If a liquid extract or tincture is used, then 20 drops twice daily should be a reasonable dosage, while allowing the patient to adjust the dose as desired. Such liquid preparations can be found in most natural foods stores, and they are easily transported and administered.

If black cohosh has any significant drug interactions or if it is contraindicated for women for whom estrogen therapy is ill advised is not known. The effects of concurrent use with hormone replacement therapy are also not well known. The Botanical Safety Handbook of the American Herbal Products Association recommends that it not be taken during pregnancy or while nursing (17). The American Herbal Pharmacopoeia (AHP) has an excellent monograph on black cohosh that should be consulted for further information (18).

CHASTE TREE FRUIT

The chaste tree fruit comes from a shrub or small tree of the Verbenaceae family that is native to southern Europe. Found growing along moist riverbanks, its scientific name is *Vitex agnus-castus*. The dried ripe fruit is sometimes called monk's pepper, agnus-castus, or simply chaste berry, stemming from the legend that ingestion of the pungent aromatic fruits helped promote chastity. The fruit, containing no less than 0.08% casticin on a dry weight basis, is the part of the plant that is most often used medicinally. The medicinal use of chaste tree fruit, albeit for injuries and inflammation, was mentioned by Hippocrates in the fourth century B.C. Plato wrote about its use as an anaphrodisiac (19).

While not well studied, chaste tree fruit is known to contain essential and fixed oils, diterpenoids, iridoid glycosides (agnuside, aucubin), and flavonoids, including casticin. Chaste tree fruit has a corpus luteum–like effect comparable to that of the LH stimulation of progesterone secretion during the luteal phase of the menstrual cycle. It increases LH and inhibits FSH release. This results in an increased progesterone release, and thus it is used to remedy luteal phase progesterone deficiency.

Chaste tree fruit's mechanism of action is believed to be the result of a dopaminergic-mediated effect on the anterior pituitary gland that reduces prolactin secretion. Recent study has demonstrated the ability of chaste tree fruit extracts to bind to dopamine D_2 receptors with activity residing in the lipophilic fraction. Opioid receptor binding activity was also found. This activity was spread across a complete range of fractions of differing polarity (20).

Chaste tree fruit and its extracts are also used to treat premenopausal progesterone decline, and, in addition, they are believed to have a galactagogue (stimulation of milk production) action. The fruit is indicated for treatment of PMS, luteal insufficiency, breast tenderness, menopausal complaints, and acne. It has been studied pharmacologically for these conditions since the 1950s. Reducing prolactin yet having a galactagogue action are paradoxical effects. The experience of herbalists is that it works well for some patients and not for others, thus operating with an overall hormonal balancing effect.

Toxicologically, chaste tree fruit has been administered to rodents at a dose of 7,000 mg per kg without an observed toxic effect. Chronic administration of 3,500 mg per kg over 5 weeks (1,400 times the human dosage) likewise produced no toxic effects. The AHP Chaste Tree Fruit Monograph lists a dozen human clinical studies on the treatment of PMS with chaste tree preparations that have been conducted since 1986. The European companies Bionorica, Madaus, Schaper and Brümmer, Strathmann AG, and Zeller Herbal Medicinal Products manufactured the tested preparations. While these are all relatively recent, numerous monitoring studies for menstrual disorder have been done on Agnolyt, produced by Madaus, in Germany since the 1930s.

Most published scientific work with chaste tree fruit preparations have been postmarketing surveillance studies. This is not out of the ordinary for herbal remedies with long histories of traditional use. Clinical trials (or phytochemical studies) of a remedy's use are not the first investigations to be conducted due to the simple fact that the remedy's use may often predate the scientific method. The first scientific investigations of use of a remedy are likely to be those of health care practitioners keeping careful track of the effects of the remedies they administer and learning from this empirical approach. Manufacturers may commission postmarket surveillance studies after a body of knowledge is built from the observation of case histories. These can be followed by increasingly rigorous trials and phytochemical evaluations (at increased costs) to test the product's safety and effectiveness, to understand its mechanism of action, and to identify active compounds.

The best double-blind, randomized, placebo-controlled clinical trial on chaste tree fruit extract to date has been conducted with a product for treatment of PMS (21). Many of the earlier observational studies included PMS among the other menstrual disorders. One tablet daily of a 20-mg dry extract product (known as Ze 440) from Zeller Herbal Medicinal Products or the matching placebo was given to 170 women (86, active; 84, placebo) over three consecutive menstrual cycles. Self-assessment items of irritability, mood alteration, anger, headache, and breast fullness were significantly improved ($P<0.001$) relative to the placebo, while bloating was unaffected by treatment.

The physicians' evaluation of the CGI scale also noted a significant improvement ($P<0.001$) for the treatment group. Additionally, the responder rate for the women taking chaste tree fruit extract was higher than that for the women on the placebo (52% versus 24%). Tolerability was good with mild severity for all events, four of which occurred in the active group and three in the placebo group.

An earlier double-blind, placebo-controlled study of chaste tree fruit for PMS treatment was negative (22), although the choice of a soy-based placebo in this study was highly questionable because hormonal effects can be elicited by soy. A third double-blind, controlled trial (23) compared Agnolyt to pyridoxine (vitamin B6) and found them to be equally effective. This is not reassuring because the efficacy of pyroxidine in the treatment of PMS is not well established.

The action of chaste tree fruit as a prolactin inhibitor has led to it being studied for the treatment of breast pain (premenstrual mastalgia). The AHP monograph reviews three randomized, double-blind, placebo-controlled studies and ten open studies supporting the efficacy of chaste tree fruit preparations for treating this condition.

Several studies in the use of chaste tree fruit preparations to treat menstrual cycle irregularities of no bleeding (secondary amenorrhea), long cycles (oligomenorrhea), and short cycles (polymenorrhea) are also presented in the

AHP monograph. More work is needed to determine chaste tree fruit's effectiveness for these uses, as well as for its reputation as a fertility-promoting agent. The hope is that the UIC/NIH Center for Botanical Dietary Supplement Research in Women's Health will shed more light on chaste tree fruit and its actions.

The dosage of chaste tree fruit is recommended as 30 to 40 mg of powdered fruit daily, 20 drops two or three times daily of a 1-to-5 (ratio of dried berries to menstruum) tincture, or another equivalent preparation. Herbalists will often dose the tincture just once a day. Higher dosages (up to 240 mg per day of the dried fruit) have also been shown to be effective. Side effects do not appear to be serious. For the practitioner willing to experiment or for patients who self-treat, chaste tree fruit appears to offer actions not found in other substances that are used to treat PMS, menstrual irregularities, and related conditions.

For such cases, one of the studied preparations that were mentioned in this chapter would be a good choice, as would a traditionally prepared alcohol-based tincture. Patients who are already amenable to complementary approaches to medical care may appreciate the hands-on work of dosing themselves with a liquid preparation. The delivered dose is easily absorbed, and the patient can titrate their dose on a drop-by-drop basis. High-quality liquid extracts of this sort are available in natural foods stores.

Chaste tree fruit preparations can offer a low-risk approach to commonly encountered menstrual cycle conditions. The author sees no reason for them not to be more widely used as an initial treatment choice. Responders may gain knowledge of an additional tool for self-care, and nonresponders retain the ability to take advantage of other treatment options.

SUMMARY AND RECOMMENDATIONS

Two commonly used botanicals, black cohosh root and rhizome and chaste tree fruit, were examined for their use in treating menopause and PMS. The history of black cohosh, a woodland plant found in the eastern United States that was used by Native Americans, was touched upon, in addition to its adoption and development into a phytopharmaceutical by European interests. Black cohosh has been officially listed in the USP, and the chapter evaluated some clinical work done with it. Although its action appears to be endocrine in nature, it has not been found to bind to or to activate estrogen receptors. Black cohosh is indicated for women's menopausal symptoms, and it has been considered a relaxing nervine to normalize female reproductive functions and for muscular pain. It is generally given in a dosage of 40 to 200 mg of dried rhizome and root or in alcohol extracts made with 40% to 60% ethanol corresponding to the same amount.

Chaste tree fruit has been presented as a European remedy that is just now finding increased North American use. It is primarily indicated for luteal insufficiency, breast tenderness, and menopausal complaints. It is often given as 30 to 40 mg of powdered fruit daily or 20 drops two to three times daily of the liquid extract tincture, although herbalists report success with once-a-day dosing.

In closing, the author would like to offer some perspective into the state of research regarding herbal products with medicinal actions. The use of rigorous clinical trials to evaluate botanical remedies in the United States is a relatively recent phenomenon. Historically, no one was in a position to fund, or to directly benefit from, the funding of such research. Only recently have the government and industry established stakes in the matter.

The sophistication of herbal extracts has increased, as has the complexity of the trials designed to assess them. Historical preparations were often simple hydroalcohol (water and alcohol) extracts taken in a liquid form. Highly controlled extraction and manufacturing procedures using consistent raw materials now produce standard tablets suitable for clinical trial purposes. However, today's clinically studied product still essentially represents the crude extracts of yesteryear because the newer extracts have not been substantively refined. They contain essentially the same broad chemical makeup as the older-style tinctures. This lack of chemical refinement is due in part to the fact that, for most herbal preparations, active materials have not been identified.

Even when active compounds have been identified, that an extract that concentrates identified active compounds at the expense of all the other naturally occurring constituents is not guaranteed to have any greater clinical efficacy then the traditionally used preparation. Until active materials are identified and the efficacy of refined extracts containing them is shown to be better than that of the traditional preparations, a dried crude extract in tablet form is probably the best candidate for clinical trial. Both chaste tree fruit and black cohosh root and rhizome are under investigation by the UIC/NIH Center for Botanical Dietary Supplement Research in Women's Health, and both have received monograph and therapeutic compendium treatment by the AHP, which may be consulted for further information.

REFERENCES

1. Shao Y, Harris A, Wang M, et al. Triterpene glycosides from *Cimifuga racemosa. J Nat Prod* 2000;63:905–910.
2. Struck D, Tegtmeier M, Harnischfeger G. Flavones in extracts of *Cimicifuga racemosa. Planta Med* 1999;63:289–290.
3. Einer-Jensen N, Zhao J, Andersen KP, Kristoffersen K. *Cimicifuga* and *Melbrosia* lack oestrogenic effects in mice and rats. *Maturitas* 1996;25:149–153.
4. Liske E, Wüstenberg P. Therapy of climacteric complaints with *Cimicifuga racemosa*: herbal medicine with clinically proven evidence. *Menopause* 1998;5:250.
5. Liu J, Burdette JE, Xu H, et al. Evaluation of estrogenic activity of plant extracts for the potential treatment of menopausal symptoms. *J Agric Food Chem* 2001;49:2472–2479.
6. Jarry H, Harnischfeger G. Studies on the endocrine efficacy of the constituents of *Cimicifuga racemosa*: 1. Influence on the serum concentration of pituitary hormones in ovariectomized rats. *Planta Med* 1995;51:46–49.
7. Jarry H, Harnischfeger G, Düker E. Studies on the endocrine efficacy of the constituents of *Cimicifuga racemosa*: 2. In vitro binding of constituents to estrogen receptors. *Planta Med* 1985;51:316–319.
8. Brücker A. Essay on the phytotherapy of hormonal disorders in women. *Med Welt* 1960;44: 2331–2333.
9. Daiber W. Climacteric complaints: success without using hormones—a phytotherapeutic agent lessens hot flushes, sweating, and insomnia. *Ärztliche Praxis* 1983;35:1946–1947.

10. Vorberg G. Therapy of climacteric complaints. *Zeitschrift Allgemeinmendizin* 1984;60:626–629.
11. Stolze H. An alternative to treat menopausal complaints. *Gyne* 1982;3:14–16.
12. Warnecke G. Influencing menopausal symptoms with a phytotherapeutic agent. *Med Welt* 1985;36: 871–874.
13. Stoll W. Phytopharmacon influences atrophic vaginal epithelium. Double-blind study: Cimicifuga vs. estrogenic substances. *Therapeuticum* 1987;1:23–31.
14. Lehmann-Willenbrock E, Riedel HH. Clinical and endrocrinological examinations concerning therapy of climacteric symptoms following hysterectomy with remaining ovaries. *Zentralbl Gynäkol* 1988;110:611–618.
15. Düker EM, Kopanski L, Jarry H, Wuttke W. Effects of extracts from *Cimicifuga racemosa* on gonadotropin release in menopausal women and ovariectomized rats. *Planta Med* 1991;57:420–424.
16. Jacobson JS, Troxel AB, Evans J, et al. Randomized trial of black cohosh for the treatment of hot flashes among women with a history of breast cancer. *J Clin Oncol* 2001;19:2739–2745.
17. McGuffin M, Hobbs C, Upton R, Goldberg A. *Botanical safety handbook*. Boca Raton: CRC, 1997: 29–30.
18. Upton R, ed. *Black cohosh rhizome,* Actaea racemosa *L. syn.* Cimicifuga racemosa *(L.) nutt. Standards of analysis, quality control, and therapeutics. American herbal pharmacopoeia and therapeutic compendium.* Santa Cruz, CA: 2002.
19. Upton R, ed. *Chaste tree fruit, Vitex agnus-castus, standards of analysis, quality control, and therapeutics. American herbal pharmacopoeia and therapeutic compendium.* Santa Cruz, CA: 2001.
20. Meier B, Berger D, Hoberg E, et al. Pharmacological activities of Vitex agnus-castus extracts in vitro. *Phytomedicine* 2000;7:373–381.
21. Schellenberg R, Kunze G, Pfaff ER, et al. Treatment for the premenstrual syndrome with agnus castus fruit extract: prospective, randomised, placebo controlled study. *BMJ* 2001;332:134–137.
22. Turner S, Mills S. A double-blind clinical trial on a herbal remedy for premenstrual syndrome: a case study. *Comp Therap Med* 1993;1:73–77.
23. Lauritzen C, Reuter HD, Repges R, et al. Treatment of premenstrual tension syndrome with Vitex agnus-castus; controlled double-blind study versus pyridoxine. *Phytomedicine* 1997;4:183–189.

12

Ginkgo Biloba Extract in Cognitive Disorders

Pierre Le Bars and Janet Kastelan

INTRODUCTION

The ginkgo biloba tree, native to China, is the last surviving species from the Ginkgoaceae family. Cooling temperatures and competition with other families of trees have most likely been responsible for the steady disappearance of this genus, which was abundant throughout the entire northern hemisphere 200 million years ago. While the biloba species was essentially extinguished from the wild, it currently remains unchanged from its ancestors and owes its survival to Chinese gardeners, who grew it for its impressive appearance, extreme resistance to pests and diseases, exceptional longevity, and valuable fruits and timber. Leaves and fruits have been used in traditional Chinese medicine for centuries, and they were introduced in European phytomedicine around the 1950s. This exceptional botanical evolution would be only a picturesque story if the modern techniques of cultivation and extraction had not been developed and had not given a new birth to this living fossil and ancient remedy. In the past 20 years, the methodical procedures of extraction and standardization have allowed the production of a highly concentrated and stable extract of ginkgo biloba (EGb) that could be systematically studied in scientific programs. Research on the extract provided replicable outcomes and consequently led to its integration in modern pharmacopoeia. Today, EGb is registered as an ethical drug in more than 50 countries around the world and is recommended for managing symptoms associated with a range of neurologic and vascular disorders, including dementia, arterial occlusive disease, retinal deficit, and tinnitus. This chapter will focus mainly on the relevant data that support its use in the treatment of cognitive disorders.

STANDARDIZATION OF GINKGO BILOBA EXTRACT

The standardization of herbal remedies is an essential condition for their scientific use, as well as a guarantee for reducing variability in treatment response. With regard to standardization, ginkgo biloba is favored over other medicinal plants because it is a lone species that can be successfully grown in plantations with a well controlled environment. Furthermore, since the leaves offer the majority of the therapeutic agents, harvest of the leaves only at a precise period in their maturation further reduces the variability of the raw material and improves the standardization of the final extraction. Methodologic procedures are used to prepare the extract from the dried leaves, with concentration ranging from 35:1 to 67:1. High stability is achieved in the ratio of the most active constituents, including the flavonoid glycosides (22% to 26%), proanthocyanidins (6% to 10%), and the terpenes—ginkgolide (2.8% to 3.4%) and bilobalide (2.6% to 3.2%). The standardization also aims to reduce the concentration of ginkgolic acids (i.e., less than 5 ppm) that are considered allergenic. Overall, about 70% of the total constituents of the extract are systematically verified to ensure the optimal ratio of the therapeutic agents and a consistent quality, regardless of the origin of the raw material. Such rigorous standardization follows a patented method with the code name extract of ginkgo biloba EGb 761 (EGb). This extract has an identical formulation and composition to the product registered in Germany under the name Tebonin forte (Schwabe Pharmaceuticals, Karlsruhe) and in France under Tanakan (Beaufour-Ipsen Pharmaceuticals, Paris). Most of the studies reviewed below tested this standardized extract of ginkgo biloba, either in total extract form or in only the constitutive fractions relevant for a particular experiment.

RATIONALE AND MODE OF ACTION

An overwhelming amount of data is currently available from basic research on ginkgo. However, selecting the relevant data to substantiate the clinical effects observed in human central nervous system (CNS) studies that test EGb is very difficult. This is due mainly to the extraordinary complexity of the extract formulation, which includes numerous agents that could interact differently with each other, generating additive, synergistic, or antagonistic effects depending on the doses, the status of the targeted tissue, and the condition of the experiment (*in vitro*, *ex vivo*, or *in vivo*). Furthermore, when EGb is administered orally in humans, some of the extract constituents may not be absorbed, while others are transformed by gastrointestinal microorganisms or are metabolized by the liver. This transformation results in an even more complex situation *in vivo* where EGb is partially converted to numerous metabolites, not all of which are active or bioavailable at the CNS level. Finally, one should keep in mind that several pharmacologic activities attributed to the total extract still can not be credited to any one specific agent or to a univocal mode of action. Currently, what is known of the effects of the whole extract surpasses what is known of its parts.

With regard to the bioavailability of EGb, the fact that in humans the terpenes (ginkgolides and bilobalide) are rapidly and totally absorbed after oral administration has been established. They reach a maximum dose-linear concentration in the blood within 1 to 2 hours with an average half-life of 3 to 4 hours, depending on the agent that is considered. The data on flavonoids are less conclusive; some reports indicate that this EGb fraction is not completely absorbed and that it undergoes an extensive transformation leading to the early release of multiple active and inactive metabolites. Using radiolabeled EGb in the rat, after oral administration, the EGb agents or their metabolites were shown to distribute broadly in the whole body (e.g., blood, liver, spleen, lung, heart, skin, vitreous humor) and, to a lesser degree, in the nervous system. A comparison between animal and human pharmacokinetic data estimates that an oral dose of 50 mg per kg for the rat roughly corresponds to a dose of 240 mg for the human. Since this human dose is commonly recommended as a total daily regimen, effects obtained with higher doses in animal studies may not be relevant for substantiating the clinical effects observed at a normal dose in humans. On the other hand, considering that the bioavailability of the active EGb agents at the CNS level has yet to be clarified, a number of effects described during *in vitro* experiments may not be observed in human pharmacology. Taking into account these caveats, four main classes of effects should be considered as follows: (a) EGb is a free radical scavenger and an antioxidant; (b) it is a platelet-activating factor (PAF) antagonist; (c) it has vasomodulation effects; and (d) it has energy-enhancing properties (1). The following attempts to delineate these actions separately; however, they are mostly interrelated *in vivo,* and some may be the end result of common underlying processes yet to be determined.

The free radical scavenging and antioxidant properties of EGb are extensively documented *in vitro*, as well as *ex vivo*. Independent of the concentration tested, EGb very efficiently scavenges hydroxyl free radicals mainly via its flavonoid fraction. Its action against superoxide anions seems to be concentration dependent and is related mostly to the terpenoid agents. The result of this synergistic interaction is that low doses of EGb are as potent as vitamin E in reducing lipid peroxidation, as has been observed with rat brain synaptosomes as well as with human lymphocytes, and they are only slightly less potent against DNA-oxidative damage. Reduction of lipid peroxidation as a result of free radical scavenging is an important aspect of the direct action of EGb against membrane insults that occur during various oxidative stresses. It may also affect the membrane fluidity and may indirectly change the functions of the bioamine receptors or transporters. Such direct and indirect actions may explain the beneficial effects of EGb in the reduction of apoptosis and in the regulation of receptor density and bioamine availability, which have been reported in numerous CNS studies and are further delineated below.

Ginkgolides are well established antagonists of PAF, which is a proinflammatory phospholipid synthesized by platelets, certain leukocytes, and endothelial cells during anaphylaxis, tissue insults, and shock. Ginkgolides specifically inhibit the binding of PAF to platelets, thus reducing thrombus formation only in relation to PAF release (ginkgolides did not show activity against adenosine diphosphate or other aggregating agents). In relatively high doses, ginkgolides can blunt PAF-induced chemotaxis, aggregation and degranulation of leukocytes, PAF-increased vascular permeability, extravasation and hemoconcentration, and PAF-induced contraction of gastrointestinal and pulmonary smooth muscles. Of the A, B, C, J, and M forms of ginkgolides, the B form was found to be the most potent PAF-antagonist. Since the total extract contains less than 1% of this ginkgolide form (A and C are the most represented), parenteral administration or extremely high oral doses of EGb may be required to reach clinically significant effects that are directly related to PAF-inhibition *in vivo*. This may explain the moderate anti-PAF effect at the peripheral level that is reported with the use of the total extract, as well as the substantial interindividual differences observed in some human studies. At the CNS level, release of PAF has been described as one of the proinflammatory processes that induce free radical production and lipid peroxidation. The PAF-inhibition of the terpenes complements the free radical scavenging action, thus reducing the oxidative stress and inflammatory responses during brain insults (e.g., inhibition of beta–amyloid–induced cell death). Such an effect is observed during hypoxia in animals receiving moderate doses of EGb (50 mg per kg orally), and it results in an increased survival time and decreased neuronal loss. Furthermore, it enhances the protection of neurons during ischemia and postischemic reperfusion phases, particularly by reducing postischemic neuronal damage at the hippocampus level.

Detailing the circulatory effects of EGb, which is polyvalent (action on the vascular wall, formed elements of the blood, heart, cerebral blood flow, etc.) and widely dependent on the experimental model, is beyond the scope of this chapter. Nevertheless, moderate and high doses of EGb, mostly via the proanthocyanidin fraction, activate the release of endothelium-derived relaxing factor (EDRF), which appears to be nitric oxide (NO). Furthermore, EGb can protect cyclic guanine monophosphate from phosphodiesterase (papaverine-like effect) and EDRF-NO from free radical attacks, thus inducing or potentiating vasorelaxation. In synergy with this proanthocyanidin effect, ginkgolides might reduce arteriolar spasm by the direct inhibition of PAF or thromboxane A_2. On the other hand, in lower doses, EGb has been shown to enhance norepinephrine-induced aortic contraction, possibly related to an increase of catecholamine release (tyramine-like action), an inhibition of catechol-O-methyl transferase, or a direct action on the α-adrenoreceptors. Collectively, these different activities qualify EGb as a vasoregulator whose final effects depend largely on the status of the vascular tone, the dose used, and its mode of administration. With regard to the CNS, EGb was shown to increase cerebral blood flow in animal models and to improve cerebral hemodynamic parameters in three open studies with patients suffering from cerebrovascular diseases.

In line with the vasomodulation properties, EGb action on cerebral metabolism depends on the normal or abnormal physiologic state of the model tested. In normal animals, moderate and high doses of EGb decrease glucose use in various brain areas. During hypoxia and ischemia, EGb restores oxidative metabolism and increases glucose consumption. During cerebral edema induced by triethyltrin, biloba was shown to be the EGb fraction that protects the cell metabolism against the uncoupling of oxidative phosphorylation, thus improving mitochondrial respiration, restoring glucose utilization, and increasing adenosine triphosphate levels. These effects on metabolism act synergistically with the free radical scavenging and/or antioxidant action, the PAF-inhibition, and the circulatory modulation that was previously mentioned to result in an increased protection against the cytotoxicity induced by various CNS insults, including those occurring during a number of degenerative diseases.

Several other CNS actions have been reported in animal models. However, a majority of these actions is indirect and secondary to the aforementioned membrane stabilization and the neuroprotective properties of the EGb constituents; these therefore will not be further developed here. An example of such an indirect effect is the EGb-increased density of neuroreceptors. This is due neither to a direct interaction with the receptor sites nor to a particular neurotransmitter system (increased density was reported for serotonin$_{1A}$ and muscarinic, as well as α-adrenergic, receptors, depending on the brain regions studied). Furthermore, it is widely dependent on the model tested, and it is most exclusively observed as a preventative effect in treated aged animal groups compared to the placebo. Nevertheless, EGb action on the glucocorticoid system and its potential anti-stress effect deserves special attention. On one hand, EGb has been shown to suppress prednisolone-induced downregulation of hippocampal type II glucocorticoid receptors, a process possibly involved in stress-induced cognitive impairment. On the other hand, the chronic administration of EGb caused a dose-dependent and reversible decrease in circulating corticosterone due to a change in the gene expression of adrenocortical mitochondrial benzodiazepine receptors. This action was considered specific at the adrenal gland level, and it was associated with a selective inhibition at the hypothalamo-pituitary level, as documented by the absence of a secondary increase of adrenocorticotropic hormone (inhibition of negative feedback). If such actions are confirmed in humans, they may shed some light on the stress-alleviating or the anxiolytic-like effects of EGb, which have been reported in some studies concomitant with the improvement of cognitive performance.

CLINICAL PHARMACOLOGY AND EFFICACY DATA

The past two decades of clinical research has produced a large body of evidence to support the efficacy of EGb in the human population. However, the very same fields that demonstrated efficacy have simultaneously yielded contradictory results. While an underpowered study or a study applying an inadequate design could occasionally explain a negative outcome, many trials meeting standard criteria nevertheless have led to inconclusive findings. An analysis of the discrepant results reveals at least three confounding factors that could be a source of discrepancy among studies as follows: (a) the characteristics of the population studied, (b) the type of outcome measurements selected, and (c) the EGb regimen tested in the trial. Each of these factors may be an important element in the success of ginkgo during the research program, as well as in clinical practice.

The following will delineate the relevant clinical outcomes and the role played by the aforementioned factors in the three CNS fields where research has demonstrated efficacy: (a) EGb-induced CNS changes, as measured by electrophysiology; (b) EGb-induced changes in memory; and (c) EGb in dementia and related cognitive disorders.

ELECTROPHYSIOLOGY

Electrophysiology is a field of interest for assessing the effect of EGb at the CNS level, particularly because electroencephalography (EEG) is extremely sensitive to changes of vigilance and because it has been extensively used to assess the pharmacodynamic effects of several CNS active agents. A change of the theta–alpha ratio or the beta and alpha bands has been considered the most adequate outcome measures for demonstrating the bioavailability and the pharmacodynamic effects of the so-called nootropic agents and cognitive activators. Agents belonging to this family usually decrease the theta–alpha ratio by either increasing alpha or decreasing theta activities. They also tend to increase slow beta activity, resulting in an overall acceleration of the EEG background.

As Table 12.1 shows, EGb may induce such EEG changes. However, the effects are not unequivocal, and they seem to differ with the characteristics of the population studied. In healthy volunteers, EGb increases the alpha and slow beta fractions of the EEG spectrum (2–5), while in patient populations, it is more prone to reduce the occurrence of slow activities (i.e., delta and theta), thus leading to a decrease of the theta–alpha ratio (6–9).

Some trials have failed to show such EEG changes and have reported conflicting findings. This discrepancy was mostly due to differences in the study populations, the EEG baseline characteristics, circadian fluctuations of electrical activities associated with spontaneous changes of vigilance, and a complex EGb dose-response relationship. An example of interference between baseline characteristics and outcome measurements can be seen in the Kunkel study (5), which failed to show a significant increase of alpha activity after 3 days of administering 160 mg of EGb to healthy volunteers. Two of the inclusion criteria were a high alpha ratio in the baseline EEG—70% of the background activity had to be spent in the alpha band—and a dominant alpha frequency, strictly between 9 and 11 Hz. These extremely selective criteria resulted in the dropout of 50% of the healthy population screened. Not surprisingly, with such a rigid preselected alpha background, EGb induced only minor changes in the alpha band (no change in the occipital areas), while significant changes could still be seen in the other frequencies. The healthy volunteers showed the expected increase of slow beta activity that reached the level of statistical significance in temporal areas when compared to the placebo. An example of multiple interference between the selection of study population, the baseline EEG, and outcome measurement is also found in the Gessner study (8), which enrolled a heterogeneous group of elderly volunteers complaining of nonspecific cognitive decline. Results based on the mean comparisons of six EEG bands did not show significant changes after receiving EGb, 120 mg per day, during a 12-week chronic dosing. However, when a more homogeneous subgroup of patients with a slow EEG background was selected (the most impaired cases), EGb induced a significant decrease of theta activity and an increase of alpha frequency, particularly during the resting EEG sessions. The authors attributed these changes to an improvement of vigilance. By performing a *post hoc* selection of the cases with the slowest EEG baseline, Gessner decreased variability and increased the magnitude of the treatment effect.

With regard to time and dose-response relationships, the EEG data remain largely elusive. As an example, Krauskoft et al. (unpublished data, see reference 1) reported a dose-related increase of alpha activity after 120, 240, 400, and 600 mg EGb, while Kunkel failed to find any dose-response relationship for 40, 80, and 160 mg per day after 3 days of chronic administration (5). Conflicting results can be related to the multiple modes of action of EGb, which change widely with the dose regimen and the experimental conditions. EGb may affect the CNS at different levels and may lead to different time-related and dose-related EEG changes. Moreover, the dose-effect relationship may or may not be linear depending on the bioassay selected in the EEG spectrum. At least four studies (Table 12.1) reported that acute single oral doses of EGb induced an increase of alpha frequency in healthy young volunteers. The effect had a very early onset (approximately 30 minutes to 1 hour after administration) and reached a peak within 2 to 4 hours. With regard to the other EGb-related EEG changes, the decrease of theta activity or the increase of slow beta activity have not been systematically reported. When they are observed, these changes seem to occur later on and only after chronic dosing (4). Selecting the alpha band as a bioassay in a pilot study testing multiple single doses of EGb (40, 120, and 240 mg), Itil et al. reported a linear dose-response relationship when the time effect was eliminated by using the area under the curve (AUC) of alpha changes (2). Although it was weak, such linearity using the AUC of alpha was also observed in the study of Le Bars et al. (2). However, in this latter trial, when the time of assessment was taken into consideration, the dose response to EGb followed a bimodal curve. In accordance with the previous studies reporting a dose-response relationship, alpha changes that occurred immediately within 3 hours after a single EGb intake were dose dependent, although not in a linear dose-related manner, and they were correlated to a decrease of drowsiness, as assessed by a significant difference from the placebo on a vigilance self-rating scale. When concomitant positive responses on EEG and the vigilance self-rating scale were used as criteria for defining an EGb response, the dose-response relationship resulted in a hyperbolic curve with leveling starting after a 120-mg single oral dose. According to the authors, such a curve predicts a ceiling effect after a 240-mg acute single dose, as well as a maximal ratio of EGb responder from 55% to 60%. Interestingly, in this study, the late EEG changes observed at 7 and 9 hours after dosing were

TABLE 12.1. Clinical trials assessing Ginkgo biloba efficacy in electrophysiology

Reference*	First author	Year	Design	Dose regimen	Population (age)	Outcome measures	Results
2	Itil TM	1996	Four-way cross-over	40, 120, 240 mg EGb 761; placebo Single oral doses	12 healthy male volunteers (18–65 yr).	22 EEG parameters, individual and group profile measured in the right occipital areas. Sum of alpha change from baseline for all brain areas.	Discrimination from placebo at 1, 2, and 3 hr for 120 mg ($P <0.05$) and 240 mg ($P <0.01$). Significant increase of alpha activity in comparison with placebo for all time periods with all EGb doses ($P <0.01$).
3	Le Bars P	1996	Four-way cross-over	80, 120, 240 mg EGb 761; placebo Single oral doses	13 healthy male volunteers (18–45 yr).	22 EEG parameters, individual and group profile. Alpha change from baseline in the right occipital. Responder rate measured by combining behavior self-rating scale for vigilance and individual EEG profile.	Discrimination from placebo at 3 hr for 120 mg ($P =0.05$) and 3 and 5 hr for 240 mg ($P <0.05$) using EEG profile or alpha changes. Dose-related effect from 1 to 3 hr ($P =0.01$). Leveling of responder rate between 120 and 240 mg.
4	Luthringer R	1995	Three-way cross-over, followed by single blind	80, 160 mg EGb 761; placebo Single oral doses Followed by 5 d single-blind, 160 mg	15 healthy male volunteers (mean age 25–35 yr).	Change in absolute and relative power of 32 brain areas compared to baseline in five major EEG bands. Event-related potentials.	Discrimination from placebo for 80 and 160 mg ($P <0.05$) at 1 hr in slow alpha and 0.5, 1, and 6 hr for fast alpha. Beta increased and theta decreased after chronic dosing.
5	Kunkel H	1993	Four-way cross-over	40, 80, 160 mg EGb 761, placebo tid for 3 consecutive d prior to testing	12 healthy male volunteers (24–29 yr) with high alpha EEG (70%).	25 EEG parameters and five frequency bands measured in frontal, temporal, and occipital areas.	Discrimination from placebo ($P <0.05$) for 80 mg mainly in temporal areas in theta and beta bands. No significant change in alpha activity.
6	Hofferberth B	1994	2 Parallel groups	240 mg (80 mg tid) EGb 761 or placebo during 24 wk	40 patients (50–75 yr) with mild dementia of the Alzheimer type. All cases analyzed.	Change in relative power of occipital areas compared to baseline in four major EEG bands; theta/alpha quotient.	Statistically significant decrease of theta activity in comparison to placebo with decrease of theta/alpha quotient ($P <0.01$).

TABLE 12.1. *Continued.*

Reference*	First author	Year	Design	Dose regimen	Population (age)	Outcome measures	Results
7	Rai GS	1991	2 Parallel groups	120 mg (40 mg tid) EGb 761 or placebo during 24 wk	31 elderly (54–89 yr) with mild to moderate dementia. 27 cases analyzed, 15 in placebo group.	Latency of auditory ERP (P300). Change in delta, theta, and alpha EEG from baseline.	Statistically significant decrease of delta activity in comparison to placebo ($P < 0.05$). No significant change in the other EEG bands and in ERP latency.
8	Gessner B	1985	3 Parallel groups	120 mg EGb 761 (40 mg tid), or 5 mg nicergoline, or placebo during 12 wk	60 elderly (57–77 yr) with age-related mild cognitive decline. 57 cases analyzed, 19 EGb, 19 placebo.	Change in absolute and relative power in occipito-central leads. Theta/alpha ratio (T/A). Exploratory analysis in subgroups based on T/A ratio and dominant frequency.	NS for any EEG changes. In the sub-group with higher T/A ratio, EGb induced a decrease of ratio with increase vigilance. In the subgroup with slower alpha, EGb increased alpha by 2 Hz.
9	Pidoux B	1983	2 Parallel groups	160 mg (80 mg bid) EGb 761 or placebo during 12 wk	14 elderly (mean age 83–87 yr) with slow alpha background. 12 cases analyzed.	Change in absolute and relative power in occipito-parietal and centro-temporal leads compared to baseline in four EEG bands. SCAG.	EGb induced a statistically significant decrease of theta activity with decrease of theta/alpha quotient ($P < 0.05$). A 29% improvement of SCAG mean score ($P < 0.05$).

All studies are randomized, double-blind, placebo-controlled trials.
*See chapter references for reference information.
Abbreviations: EEG, electroencephalogram; EGb, extract of Ginkgo biloba EGb 761; ERP, event-related potential; NS, not significant; SCAG, Sandoz Clinical Assessment Geriatric scale.

not dose dependent, nor were they correlated to significant changes in vigilance. This late effect of EGb was more in line with the outcomes of trials measuring EEG after multiple dosing or chronic EGb regimens, as seen in the Kunkel trial.

The apparent complexity of the effects of EGb on the human EEG might reflect different bioavailability and modes of action of its constituents. As the previous section reported, EGb effect may be expressed differently depending on the status of the targeted organ and the varying interactions between its active agents and metabolites. Early studies attempted to explore the EEG changes induced by subfractions isolated from the extract, such as flavonoids and terpenes. However, this pioneer work led to inconclusive results, and further research is needed to substantiate the EEG pharmacodynamic effects of these EGb subfractions and to clarify their clinical relevance.

MEMORY AND NEUROPSYCHOLOGY

Memory and neuropsychologic testing provide a favorable domain in which to assess EGb efficacy on cognitive processes and to delineate the influence of the following two confounding factors: (a) the characteristics of the population studied and (b) the adequate selection of outcome measurements. In the studies summarized in Table 12.2, efficacy was systematically demonstrated when the study population consisted of the elderly or of subjects who were cognitively impaired at baseline, and it was rarely observed when the subjects were a group of young healthy volunteers (11–17). Assessments measuring accuracy and speed, which are mostly related to working memory, were more successful for observing the EGb effect than the assessments measuring long-term storage and retrieval abilities (delayed recall and recognition), regardless of study population. EGb seems to enhance complex attention, the speed of information processing, and the rate of working memory. Performance tests using response times as outcome measurements are particularly desirable and are sensitive enough to assess these cognitive domains. This may explain why the EGb effect was observed most on scanning speed (10,12), word recognition time (17), the rate of information processing, and the duration of present time (14) or time for dual coding (13). Warot et al. (11) reported a striking positive effect of EGb on a memory test that assessed the immediate recall of 20 pictures. However, the difference in the amount of material recalled was not due to an increase of performance in the EGb group (mean recall of 15.5 pictures at baseline versus 15.6 pictures 1 hour after the administration of 600 mg EGb) but rather to a statistically significant decrease of performance in the placebo group (15.7 pictures at baseline versus 13 at the 1 hour session). As a conclusion of their study, these authors suggested that EGb might have a preventative, rather than a memory-enhancing, effect. However, considering the healthy population enrolled in the trial and the short duration of the treatment, this preventative potential remains hypothetical.

In comparison with healthy subjects, the same type of effect with a greater treatment size was observed in groups of patients complaining of cognitive decline. Wesnes et al. (17) reported a significant increase in the speed of performance after 12 weeks of treatment with EGb, while no significant change was noted on the amount of words recognized. The study of Israel et al. (16) confirmed that EGb specifically improves attention and mental fluency and also minimally enhances general memory (recall). Finally, Rai et al. (7) demonstrated EGb efficacy on the speed of a classification task but not on the digit recall test.

The adequate dosage of EGb for achieving efficacy in these cognitive domains varied widely with the population studied and the treatment regimen used (single or multiple dosing and acute or chronic treatment). Overall, in healthy subjects, high doses (up to 600 mg) generally seemed to be required in order to achieve efficacy when acute single doses were tested. This was further substantiated in a recent study showing that a 120-mg single dose was more efficient in improving the Sternberg reaction time (i.e., scanning time in working memory) than was 50 mg given three times a day (150 mg daily dose) (11). On the other hand, no further benefit was observed by increasing the dose to a 240 mg, acute single regimen. At present, however, the optimal doses to achieve efficacy and the delineation of the dose-response relationship have not yet been determined in the patient population. Furthermore, if EGb effect is to be considered more in terms of the improvement of attention, working memory, and processing speed, additional research comparing the effects of multiple and different EGb regimens in the elderly with mild cognitive decline, as well as in impaired youngsters, should be considered.

CLINICAL STUDIES IN DEMENTIA AND RELATED DISORDERS

The majority of the clinical trials performed with EGb before 1989 were undertaken in Europe and used as inclusion criteria the diagnosis of cerebral insufficiency, which does not have an analogue in the current classification of disease (*International classification of disease,* 10th edition, [ICD-10] or *Diagnostic and statistical manual of mental disorders*, fourth edition, [DSM-IV]). This syndrome includes signs and symptoms very similar to those integrated in the so-called age-associated memory impairment syndrome. However, it could also have covered incipient dementia, as well as a mood-affective disorder that is not otherwise specified. A review of the literature at large by Kleijnen and Knipschild summarized the findings obtained in such patient populations (18). Of the 40 trials reviewed, 20 were double-blind studies, and eight met the minimum criteria to be considered an adequate randomized clinical trial (RCT). All the studies used 100 to 160 mg per day of EGb in chronic doses and reported significant improvements of the clinical global impression after a minimum 6-week to 12-week treatment. The responder rate varied from

TABLE 12.2. *Clinical trials assessing Ginkgo biloba efficacy on memory*

Reference*	First author	Year	Design	Dose regimen	Population (age)	Outcome measures	Results
10	Rigney U	1999	Five-way cross-over	120 mg, 50 mg tid, 240 mg, 100 mg tid, placebo; 2-Day oral doses	36 Healthy volunteers (30–59 yr). 31 cases analyzed.	CFF (vigilance), Choice RT, Stroop test, Sternberg test (memory scanning). Immediate and delayed word recall. Digit symbol substitution. Behavior rating scale.	NS for CFF, CRT, Stroop test, immediate and delayed recall, behavior rating scale, and digit symbol substitution. Time for Sternberg test was improved with 120, 240 mg and 100 mg tid (P <0.02).
11	Warot D	1991	Three-way cross-over	600 mg EGb 761, 600 mg Ginkgo, placebo; Single oral doses	12 Healthy female volunteers (19–30 yr).	CFF (vigilance), Choice RT, Sternberg test (memory scanning). Recall and recognition of images. Subjective ratings of drug effect.	NS for CFF, CRT, Sternberg test, and subjective ratings. Significant difference in image recalled (P =0.03) related to decrease with placebo (no change with EGb 761).
12	Subhan Z	1984	Four-way cross-over	120, 240, 600 mg EGb 761, placebo; Single oral doses	8 Healthy female volunteers (25–40 yr).	CFF (vigilance), Choice RT, Sternberg test. Subjective ratings of drug effect.	NS for CFF, CRT, number recognized in Sternberg test and subjective ratings. Time for Sternberg test was improved with 600 mg (P <0.001).
13	Allain H	1993	Three-way cross-over	320, 600 mg EGb 761, placebo; Single oral doses	18 Elderly (60–80 yr) with mild cognitive impairment.	Correct drawings and word recall. D/W differences in recall. Presentation time with dual coding.	Significant shift of dual coding (P <0.05) between placebo (1920 ms) and 320 or 600 mg of EGb 761 (960 ms). NS for correct drawings or word recall, or D/W recall differences.
14	Grassel E	1992	Multicenter, 2 parallel groups	160 mg (80 mg bid) EGb 761 or placebo during 24 wk	72 Patients (64 ± 8 yr) with cerebrovascular insufficiency and mild cognitive impairment. 53 Cases analyzed; 24 placebo, 29 EGb.	STM with processing speed and time of information accessibility. Basic learning rate (long-term retention). All measures were standardized and provided in M-IQ units.	STM increased significantly in EGb group (93.5 to 107.5 IQ) and was significantly different from placebo (93.8 to 95.8 IQ) after 24 wk (P =0.018). Differences in basic learning rate were NS.

TABLE 12.2. *Continued.*

Reference*	First author	Year	Design	Dose regimen	Population (age)	Outcome measures	Results
15	Hofferberth B	1989	2 Parallel groups	120 mg (40 mg tid) EGb 761 or placebo during 8 wk.	36 Patients (53–69 yr) with cerebrovascular insufficiency and/or mild cognitive impairment. 36 Cases analyzed.	Saccadic eye movement test (duration and latency). Vienna test (choice RT and % of correct responses). Trail making (executive function).	In the EGb group, saccade was significantly improved for duration (from 162 to 117 ms, $P <0.01$) and latency (from 249 to 196 ms; $P <0.01$); EGb normalized RT and % correct responses ($P <0.01$); Trail making time decreased from 40 sec to 27 sec ($P <0.01$).
16	Israel L	1987	4 Parallel groups	160 mg (80 mg bid) EGb 761 or placebo with or without memory training during 12 wk.	80 Elderly (50–83 yr) with mild cognitive impairment (MMSE 20-26). 5 Cases excluded from the analysis.	Global memory factor, attention-working memory, verbal learning rate, mental fluency and speed.	Global memory factor and verbal learning were not affected by EGb, while attention ($P <0.01$) and mental fluency ($P <0.005$) significantly improved in comparison to placebo.
17	Wesnes K	1987	2 Parallel groups	120 mg (40 mg tid) EGb 761 or placebo during 12 wk.	58 Elderly (62–85 yr) with mild cognitive impairment. 54 Cases analyzed, 27 in each group.	Immediate word recall, number matching task, rapid visual processing task, and choice RT. Digit symbol substitution. Delayed word recognition. Behavior rating scale.	In comparison with placebo, significant differences from baseline were found with EGb in number matching (correct detection, $P =0.02$; speed, $P =0.06$) and in speed of word recognition ($P =0.026$).

All studies were randomized, double-blind, placebo-controlled trials.

*See chapter references for reference information.

Abbreviations: CFF, critical flicker fusion; D/W, drawing versus word; EGb, extract of Ginkgo biloba EGb 761; M-IQ, memory-intelligence quotient; MMSE, mini-mental status examination; NS, not significant; RT, reaction time; STM, short-term performance.

20% to 70% depending on the study. Results obtained in such a nonspecific diagnosis framework, however, may not necessarily apply for pure cognitive disorders, and they are difficult to integrate today in a review of EGb efficacy.

A later review of the literature by Letzel (19) exclusively selected EGb studies enrolling patient populations with a diagnosis of cognitive disorder. Of 25 randomized, double-blind, placebo-controlled EGb studies available at that time, eight explicitly included demented patients, and three applied standard inclusion criteria of dementia using DSM-III-R. Overall, 23 studies reported a statistically significant difference favorable to EGb on at least one of the three levels of assessment as follows: clinical global impression, psychometric, or social behavior and daily living. Of the 18 studies that included simultaneous assessments of the clinical global impression and the psychometric, ten demonstrated that the EGb effect could be discriminated from the placebo at a statistical level of significance. When only dementia was considered as the population of interest, seven of the eight trials available reported a significant treatment effect. Five of these trials showed positive results simultaneously in at least two levels of assessment (clinical global impression and psychometric). With regard to safety, no significant difference was found between EGb and the placebo. Of a whole study population of 739 patients, the most frequent events were gastrointestinal (19 patients or 2.6%), headache (seven patients or 0.9%), sleep disturbances and dizziness (three patients or 0.4%), and skin eruptions (two patients or 0.3%).

Since the review of Letzel, the efficacy of EGb has been further supported by the results obtained from a multicenter randomized clinical trial conducted in the United States, which enrolled 327 patients with Alzheimer disease (AD) or multiinfarct dementia (20). While the largest study conducted in Europe used 240 mg of EGb per day during 24 weeks and focused on dementia of mild-to-moderate severity (21), the North American study (20) tested 120 mg per day during 52 weeks and included patients showing a broader range of impairment, as assessed by Mini Mental State Examination scores ranging from 9 to 26 and Global Deterioration Scale scores of 3 to 6. At the 52-week endpoint, the group that received EGb did not show a significant worsening on the psychometric scale (a cognitive subtest of the Alzheimer's Disease Assessment Scale), whereas the placebo group showed a worsening of 1.5 points, resulting in a statistically significant difference favoring EGb (1.4 points, P=0.04). On the Geriatric Evaluation by Relative's Rating Instrument scale, which was used by the caregivers to assess daily living and social behavior, mild improvement was observed for the EGb group, whereas the placebo group worsened. The mean treatment effect of 0.14 points showed a statistically significant benefit for EGb (P=0.004). No difference was found, however, on the Clinical Global Impression (CGI).

To facilitate a historical comparison between EGb studies, a *post hoc* intent-to-treat analysis using a 6-month endpoint was recently performed on the North American data set (22). A summary of the outcomes of these analyses is provided in Table 12.3, along with those from the trials of Hofferberth (6) and

Kanowski et al. (21) because they may be considered the most representative of the European data. Comparison of the North American results with those reported in the German studies might suggest that an increased EGb dose would result in an increased treatment effect. After a similar treatment duration (24 weeks), the group in the Kanowski study treated with 240 mg EGb showed a positive outcome on the CGI and a higher percentage of improved patients. In the EGb group, 38% of the patients reached the highest cutoff point on the cognitive scale versus 26% in the North American study. Both showed a similar placebo response (17% to 18%). The increase in the responder rate, however, does not seem to be linear with the increase of dosage. In other words, doses higher than 240 mg may not significantly increase the treatment size. This pattern of response was previously predicted by the EEG results (3). Ultimately, a control study with multiple doses of EGb would be needed to clarify the dose-response relationship and to help delineate the optimal regimen to obtain symptomatic improvement in dementia.

CONCLUSION

Standardization of EGb has been successfully achieved, and scientific evidence is available to delineate some of its actions in humans. Effects at the CNS level have been objectively demonstrated by the use of neuropsychologic tests and electrophysiologic assessments. Finally, EGb efficacy has been reasonably substantiated by the positive outcomes of several clinical trials in groups of patients suffering with dementia. Except for the risk of hemorrhage in patients who take anticoagulants, have bleeding disorders, or must undergo surgery (23–29), EGb appears to be very safe.

Many trials have yielded discrepant findings, which can be explained by the interference of confounding factors. To guarantee successes in future research, as well as in medical interventions, the following three factors should be controlled. First, the population of interest should show an objective cognitive impairment at baseline. Second, in the selection of outcome measurements, one should add to the broad assessments of cognition timed tests that measure attention and working memory in particular (e.g., Syndrome Kurtz test or Sternberg test). Third, treatment should explore multiple EGb regimens with a maximal single dose equal to 120 mg; daily doses higher than 240 mg may eventually be required to achieve an optimal response in some patients depending on the domain of impairment.

Considering the possible modes of action of EGb, preventative effects may be expected. Thus, future trials with special designs to assess a possible change in the course of CNS pathophysiologic processes would be important for delineating fully the role this special extract of ginkgo biloba can play in modern pharmacopoeia.

Ginkgo's potential role in the management of antidepressant-induced sexual dysfunction is reviewed in Chapter 13.

TABLE 12.3. *Clinical trials assessing Ginkgo biloba efficacy in Alzheimer disease and vascular dementia*

Reference*	First author	Year	Design	Dose	Population	Outcome measures	Results
6	Hofferberth B	1994	2 Parallel groups	240 mg (80 tid) EGb 761 or placebo during 24 wk	40 Inpatients (50–75 yr) with dementia of the Alzheimer type. 21 EGb, 19 placebo. All cases analyzed.	SKT (attention and memory). SCAG. Subjective ratings of drug effect (global impression of physician). (Choice RT, EEG, and saccadic eye movement test).	SKT: Improvement for EGb (from 17 to 12 points); 50% of EGb group improved by 5 pts versus 0% placebo ($P < 0.001$). SCAG: Improvement on 13/18 items and all 5 subscales (6 items reached a descriptive $P < 0.01$). Global impression was favored to EGb ($P < 0.05$) with 16/21 patients much improved (76%) versus 0% placebo.
20	Le Bars P	1997	2 Parallel groups	120 mg (40 tid) EGb 761 or placebo during 52 wk	327 Outpatients (69 ± 10 yr) with mild to moderate AD or vascular dementia. 137 Reached 52 wk. 309 Analyzed (ITT).	ADAS-Cog (mental status). CGI. GERRI (social behavior). Therapy response was defined *a posteriori*: 4 pts ADAS-Cog and 0.2 pts improvement on GERRI.	ADAS: 1.4 pts difference favorable to EGb ($P = 0.04$) with 27% EGb responders versus 13% placebo. ($P < 0.01$). CGI was NS. GERRI: 0.14 pts difference favorable to EGb ($P < 0.01$) with 37% EGb responders versus 23% placebo.

TABLE 12.3. *Continued.*

Reference*	First author	Year	Design	Dose	Population	Outcome measures	Results
21	Kanowski S	1996	2 Parallel groups	240 mg (120 bid) EGb 761 or placebo during 24 wk	222 Outpatients (70 ± 10 yr) with mild to moderate AD or vascular dementia. 216 Randomized, 156 analyzed.	SKT (attention and memory). CGI. NAB (social behavior). Therapy response was defined *a priori*: at least 4 pts SKT and 2 pts CGI or NAB.	SKT: 38% EGb responders versus 18% placebo (*P* <0.05). CGI: 32% EGb responders versus 17% placebo (*P* <0.05). NAB: 33% EGb responders versus 23% placebo (*P* =0.09, NS).
22	Le Bars P	2000	2 Parallel groups	120 mg (40 tid) EGb 761 or placebo during 26 wk	327 Outpatients (69 ± 10 yr) with mild to moderate AD or vascular dementia. 244 Reached 26 wk. 309 Analyzed (ITT).	ADAS-Cog (mental status). CGI. GERRI (social behavior). Therapy response was defined *a posteriori*: 4 pts ADAS-Cog and 0.2 pts improvement on GERRI.	ADAS: 1.3 pts difference favorable to EGb (*P* =0.04) with 26% EGb responders versus 17% placebo (*P* =0.04). CGI was NS. GERRI: 0.12 pts difference favorable to EGb (*P* <0.01) with 30% improved and 17% worsened EGb patients versus 25% and 37% placebo, respectively.

All studies are randomized, double-blind, placebo-controlled trials.
*See chapter references for reference information.
Abbreviations: AD, Alzheimer disease; ADAS-Cog, Alzheimer Disease Assessment Scale, Cognitive subtest; CGI, Clinical Global Impression; EGb, extract of Ginkgo biloba; GERRI, Geriatric Evaluation by Relative's Rating Instrument; ITT, Intent-to-treat; NAB, Nurnberger Alters-Beobachtungsskala; NS, not significant; SCAG, Sandoz Clinical Assessment Geriatric scale; SKT, Syndrome-Kurztest.

REFERENCES

1. DeFeudis FV, ed. *Ginkgo biloba extract (EGb 761): from chemistry to the clinic.* Wiesbaden, Germany: Ullstein Medical, 1998.
2. Itil TM, Emin E, Tsambis E, et al. Central nervous system effect of ginkgo biloba, a plant extract. *Am J Ther* 1996;3:63-73.
3. Le Bars P, Itil TM, Salzman C, et al. QEEG for dose-finding of new psychotropics and antidementia drugs. In: Kimura J, Shibasaki H, eds. *Recent advances in clinical neurophysiology.* Amsterdam: Elsevier, 1996:780–783.
4. Luthringer R, d'Arbigny P, Macher JP. Ginkgo biloba extract (EGb 761), EEG and event-related potentials mapping profile. In: Christen Y, Courtois Y, Droy-Lefaix MT, eds. *Advances in ginkgo biloba extract research*, Vol. 4. Effects of ginkgo biloba extract (EGb 761) on aging and age-related disorders. Paris: Elsevier, 1995:107–118.
5. Kunkel H. EEG profile of three different extractions of ginkgo biloba. *Neuropsychobiology* 1993;27: 40–45.
6. Hofferberth B. The efficacy of EGb 761 in patients with senile dementia of the Alzheimer type, a double-blind, placebo-controlled study on different levels of investigation. *Human Psychopharmacol* 1994;9:215–222.
7. Rai GS, Shovlin C, Wesnes KA. A double-blind, placebo controlled study of ginkgo biloba extract (tanakan) in elderly outpatients with mild to moderate memory impairment. *Curr Med Res Opinion* 1991;12:350–355.
8. Gessner B, Voelp A, Klasser M. Study of the long-term action of ginkgo biloba extract on vigilance and mental performance as determine by means of quantitative pharmaco-EEG and psychometric measurements. *Arzneim Forsch Drug Res* 1985;35:1459–1465.
9. Pidoux B, Bastien C, Niddam S. Clinical and quantitative EEG double-blind study of ginkgo biloba extract (GBE). *J Cereb Blood Flow Metab* 1983;3:S556–S557.
10. Rigney U, Kimber S, Hindmarch I. The effect of acute doses of standardized ginkgo biloba extract on memory and psychomotor performance in volunteers. *Phytother Res* 1999;13:408–415.
11. Warot D, Lacombez L, Danjou P, et al. Comparative effects of Ginkgo biloba extract on psychomotor performance and memory in healthy volunteers (in French). *Therapie* 1991;46:33–36.
12. Subhan Z, Hindmarch I. The pharmacological effects of ginkgo biloba extract in normal healthy volunteers. *Int J Clin Pharm Res* 1984;4:89–93.
13. Allain H, Raoul P, Lieury A, et al. Effect of two doses of ginkgo biloba extract (EGb 761) on the dual-coding test in elderly subjects. *Clin Ther* 1993;15:549–558.
14. Grassel E. The influence of ginkgo biloba extract on mental performance, a double blind study under computerized measurement conditions in patient with cerebral insufficiency (in German). *Fortschr Med* 1992;110:73–76.
15. Hofferberth B. Effect of ginkgo extract on neurophysiological and psychometric findings in patients with cerebro-organic syndrome (in German). *Arzneim Forsch Drug Res* 1989;39:918–922.
16. Israel L, Dell'Accio E, Martin G, Hugonot R. Ginkgo biloba and memory training programs. Comparative assessment on elderly out-patients (in French). *Psychol Med* 1987;19:1431–1439.
17. Wesnes K, Simmons D, Rook M, Simpson P. A double-blind placebo-controlled trial of tanakan in the treatment of idiopathic cognitive impairment in the elderly. *Human Psychopharmacol* 1987;2:159–169.
18. Kleijnen J, Knipschild P. Ginkgo biloba for cerebral insufficiency. *Br J Clin Pharmacol* 1992;34: 352–358.
19. Letzel H, Haan J, Feil WB. Nootropics: efficacy and tolerability of products from three active substance classes. *J Drug Dev Clin Pract* 1996;8:77–94.
20. Le Bars PL, Katz MM, Berman N, et al. A placebo-controlled, double-blind, randomized trial of an extract of ginkgo biloba for dementia. *JAMA* 1997;278:1327–1332.
21. Kanowski S, Herrmann WM, Stephan K, et al. Proof of efficacy of ginkgo biloba special extract EGb 761 in outpatients suffering from mild to moderate primary degenerative dementia of the Alzheimer type or multi-infarct dementia. *Pharmacopsychiatry* 1996;29:47–56.
22. Le Bars PL, Kieser M, Itil KZ. A 26-week analysis of a double-blind, placebo-controlled trial of the ginkgo biloba extract EGb 761 in dementia. *Dement Geriatr Cogn Disord* 2000;11:230–237.
23. Smith PF, Maclennan K, Darlington CL. The neuroprotective properties of the ginkgo biloba leaf: a review of the possible relationship to platelet-activating factor (PAF). *J Ethnopharmacol* 1996;50: 131–139.
24. Ang-Lee MK, Moss J, Yuan CS. Herbal medicines and perioperative care. *JAMA* 2001;286:208–216.

25. Pribitkin ED, Boger G. Herbal therapy: what every facial plastic surgeon must know. *Arch Facial Plast Surg* 2001;3:127–132.

26. Fessenden JM, Wittenborn W, Clarke L. Gingko biloba: a case report of herbal medicine and bleeding postoperatively from a laparoscopic cholecystectomy. *Am Surg* 2001;67:33–35.

27. Benjamin J, Muir T, Briggs K, Pentland B. A case of cerebral haemorrhage-can ginkgo biloba be implicated? *Postgrad Med J* 2001;77:112–113.

28. Evans V. Herbs and the brain: friend or foe? The effects of ginkgo and garlic on warfarin use. *J Neurosci Nurs* 2000;32:229–232.

29. Heck AM, DeWitt BA, Lukes AL. Potential interactions between alternative therapies and warfarin. *Am J Health Syst Pharm* 2000;57:1221–1227.

PART IV

Polypharmacy and
Side Effects Management

13

Polypharmacy and Side Effects Management with Natural Psychotropic Medications

David Mischoulon

INTRODUCTION

With the increasing numbers of psychotropic agents that are available, psychiatrists often find themselves practicing polypharmacy, a strategy that involves the use of medications with—usually—complementary mechanisms of action. This approach may be used to treat a single condition aggressively, to treat coexisting conditions or symptom clusters, or to counteract the adverse effects from one psychotropic agent. For example, patients with very severe depression may require the administration of two or more antidepressant agents with complementary mechanisms of action (e.g., selective serotonin reuptake inhibitors [SSRI] plus bupropion), patients with anxious depression may benefit from the combination of antidepressants with anxiolytics, and patients experiencing sexual dysfunction from SSRIs may benefit from the addition of bupropion, and so on.

While augmentation and combination strategies with registered psychotropic agents have been studied in research settings and have been reviewed in the literature (1), a paucity of data exists regarding the effectiveness, safety, and drug-drug interactions of combinations of natural psychotropic agents, either with other natural remedies or with registered medications.

Increasing numbers of individuals nowadays are choosing to self-medicate with natural over-the-counter treatments, often without informing their physician (2–4). Patients may use these remedies in combination with prescription medications or with other natural medications. As the preceding chapters illustrate, information is limited about adverse drug-drug interactions with natural psychotropic agents; but reports of adverse interactions have been increasing, and safety is therefore a major consideration. Despite the risks of over-the-counter polypharmacy, many patients have benefited from taking a natural medication in conjunction with a registered medication or with other natural remedies. For example, some formulations of the antidepressant St. John's wort also contain kava for added anxiolysis (5). Clinicians should therefore routinely ask their patients about their natural medication use and should discuss the risks and benefits of polypharmacy with natural agents.

Given the importance and widespread use of augmentation and combination strategies in psychopharmacology (6,7), establishing a framework for polypharmacy with natural remedies as part of the patient's regimen is worthwhile. Using the available data on natural medications and the clinician's experience with registered medications, developing some reasonable strategies for approaching the patient who may require (or desire) polypharmacy with natural remedies is possible. As with registered medications, the clinician can, in theory, use natural remedies in combination with other natural or even registered medications to treat concurrent disorders, to obtain a more robust effect on one disorder, or to counteract the adverse effects of a concomitant medication. A few such strategies will be outlined in this chapter. The reader should bear in mind that the combination strategies considered here are largely speculative and do not have solid research data to support or reject their use. Caution should always be exercised when considering polypharmacy with alternative medications.

MANAGEMENT OF SEXUAL DYSFUNCTION SECONDARY TO ANTIDEPRESSANTS

Ginkgo Biloba

Ginkgo biloba (reviewed in detail in Chapter 12) has been recently proposed as having a potential role in the treatment of antidepressant-induced sexual dysfunction (8,9). In one open trial, 63 patients with sexual dysfunction secondary to various antidepressants of different classes (e.g., SSRIs, serotonin-norepinephrine reuptake inhibitors [SNRIs], tricyclic antidepressants, and monoamine oxidase inhibitors) (9) received ginkgo in conjunction with their usual antidepressant. Results suggested the effectiveness of ginkgo in the alleviation of sexual dysfunction, with 91% of women and 76% of men reporting improvement in all aspects of the sexual cycle (desire, excitement, orgasm, and resolution). The effective dosages were between 60 and 180 mg twice daily, which are lower than those often used for cognitive enhancement. The mechanism for improvement in sexual function is unclear, but current thought is that it involves ginkgo's interaction with platelet activating factor, prostaglandins, peripheral vasodilatation, and central serotonin and norepinephrine receptor activity.

Apart from the risk of hemorrhage in people who take anticoagulants (10), ginkgo appears to be safe to combine with other medications. Ginkgo may be a useful addition for patients who are experiencing antidepressant-induced sexual dysfunction and who have not been helped by more conventional agents, such as sildenafil or yohimbine. The full extent of ginkgo's role in the management of this common side effect remains to be clarified.

Maca

Maca (*Lepidium meyenii*) is a root vegetable (tuber) that grows in the mountains of Peru (11,12). Little is known about the origins of maca (also called Peruvian ginseng, as well as several other names), but native Peruvians have been known to use maca as a food since before the time of the Incas (11). The historical uses of maca include nutritional supplementation in a harsh environment, as well as enhancing fertility and sexual potency. When the Spanish arrived in Peru in 1526, they were advised by locals to feed their horses maca to keep them well nourished and to maintain their fertility (13). Impressed by the results, the Spaniards reasoned that maca might promote sexual function in humans. While such claims have not been substantiated by well designed clinical studies, the herb's chemical composition appears consistent with, among other functions, a role as a sexual enhancer.

The maca root contains a wide variety of essential substances, including amino acids and proteins; complex carbohydrates; minerals, such as calcium, phosphorus, zinc, magnesium, iron and iodine; vitamins B_1, B_2, B_{12}, C, and E; fatty acids, including linolenic, palmitic, and oleic acids; steroidal glycosides (sterols); alkaloids; beta-ecdysone; p-methoxybenzyl isothiocyanate (suggested to function as an aphrodisiac); saponins; tannins; and glucosinolates (which may enhance fertility) (13–18).

Today, maca is growing in popularity due to claims of energizing effects, fertility enhancement, and aphrodisiac qualities. Other uses for maca include the alleviation of menstrual irregularities and female hormonal imbalances, including menopause symptoms and chronic fatigue syndrome (11,19). In traditional Peruvian herbal medicine, maca is also used as an immunostimulant; as a memory enhancer; and for treating various medical conditions, including anemia, tuberculosis, and stomach cancer (11,19,20).

The maca tuber can be consumed fresh or dried. The dried roots can be stored for years and can be later baked, roasted, or boiled in water or milk to make a porridge. In addition, maca is often made into a sweet drink called maca chicha (13–15). In traditional Peruvian medicine, maca powder is delivered at doses of 5 to 20 g in tablets or capsules, stirred into water or juice, or sprinkled over the food twice daily. Maca is also consumed as mazzamora, a porridge-type preparation that may contain up to 60 g of the root. In the United States and elsewhere, maca is sold in drug stores and health food stores in capsule form. Most commercially available preparations of maca contain about 500 mg of ground tuber in each capsule. Recommended dosages range from 3 to 6 g per day, but no consensus has been reached on the ideal therapeutic dose of maca.

Despite its popularity, virtually no systematic human research has been done on maca as a potential treatment for antidepressant-induced sexual dysfunction or for sexual dysfunction in general. In animal studies, maca consumption increases strength and sexual activity (21,22). Most human data are in the form of case vignettes or anecdotal evidence, some of which make dramatic claims. So far, maca has shown no toxicity and no adverse pharmacologic effects. Pregnant or nursing women are nonetheless advised by manufacturers to seek the advice a physician before using maca. Likewise, the recommendation is that maca be avoided in men with elevated prostate-specific antigen or a history of prostate cancer and in women with a history of breast cancer or other hormonal cancers.

Given the lack of systematic data to support the use of maca as a sexual enhancer, offering any specific recommendations at this time is difficult. Since a variety of registered medications are widely used to ameliorate antidepressant-induced sexual dysfunction (e.g., sildenafil, yohimbine, and bupropion), maca may be considered in individuals who have unsuccessfully tried registered aphrodisiacs or who have a strong interest in natural remedies.

MANAGEMENT OF WEIGHT GAIN SECONDARY TO PSYCHOTROPIC MEDICATIONS

Although obesity is generally managed by primary care physicians or by nutritionists, psychiatrists are often called upon to address this problem in patients who gain weight as a side effect from the various psychotropic medications.

Given the increasing numbers of overweight individuals, the weight loss and weight management industry has been growing dramatically in the United States and worldwide. Literally dozens of weight loss programs and diets go in and out of vogue each year, as well as a plethora of over-the-counter medications that promise easy and rapid weight loss. The recent years have even seen the emergence of a few anorexiants, such as orlistat and sibutramine, which are approved by the United States Food and Drug Administration as weight loss promoters to be used as part of a comprehensive weight loss program. However, these medications do not provide an easy ride to weight loss because patients are still required to increase physical activity and to exercise self-control when eating. As a result, many people are still searching for the ideal weight loss remedy—one that can allow them to eat anything they want and still lose weight.

A comprehensive review of available weight loss products is beyond the scope of this chapter. However, the following observations are worth noting.

1. Despite the wide use of alternative treatments for weight loss, minimal support for their effectiveness is found in the peer-reviewed literature. For example, Allison et al. (23) reviewed 18 anti-obesity/fat-reducing methods and products. Of these, none was demonstrated to be safe and effective in at least two double-blind, randomized, placebo-controlled studies performed by more than one independent research group. The authors noted that while preliminary data may warrant further study, the claims of effectiveness are largely premature.

2. Many weight loss studies observe patients for relatively short periods (less than 1 year). While some benefit may be reported, whether the weight loss is maintained for longer periods is not clear, particularly once the patients leave the study setting and lose the structure and support provided by the regular visits to the clinic.

3. Safety is a particularly important issue to consider when evaluating weight loss treatments. While most claim to be natural and safe, many of them contain

natural but powerful stimulants, such as ma-huang, which can cause toxic reactions when taken in high doses (24).

4. A review of various well established weight loss programs (Gadde et al., unpublished information) suggested that even among the most successful programs, the average weight loss obtained is only 10% of the initial body weight. This is particularly sobering, when one considers that the average person would have to be no more than 10 to 15 pounds overweight to be able to return to their normal weight in such a program. In the psychiatric setting, these programs may prove valuable to the individual who gains a relatively small amount of weight as a side effect from psychotropic agents. However, for those individuals with more severe weight gain (as is often seen with mood stabilizers and antipsychotic agents), the modest benefit may prove disappointing.

Whatever the cause of weight gain, clearly no shortcut to weight loss exists at this time. The best recommendation for psychiatrists is to warn their patients about the risks and limited effectiveness of weight-loss pills. A better approach may be to recommend a more reasonable program of diet and exercise (preferably with the assistance of the patient's primary care physician) or to consider modifying the patient's medication regimen, if feasible.

OTHER EXAMPLES OF POSSIBLE COMBINATIONS OF NATURAL MEDICATION

In cases where coexisting illness—such as anxious depression or bipolar depression—is found, several combinations of natural medications exist that may theoretically provide the alleviation of a broader range of symptoms. Several such combinations are illustrated in Table 13.1, and some representative examples are listed below.

1. Ginkgo may be combined with antidepressant agents in cases where antidepressant-induced sexual dysfunction occurs.
2. Hypericum may be combined with valerian (or melatonin) for depression with insomnia.
3. Hypericum may be combined with kava for depression with generalized anxiety.
4. Omega-3 fatty acids (FAs) may be combined with hypericum for bipolar depression. The mood-stabilizing effect of the omega-3 could protect from cycling. However, until the effectiveness of omega-3 FAs is better characterized, concomitant treatment with a standard mood stabilizer (e.g., lithium) should be administered.
5. Omega-3 FAs may be combined with omega-6 FAs for schizoaffective disorder to control some mood and psychotic symptoms, although these are usually an add-on to standard antipsychotic agents or mood stabilizers.
6. Inositol may be combined with clonazepam or other benzodiazepines for treatment of refractory panic attacks.

TABLE 13.1. Examples of possible combination strategies with natural medications

Medications	DHEA	Fatty acids	Ginkgo	Inositol	Kava	Melatonin	PEA	SAMe	SJW	Valerian
DHEA	MDD + Bulimia	Bipolar* depression + Dementia	MDD + Dementia	MDD + OCD + Panic + Bulimia + Dementia	MDD + Anxiety + Dementia	MDD + Insomnia + Dementia	Severe MDD + Dementia	Severe MDD + Dementia	Severe MDD + Dementia	MDD + Insomnia + Dementia
Omega fatty acids	—	—	BPD* + Psychosis + Dementia	Bipolar* depression + Psychosis + OCD + Bulimia	BPD* + Psychosis + Anxiety	BPD* + Psychosis + Insomnia	Bipolar* depression + Psychosis	Bipolar* depression + Psychosis	Bipolar* depression + Psychosis	BPD* + Psychosis + Insomnia
Ginkgo biloba	—	—	Dementia + Sex dys	MDD + OCD + Panic + Dementia + Sex dys + Bulimia	Anxiety + Dementia + Sex dys	Insomnia + Dementia + Sex dys	MDD + Dementia + Sex dys	MDD + Dementia + Sex dys	MDD + Dementia + Sex dys	Insomnia + Dementia + Sex dys
Inositol	—	—	—	MDD + OCD + Panic + Bulimia	Anxiety + MDD + OCD + Panic + Bulimia	Insomnia + MDD + OCD + Panic + Bulimia	MDD + OCD + Panic + Bulimia	MDD + OCD + Panic + Bulimia	MDD + OCD + Panic + Bulimia	Insomnia + MDD + OCD + Panic + Bulimia
Kava	—	—	—	—	Anxiety	Insomnia + Anxiety	MDD + Anxiety	MDD + Anxiety	MDD + Anxiety	Insomnia + Anxiety
Melatonin	—	—	—	—	—	Insomnia	MDD + Insomnia	MDD + Insomnia	MDD + Insomnia	Severe insomnia
PEA	—	—	—	—	—	—	MDD	Severe MDD	Severe MDD	Insomnia + MDD
SAMe	—	—	—	—	—	—	—	MDD	Severe MDD	Insomnia + MDD
SJW	—	—	—	—	—	—	—	—	MDD	Insomnia + MDD
Valerian	—	—	—	—	—	—	—	—	—	Insomnia

*Patients with bipolar disorder should probably be treated with concomitant standard mood stabilizers, such as lithium.

Abbreviations: BPD, bipolar disorder; DHEA, dehydroepiandrosterone; MDD, major depressive disorder; OCD, obsessive-compulsive disorder; PEA, phenylethalamine; SAMe, S-adenosyl-L-methionine; Sex dys, sexual dysfunction; SJW, St. John's wort.

While adverse interactions appear to be relatively uncommon with natural medications, clinicians must recognize the importance of warning patients about the lack of data on the risks of using these remedies in combination with other medications. As the various chapters reviewed, documented interactions between alternative and registered medications have occurred, some of which can be of grave consequence (Table 13.2). Examples include the combination of ginkgo with anticoagulant agents, as well as hyperforin's (St. John's wort) induction of CYP-3A4 expression (25), which may result in interactions between hypericum products and warfarin, cyclosporin, oral contraceptives, theophylline, fenprocoumon, digoxin, and indinavir, leading to reduced therapeutic activity (26–29). A good rule of thumb, therefore, is to manage these medications with the same care and respect given to registered medications.

TABLE 13.2. *Summary of interactions and suggestions for combination*

Medication	Summary of interactions, suggestions for combination
Black cohosh	Probably safe to combine with other psychotropics.
Chaste tree berry	Probably safe to combine with other psychotropics.
DHEA	Probably safe to combine with other psychotropics; care should be taken with patients on other hormonal preparations.
Ginkgo biloba	Avoid combinations with anticoagulants, as hemorrhage may occur. Probably safe to combine with other psychotropics.
Homeopathy	Probably safe to combine with other psychotropics, but need to be aware of all components of specific preparations; amounts used in homeopathy are likely too small to result in significant interactions.
Inositol	Probably safe to combine with other psychotropics.
Kava	Probably safe to combine with other psychotropics.
	Be careful with patients on benzodiazepines, as excess sedation may occur.
	Be careful with patients on multiple medications and/or underlying medical illness, as long-term toxicities may result.
Melatonin	Interactions may occur with valproic acid and serotonergic and noradrenergic drugs.
	Avoid in individuals taking steroids or sertraline, as immune suppression or retinal problems may occur.
Omega fatty acids	Probably safe to combine with other psychotropics.
PEA	Probably safe to combine with other psychotropics; usually combined with MAO-B inhibitors to prevent breakdown.
	Tricyclic antidepressants may increase PEA concentration.
	Lithium may decrease PEA concentration.
SJW	Avoid in combination with SSRIs, MAOIs, and other antidepressants, as serotonin syndrome may result.
	Use with care in bipolar depression and always with a standard mood stabilizer; otherwise, cycling may occur.
	Probably safe to combine with anxiolytics.
SAMe	Probably safe to combine with other psychotropics.
Valerian	Probably safe to combine with other psychotropics.

Abbreviations: DHEA, dehydroepiandrosterone; MAO, monoamine oxidase; PEA, phenylethylamine; SAMe, S-adenosyl-L-methionine; SJW, St. John's Wort; SSRI, selective serotonin reuptake inhibitors.

CONCLUSION

Polypharmacy, either for the more aggressive management of clinical symptoms or for the alleviation of side effects, is a challenging area of alternative psychopharmacology, as well as of psychopharmacology in general. As the book illustrates, relatively little is currently known about the effectiveness and safety of combination strategies with natural medications. As more data on these treatments begin to emerge, the improved understanding of approaches to treatment will allow clinicians to make more effective recommendations for patients. For now, one hopes that the ideas put forth in this chapter will provide a framework for the clinician who is faced with the prospect of alternative polypharmacy.

REFERENCES

1. Rosenbaum JF, Fava M, Nierenberg AA, Sachs G. Treatment-resistant mood disorders. In: Gabbard GO, ed. *Treatments of psychiatric disorders*, 2nd ed. Vol. 1. Washington, D.C.: APPI, 1995:1276–1328.
2. Smith M, Buckwalter KC. Medication management, antidepressant drugs, and the elderly: an overview. *J Psychosoc Nurs Ment Health Serv* 1992;30:30–36.
3. Corcoran ME. Polypharmacy in the older patient with cancer. *Cancer Control* 1997;4:419–428.
4. Barat I, Andreasen F, Damsgaard EM. The consumption of drugs by 75-year-old individuals living in their own homes. *Eur J Clin Pharmacol* 2000;56:501–509.
5. Fisher P. The wheat and chaff in alternative medicine. *Lancet* 1997;349:1629.
6. Linde K, Ramirez G, Mulrow CD, et al. St. John's wort for depression-an overview and meta-analysis of randomized clinical trials. *BMJ* 1996;313:253–258.
7. Mischoulon D, Nierenberg AA, Kizilbash L, et al. Strategies for management of depression refractory to SSRI treatment: a survey of clinicians. *Can J Psychiatry* 2000;45:476–481.
8. Cohen A. Treatment of antidepressant-induced sexual dysfunction: a new scientific study shows benefits of ginkgo biloba. *Healthwatch* 1996;5.
9. Cohen A. *Ginkgo biloba for drug-induced sexual dysfunction* [abstract 35]. In: Syllabus and Proceedings Summary, American Psychiatric Association Annual Meeting, San Diego, 1997:5.
10. Smith PF, Maclennan K, Darlington CL. The neuroprotective properties of the ginkgo biloba leaf: a review of the possible relationship to platelet-activating factor (PAF). *J Ethnopharmacol* 1996;50:131–139.
11. Rea J. Raices andinas: maca. In: Bermejo H, Leon JE, eds. *Cultivos marginados, otra perspectiva de 1492*. 1992.
12. King S. *Ancient buried treasure of the Andes*. Garden, 1986.
13. Report of an Ad Hoc Panel of the Advisory Committee on Technical Innovation, Board on Science and Technology for International Development, National Research Council, 1989. Lost crops of the Incas: little known plants of the Andes with promise for worldwide cultivation.
14. Johns T. The anu and the maca. *J Ethnobiol* 1981;1:208–212.
15. Quiros C, et al. Physiological studies and determination of chromosome number in maca, *Lepidium meyenii*. *Econ Bot* 1996;50:216–223.
16. Leon J. The maca (*Lepidium meyenii*) a little known food plant of Peru. *Econ Bot* 1964;18:122–127.
17. Chacon RC. *Estudio fitoquimico de Lepidium meyenii*. Dissertation, University Nacionale Mayo de San Marcos, Peru, 1994.
18. Dini A, et al. Chemical composition of *Lepidium meyenii*. *Food Chem* 1994;49: 347–349.
19. Steinberg P. *Phil Steinberg's cat's claw news*. 1994:1.
20. Gomez A. Maca, es alternativa nutricional para el ano 2000. *Informe Ojo Salud* 1997:58.
21. Cicero AF, Bandieri E, Arletti R. *Lepidium meyenii* improves sexual behaviour in male rats independently from its action on spontaneous locomotor activity. *J Ethnopharmacol* 2001;75:225–229.
22. Zheng BL, He K, Kim CH, et al. Effect of a lipidic extract from lepidium meyenii on sexual behavior in mice and rats. *Urology* 2000;55:598–602.
23. Allison DB, Fontaine KR, Hesjka S, et al. Alternative treatments for weight loss: a critical review. *Crit Rev Food Sci Nutr* 2001;41:1–28.

24. Sardina J. Misconceptions and misleading information prevail—less regulation does not mean less danger to consumers: dangerous herbal weight loss products. *J Law Health* 1999–2000;14:107–132.
25. Moore LB, Goodwin B, Jones SA, et al. St. John's wort induces hepatic drug metabolism through activation of the pregnane X receptor. *Proc Natl Acad Sci U S A* 2000;97:7500–7502.
26. Fugh-Berman A. Herb-drug interactions. *Lancet* 2000;355:134–138
27. Baede-van Dijk PA, van Galen E, Lekkerkerker JF. [Drug interactions of Hypericum perforatum (St. John's wort) are potentially hazardous]. *Ned Tijdschr Geneeskd* 2000;144:811–812.
28. Miller JL. Interaction between indinavir and St. John's wort reported. *Am J Health Syst Pharm* 2000; 57:625–626.
29. Piscitelli SC, Burstein AH, Chaitt D, et al. Indinavir concentrations and St John's wort. *Lancet* 2000; 355:547–548.

PART V

Afterword

14

Afterword

David Mischoulon and Jerrold F. Rosenbaum

"I only know that I know nothing."
—Socrates

This volume illustrates the fact that natural medications represent an exciting and rapidly growing field in the treatment of psychiatric disorders. Natural remedies in the United States have gone from being part of a small subculture to achieving mainstream use and acceptability in the population at large. In many clinical settings, these medications are regularly used as secondary agents, either as an alternative to conventional medications or as adjunctive treatment, and in some instances, even as the first line of treatment.

Anecdotal data and case reports in the psychiatric literature are compelling; the studies that have been published so far are promising; and new natural treatments continue to emerge every day, each with a promise of improving mental well-being. Excitement and controversy inevitably follow the appearance of such new treatments, and their effectiveness and safety continues to be a topic of sometimes heated debate. One could often say, in line with the old Chinese curse, that psychiatry is now living in interesting times, and indeed, the rise of natural psychotropic agents has been a major contributor to the oscillating state of affairs.

But a curse may often turn out to be a blessing in disguise. In time, these treatments may indeed occupy a key place in the psychiatrist's pharmacologic armamentarium and may even attain equal status with current registered medications. But before these medications can be deemed appropriate and recommended as effective and safe first-line or second-line treatments, more systematic, placebo-controlled studies on adequately sized patient samples need to be carried out.

The National Institutes of Health and the National Institute of Mental Health have acknowledged the importance of studying the effectiveness and safety of these medications and have begun to support larger-scale clinical trials using both a placebo and registered agents as active comparators (1,2). Several multi-center studies on natural medications, such as St. John's wort, kava, and the like,

Portions of this chapter were previously published by the authors in modified form in Mischoulon D, Rosenbaum JF. The use of natural medications in psychiatry: a commentary. *Harv Rev Psychiatry* 1999;6:279–283 (used with permission).

are underway in different academic institutions across the country. The hope is that these studies will address the knowledge gaps illustrated in this volume. For now, the medical community still needs to acknowledge its relative ignorance about these medications and remain humble in the face of their mystery. With that in mind, the authors make the following recommendations for practitioners:

1. Practitioners should routinely inquire about their patients' use of alternative medications and should encourage their patients to feel comfortable in discussing them (3). Nevertheless, they should also proceed with caution (3) when faced with a patient who expresses an interest in taking a natural medication. Above all, one must emphasize to patients that these medications are still relatively untested with regard to formal studies and scientific data.

2. In the absence of more conclusive data, the authors believe that two kinds of patients may be considered good candidates for natural remedies. The first is the mildly symptomatic patient with a strong interest in natural remedies; for such a patient, a delay in adequate treatment would not be devastating. At the other extreme, the patient who has failed multiple trials of more conventional medications or who is particularly intolerant of side effects would have little to lose by trying natural remedies. However, these patients are often the most difficult to treat, and alternative agents appear to be most suitable for the mildly ill (4).

3. Finally, care must be taken with the patient who is taking multiple medications because still relatively little is known about drug-drug interactions and toxicities. Combinations of alternative medications with other alternative medications or with registered medications should be used with extreme caution, although anecdotes suggest usefulness for some difficult-to-treat patients.

Much has been learned about natural remedies in the past century, particularly in the past few years. And much more still exists to be learned.

REFERENCES

1. National Institutes of Health Office of Alternative Medicine. *Alternative medicine: expanding medical horizons*. Rockville, MD: National Institutes of Health, 1992.
2. National Institutes of Health Office of Alternative Medicine. *General information on sponsored research*. Rockville, MD: National Institutes of Health, 1997.
3. Eisenberg DM. Advising patients who seek alternative medical therapies. *Ann Intern Med* 1997;127:61–69.
4. Schulz V, Hansel R, Tyler VE. *Rational phytotherapy: a physicians' guide to herbal medicine*, 4th ed. Berlin: Springer, 2001.

Appendices

Appendix A

Summary of the Different Natural Medications: Indications, Dosages, and Adverse Effects

TABLE A.1. *Different natural medications: Indication, doses, and adverse effects*

Medication	Active components	Putative indications	Possible mechanisms of action	Suggested dosages	Adverse events
Black cohosh (*Cimicifuga racemosa*)	Triterpenoids, isoflavones, aglycones	Menopausal symptoms	Suppression of luteinizing hormone	40–200 mg/d	GI upset, dizziness, headache, weight gain
Chaste tree berry (*Vitex agnus castus*)	Diterpenoids, iridoid glycosides (agnuside, aucubin), flavonoids (casticin)	Premenstrual symptoms	Prolactin inhibition, interaction with dopaminergic receptors	20–400 mg/d	None
Dehydroepian-drosterone	Adrenal gland steroid hormone	Depression and dementia	GABA antagonism, NMDA potentiation, increase in brain serotonin and dopamine activity	5–100 mg/d in bid–tid dosing	Acne, irritability, insomnia, headaches, menstrual irregularities, increased ocular pressure, palpitations
Fatty acids	Essential fatty acids (primarily omega-6 and omega-3)	Depression (docosahexanoic acid–omega-3) Mania (omega-3 fatty acid mix) Psychosis (omega-3 and omega-6)	Inhibition of membrane signal transduction	200–3,000 mg/d (doses vary)	GI upset
Folic acid Ginkgo biloba	Vitamin Flavonoids, terpene lactones	Depression Dementia Sexual dysfunction-secondary to anti-depressants	Neurotransmitter synthesis Nerve-cell stimulation and protection, membrane/ receptor stabilization, free radical scavenging, PAF inhibition	200–400 µg/d 120–240 mg/d in bid–tid dose	None Mild GI upset, headache, irritability, dizziness, possible bleeding in individuals with bleeding disorders or in those who take anticoagulants
Homeopathy	Various herbs and minerals	Various disorders	Unknown	Varies with preparation	Mild transient worsening of target symptoms
Inositol	Second messenger precursor	Depression, panic, OCD, bulimia	Second messenger synthesis Sensitization of serotonin receptors	12–18 g/d	GI upset, dizziness, insomnia, sedation, headache
Kava (*Piper methysticum*)	Kavapyrones, kavalactones	Anxiety	Central muscle relaxant, anticonvulsant, GABA receptor binding	60–300 mg/d	GI upset, allergic skin reactions, headaches, dizziness, ataxia, hair loss, visual problems, respiratory problems, kava dermopathy

TABLE A.1. *Continued.*

Medication	Active components	Putative indications	Possible mechanisms of action	Suggested dosages	Adverse events
Melatonin	Pineal gland hormone	Insomnia	Circadian rhythm regulation in suprachiasmatic nucleus	0.1–0.3 mg/d (sometimes higher)	Sedation, confusion, inhibition of fertility, decreased sex drive, hypothermia, retinal damage
Phenylethylamine	Neurohormone, amino acid derivative	Depression	Catecholamine release	10–60 mg/d, with 5–10 mg/d selegiline	Mild anorexia
S-adenosyl-L-methionine	Amino acid derivative	Depression	Methyl donor in neurotransmitter synthesis	200–1,600 mg/d (sometimes higher)	Mania in bipolar patients
St. John's wort (*Hypericum perforatum*)	Hypericin, hyperforin, polycyclic phenols, pseudohypericin	Depression	Cytokine production Decreased serotonin receptor density Decreased neurotransmitter reuptake MAOI activity	900–1,200 mg/d in bid–tid dosing	Dry mouth, dizziness, constipation, phototoxicity, serotonin syndrome when combined with SSRIs Adverse interactions with warfarin, cyclosporin, oral contraceptives, theophylline, fenprocoumon, digoxin, an indinavir
Valerian (*Valeriana officinalis*)	Valepotriates, sesquiterpenes	Insomnia	Decrease GABA breakdown	450–600 mg/d	Mania in bipolar patients Blurry vision, dystonias, hepatotoxicity (?), headaches, mutagenicity (?)
Vitamin B₁₂	Vitamin	Depression	Neurotransmitter synthesis	6 µg/d	None

Abbreviations: GABA, γ-aminobutyric acid; GI, gastrointestinal; MAOI, monoamine oxidase inhibitor; NMDA, *N*-methyl-D-aspartate; OCD, obsessive-compulsive disorder; PAF, platelet-activating factor; SSRIs, selective serotonin reuptake inhibitors.

Appendix B

Examples of Possible Combination Strategies with Natural Medications

TABLE B.1. *Possible combination strategies for natural medications*

Medications	DHEA	Fatty acids	Ginkgo	Inositol	Kava	Melatonin	PEA	SAMe	SJW	Valerian
DHEA	MDD + dementia	Bipolar depression + dementia	MDD + dementia	MDD + OCD + panic + dementia + bulimia	MDD + anxiety + dementia	MDD + insomnia + dementia	Severe MDD + dementia	Severe MDD + dementia	Severe MDD + dementia	MDD + insomnia + dementia
Omega fatty acids	—	BPD + psychosis	BPD + psychosis + dementia	Bipolar depression + psychosis + OCD + bulimia + panic	BPD + psychosis + anxiety	BPD + psychosis + insomnia	Bipolar depression + psychosis	Bipolar depression + psychosis	Bipolar depression + psychosis	BPD + psychosis + insomnia
Ginkgo biloba	—	—	Dementia + sex dys	MDD + OCD + panic + dementia + sex dys + bulimia	Anxiety + dementia + sex dys	Insomnia + dementia + sex dys	MDD + dementia + sex dys	MDD + dementia + sex dys	MDD + dementia + sex dys	Insomnia + dementia + sex dys
Inositol	—	—	—	MDD + OCD + panic + bulimia	Anxiety + MDD + OCD + panic + bulimia	Insomnia + MDD + OCD + panic + bulimia	MDD + OCD + panic + bulimia	MDD + OCD + panic + bulimia	MDD + OCD + panic + bulimia	Insomnia + MDD + OCD + panic + bulimia

continued.

TABLE B.1. *Conitnued.*

Medications	DHEA	Fatty acids	Ginkgo	Inositol	Kava	Melatonin	PEA	SAMe	SJW	Valerian
Kava	—	—	—	—	Anxiety	Insomnia + anxiety	MDD + anxiety	MDD + anxiety	MDD + anxiety	Insomnia + anxiety
Melatonin	—	—	—	—	—	Insomnia	MDD + insomnia	MDD + insomnia	MDD + insomnia	Severe insomnia
PEA	—	—	—	—	—	—	MDD	Severe MDD	Severe MDD	Insomnia + MDD
SAMe	—	—	—	—	—	—	—	MDD	Severe MDD	Insomnia + MDD
SJW	—	—	—	—	—	—	—	—	MDD	Insomnia + MDD
Valerian	—	—	—	—	—	—	—	—	—	Insomnia

Abbreviations: BPD, bipolar disorder; DHEA, dehydroepiandrosterone; MDD, major depressive disorder; OCD, obsessive-compulsive disorder; PEA, phenylethylamine; SAMe, S-adenosyl-L-methionine; sex dys, sexual dysfunction; SJW, St. John's wort.
Patients with bipolar disorder should probably be treated with concomitant standard mood stabilizers, such as lithium.

Appendix C

Summary of Interactions and Suggestions for Combination

TABLE C.1. *Summary of interactions and combination strategies*

Medication	Summary of interactions, suggestions for combination
Black cohosh	Probably safe to combine with other psychotropics.
Chaste tree berry	Probably safe to combine with other psychotropics.
DHEA	Probably safe to combine with other psychotropics; care should be taken with patients on other hormonal preparations.
Ginkgo biloba	Avoid combinations with anticoagulants, as hemorrhage may occur; probably safe to combine with other psychotropics.
Homeopathy	Probably safe to combine with other psychotropics, but need to be aware of all components of specific preparations; amounts used in homeopathy are likely too small to result in significant interactions.
Inositol	Probably safe to combine with other psychotropics.
Kava	Probably safe to combine with other psychotropics; be careful with patients on benzodiazepines, as excess sedation may occur; be careful with patients on multiple medications or underlying medical illness, as long-term toxicities are associated.
Melatonin	Interactions may occur with valproic acid, serotonergic, and noradrenergic drugs; avoid in individuals taking steroids or sertraline, as immune suppression or retinal problems can occur.
Omega fatty acids	Probably safe to combine with other psychotropics.
PEA	Probably safe to combine with other psychotropics; usually combined with MAO-B inhibitors to prevent breakdown; tricyclic antidepressants may increase PEA concentration; lithium may decrease PEA concentration.
SAMe	Probably safe to combine with other psychotropics.
SJW	Avoid in combination with SSRIs, MAOIs, and other antidepressants, as serotonin syndrome may result; use with care in bipolar depression and always with a standard mood stabilizer, or cycling may occur; probably safe to combine with anxiolytics.
Valerian	Probably safe to combine with other psychotropics.

Abbreviations: DHEA, dehydroepiandrosterone; MAO-B, monoamine oxidase type B; MAOIs, monoamine oxidase inhibitors; PEA, phenylethylamine; SAMe, S-adenosyl-L-methionine; SJW, St. John's wort; SSRIs, selective serotonin reuptake inhibitors.

Subject Index

Note: Page numbers followed by *f* indicate figures; those followed by *t* indicate tables.